Vaccination Controversies

Recent Titles in the

CONTEMPORARY WORLD ISSUES
Series

Tax Reform: A Reference Handbook, Second Edition
James John Jurinski

Child Soldiers: A Reference Handbook
David M. Rosen

Medical Tourism: A Reference Handbook
Kathy Stolley and Stephanie Watson

Women and Crime: A Reference Handbook
Judith A. Warner

World Sports: A Reference Handbook
Maylon Hanold

Entertainment Industry: A Reference Handbook
Michael J. Haupert

World Energy Crisis: A Reference Handbook
David E. Newton

Military Robots and Drones: A Reference Handbook
Paul J. Springer

Marijuana: A Reference Handbook
David E. Newton

Religious Nationalism: A Reference Handbook
Atalia Omer and Jason A. Springs

The Rising Costs of Higher Education: A Reference Handbook
John R. Thelin

The Animal Experimentation Debate: A Reference Handbook
David E. Newton

Books in the **Contemporary World Issues** series address vital issues in today's society such as genetic engineering, pollution, and biodiversity. Written by professional writers, scholars, and nonacademic experts, these books are authoritative, clearly written, up-to-date, and objective. They provide a good starting point for research by high school and college students, scholars, and general readers as well as by legislators, businesspeople, activists, and others.

Each book, carefully organized and easy to use, contains an overview of the subject, a detailed chronology, biographical sketches, facts and data and/or documents and other primary source material, a directory of organizations and agencies, annotated lists of print and nonprint resources, and an index.

Readers of books in the **Contemporary World Issues** series will find the information they need in order to have a better understanding of the social, political, environmental, and economic issues facing the world today.

CONTEMPORARY WORLD ISSUES

Science, Technology, and Medicine

Vaccination Controversies

A REFERENCE HANDBOOK

David E. Newton

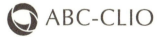 ABC-CLIO

Santa Barbara, California • Denver, Colorado • Oxford, England

Library of Congress Cataloging-in-Publication Data

Newton, David E.
   Vaccination controversies : a reference handbook / David E. Newton.
      pages cm. — (Contemporary world issues)
   Includes bibliographical references and index.
   ISBN 978-1-61069-311-0 (hardcopy : alk. paper) —
ISBN 978-1-61069-312-7 (ebook)   1. Vaccination—Handbooks, manuals, etc.   2. Vaccines—Handbooks, manuals, etc.
3. Immunization—Handbooks, manuals, etc.   I. Title.
   RA638.N495   2013
   614.4'7—dc23   2012048155

ISBN: 978-1-61069-311-0
EISBN: 978-1-61069-312-7

17   16   15   14   13   1   2   3   4   5

This book is also available on the World Wide Web as an eBook.
Visit www.abc-clio.com for details.

ABC-CLIO, LLC
130 Cremona Drive, P.O. Box 1911
Santa Barbara, California 93116-1911

This book is printed on acid-free paper ∞

Manufactured in the United States of America

List of Tables, xiii
Preface, xv

1   BACKGROUND AND HISTORY, 3

Infectious Diseases in History, 4
    Epidemics in Early Human History, 7

The Nature of Infectious Diseases, 14

Major Infectious Diseases, 16
    Smallpox, 18
    Poliomyelitis, 21
    Dengue Fever, 23
    Hepatitis C, 25

The Human Immune System, 26
    Primary Immune Response, 27
    Secondary Immune Response, 30

Vaccination, 31
    The Language of Vaccinology, 32

The History of Vaccination, 38
    Variolation, 38
    From Variolation to Vaccination, 42

References, 47

2   PROBLEMS, C**ONTROVERSIES, AND** S**OLUTIONS,** 57

A Brief History of Opposition to Vaccination, 58
    The English Vaccination Laws, 61
    Anti-Vaccinationism in the United States, 65
    Vaccination Laws in the United States, 73
    Vaccination Laws Worldwide, 77
    Vaccination Epidemics, 78
        Kyoto, Japan: 1948, 81
        Complications Resulting from DTP
        Vaccinations: Mid-1970s, 81
        Polio: 1955, 82
        Rotavirus: 1999, 83

The Legal Status of Vaccination, 84

Modern Anti-Vaccinationism, 85
    Vaccines Cause Illness, 86
        The Vaccine-Autism Link, 90
        Vaccines and Gulf War
        Syndrome, 93
    Vaccines Do Not Work, 95
    Big Business and Big Government, 98
    Alternatives to Vaccination, 101
    Too Aggressive Vaccination Schedules, 103
    Threats from Thimerosal and Adjuvants, 105
        Aluminum Compounds, 106
        Squalene, 108
    Old Wine in New Bottles, 110
    The Human Papillomavirus Vaccine, 111
    Where to from Here? 114

References, 115

3   PERSPECTIVES, 133

HPV Vaccine for All, *Bob Roehr,* 133
    HPV Diseases, 135
    Other Benefits, 136

Further Reading, 137

HPV Vaccine Mandates: Little Benefit, Real Harm, *Diane M. Harper*, 137

Vaccine Shortages—A Perspective, *Dean A. Haycock*, 141

References, 144

Sounds of Death: Whooping Cough and Vaccine Refusal, *Benjamin Radford*, 144

Anti-Vaccination Fears, 146

References, 147

Vaccination Doubts, *Louise Kuo Habakus*, 148

References, 153

Federal Law and Mandatory Vaccination, *Stephen Lendman*, 154
    Massachusetts May Be a Forerunner of What's to
        Come, 157

References, 157

Hepatitis B Vaccine and Multiple Sclerosis, *Joan R. Callahan*, 158
    Consequences, 161
    What Went Wrong?, 161

Further Readings, 162

4   PROFILES, 167

Baruch S. Blumberg (1925–2011), 167

Dale and Betty Bumpers Vaccine Research Center, 170

Every Child By Two, 172

Ian Frazer (1953–), 175

Maurice Hilleman (1919–2005), 177

Immunization Action Coalition, 180

Edward Jenner (1749–1823), 182

Albert Z. Kapikian (1930–), 185

Pearl Kendrick (1890–1980) and
Grace Eldering (1901–1988), 187

Shibasaburo Kitasato (1852–1931), 190

Douglas R. Lowy and John T. Schiller, 192

Jacques Miller (1931–), 195

National Vaccine Information Center, 197

Ruth S. Nussenzweig (1928–), 200

Paul A. Offit (1951–), 202

Louis Pasteur (1822–1895), 205

Stanley A. Plotkin (1932–), 208

Gaston Ramon (1886–1963), 210

Benjamin A. Rubin (1917–2010), 213

Albert Sabin (1906–1993), 215

Jonas Salk (1914–1995), 218

Viera Scheibner (1935–), 221

Vaccine Education Center, 223

Vaccination Risk Awareness
Network, Inc., 225

Emil von Behring (1854–1917), 227

Andrew Wakefield (1957–), 229

Lady Mary Wortley Montagu (1689–1762), 232

5 DATA AND DOCUMENTS, 237

Data, 237
  Table 5.1: National and State Vaccination
    Coverage among Children Aged 19–35
    Months—United States, 2010, 238
  Table 5.2: Recommended Immunization
    Schedule, 241
  Table 5.3: Approved Vaccines and Their
    Effectiveness, 242
  Table 5.4: Coverage of Two Major Vaccination
    Schedules Worldwide, 1980–2010, 244

Documents, 250
  Letter from Lady Mary Wortley Montagu about
    Variolation in Turkey (1717), 250
  Boylston's Inoculation Efforts in Colonial Boston
    (1726), 251
  An Act to Secure General Vaccination
    (1855), 253
  Jacobson v. Massachusetts, 197 U.S. 11
    (1905), 255
  Poliomyelitis Vaccination Assistance Act, P.l. 377
    Chapter 863 (1955), 258
  Vaccination Assistance Act of 1962 (42 USC Sec.
    247b), 259
  National Childhood Vaccine Injury Act of 1986
    (Public Law 99-660), 261
  Measles Eradication Program (1996), 265
  Project Bioshield Act, P.l. 108-276
    (2004), 267
  Project Bioshield Assessment (2007), 269
  Executive Order RP65 (State of Texas)
    (2007), 271
  Texas House Bill 1098 (2007), 274
  *Cedillo and Cedillo vs. Secretary of Health and
    Human Services* (2010), 275

Frequently Asked Questions about Thimerosal
(Ethylmercury) (2011), 276
Exemption from Vaccination, 279

6   RESOURCES, 283

Books, 283

Periodicals, 296

Reports, 306

Internet Resources, 306

7   CHRONOLOGY, 325

Glossary, 339
Index, 345
About the Author, 353

Table 1.1   Important Epidemics in Human History, 10

Table 1.2   Nations with the Highest Percent of People
                 Infected with HIV, 2009, 13

Table 1.3   Worst Infectious Diseases
                 Worldwide, 2008, 17

Table 1.4   First Discovery of Vaccines, 47

Table 5.1   National and State Vaccination Coverage
                 among Children Aged 19–35 Months—
                 United States, 2010, 238

Table 5.2   Recommended Immunization Schedule, 241

Table 5.3   Approved Vaccines and Their
                 Effectiveness, 242

Table 5.4   Coverage of Two Major Vaccination
                 Schedules Worldwide, 1980–2010, 244

Infectious diseases have been an integral part of human civilization for at least 5,000 years, and possibly much longer. Historians have found evidence of the existence of diphtheria, leprosy, smallpox, and tuberculosis in the oldest written records available and in modern medical investigations of early skeletons. Scars, characteristic of smallpox, for example, have been found in mummies that date to the 18th dynasty in Egypt (ca. 1550–ca. 1292 BCE), and the pharaoh Ramses V is generally thought to have died from smallpox in 1157 BCE.

Of course, infectious diseases are not simply a problem from ancient human history; such diseases are still widespread throughout the world today, accounting, according to some estimates, for more than 300 million illnesses and 5 million deaths annually. A short list of those diseases includes African trypanosomiasis ("sleeping sickness"), transmitted by the tsetse fly; cholera, transmitted through contaminated drinking water; cryptosporidiosis, a water-borne disease; dengue, transmitted by the *Aedes aegypti* mosquito; hepatitis A, B, and C, all caused by viruses; HIV/AIDS, currently one of the most devastating diseases in the world; malaria, arguably the single most serious infectious disease in the world today; and onchocerciasis ("river blindness"), caused by the larvae of the parasitic worm *Onchocerca volvulus.*

For most of human history, medical science had relatively little success in dealing with infectious diseases. Next to nothing was known about their causes or about methods that could be used to treat a person who had contracted an infectious disease. And only the most rudimentary knowledge was available about the prevention of an infectious disease, calling on procedures that were sometimes as likely to cause a disease as to prevent it. As a consequence, once an infectious disease broke out in a region, it often spread uncontrollably throughout that region, resulting in widespread epidemic that killed thousands of men, women, and children. An epidemic that spread through Athens from 430 to 426 BCE, for example, is thought to have killed at least half of the city's population. (The disease involved has still not been positively identified.)

One general principle on which preventative procedures were (and are) based was known at least as early as about 1500 BCE. According to that principle, a person who has once been exposed to an infectious disease and survived is much less likely to contract that disease again in the future. And with the understanding of that principle was born the practice of immunization, a practice in which infectious materials taken from one person, animal, or other source are inserted into the body of a second person. The immune system of that second person then reacts to the infectious material and prepares itself for some possible later attack by the same infectious organism. The precise method by which this procedure is employed has changed over the centuries, but the underlying principle is much the same in the second decade of the 21st century as it was in the 15th century BCE. Today, we call that procedure *immunization* or *vaccination*. Vaccination has been almost unbelievably successful in limiting many infectious diseases and wiping out a handful of those diseases. For example, one of the most devastating of all infectious diseases, smallpox, is no longer found naturally anywhere in the world. It exists only in the form of laboratory samples stored in two locations in the United States and Russia.

The purpose of this book is to provide a general introduction to the subject of vaccination. Chapter 1 provides a history of infectious diseases and the methods that have been developed to prevent those diseases by the use of vaccination. The chapter also provides a brief introduction to the science of immunology, the mechanism by which bodies recognize and respond to foreign invading agents, such as bacteria and viruses. This subject applies equally to all animals, including cats, dogs, horses, cows, and other domestic and wild animals as it does to humans. Indeed, the subject of vaccination is of critical importance in veterinary medicine and wildlife management. This book does not, however, deal with that aspect of the subject, and focuses, instead, on the history, technology, and issues associated with vaccination among humans.

At first glance, vaccination would appear to be an unalloyed blessing for humans, providing a simple and relatively inexpensive way of protecting individuals from diseases that can range from the unpleasant and inconvenient to the debilitating and fatal. But the history of vaccinations is not that simple. Indeed, from almost the moment that the principles of vaccination were discovered, there have been concerns raised about the practice: Is it safe for people to be infected artificially with vaccines? Are the risks of the procedure worth the benefits gained? Should individuals be *required* to be vaccinated against certain diseases, even if they have personal objections to the practice? Are all vaccines equally necessary, or should some be mandatory and others optional? Chapter 2 of this book reviews some of the issues that have arisen with regard to the use of vaccination to protect individuals from infectious diseases, issues that have existed in the past and those that are still being debated.

The major purpose of this book is to provide the reader with sufficient background information and resources to carry out additional research on the topic of vaccination. In addition to the history and background provided in the first two chapters, the book contains the viewpoint of experts on various topics in the field of vaccinology (Chapter 3); profiles of important individuals and organizations in the field of vaccinology, both in the past and the present (Chapter 4); a collection of laws, court decisions, official pronouncements, and other documents, as well as some relevant data on vaccination (Chapter 5); a list of print and electronic resources on the subject of vaccination (Chapter 6); a chronology of important events in the history of vaccinology (Chapter 7); and a glossary of important terms in the field of vaccinology.

Vaccination Controversies

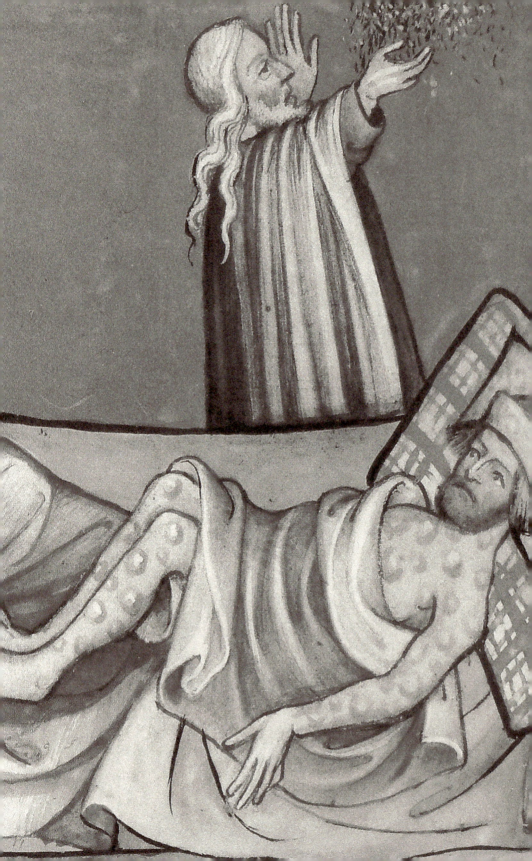

Mei Wah watched as her daughter got sicker, almost by the hour. She recognized the signs of the illness well enough: It was The Scourge. Four children in the royal household had already died of the illness this week. And there was nothing Mei Wah could do to help her child, except to make her comfortable. Her only real choice was to pray to the spirits. Prayers sometimes helped, but, more often, they made no difference. And the children who survived The Scourge were often horribly scarred. If Mei Wah's daughter did survive The Scourge, she might well be so badly scarred that she would never find a husband.

Mei Wah knew that a treatment was available to prevent The Scourge. The Emperor had seen that his four sons had all received the treatment. Sometimes the treatment did not work, and a child did get The Scourge. But far more often it *did* work, and a child was protected from the terrible illness. The treatment would not have helped any of Mei Wah's children, however. It was available, first of all, only to male children; female children were expendable. In any case, it was available only to sons of the Emperor. It was never given to other members of the royal household and certainly not to common people.

Detail from a miniature from the Swiss Toggenburg Bible (1411) depicting a man suffering from the blisters of the Black Death, the bubonic plague that swept Europe in the Middle Ages. (Corbis)

Infectious Diseases in History

Infectious diseases have been the scourge of human societies almost since the beginning of recorded time. Mei Wah's story could have been set in the 19th century, when preventative treatments for The Scourge (what we now call smallpox) were already available. Or, it could have been set, with different characters. Tracing the earliest history of infectious diseases is a challenging task. There are, of course, no photographs that show the diseases from which people suffered, and there are relatively few drawings or written descriptions of those diseases until well into the first millennium of the common era. Yet, medical detectives have made some interesting discoveries about the presence of diseases such as smallpox, tuberculosis, malaria, and leprosy in Asia and the Middle East as far back as the second millennium BCE. As an example, a research team led by American epidemiologist Donald R. Hopkins undertook a detailed analysis of the pharaoh Ramses V's mummy in 1979. As early as 1898, when the mummy was first discovered, some experts suspected that the rashes seen on the mummy's remains were caused by an attack of smallpox and that the disease may have killed the Egyptian ruler. Hopkins' team looked for remnants of the variola virus that causes smallpox in an effort to prove that hypothesis. They were unsuccessful in finding evidence of the virus, but their examination led them to conclude that the ruler had, indeed, suffered from the dreaded disease. Hopkins concluded his report on the team's research by observing that "after seeing at first hand the rash on this remarkable mummy, I am almost as convinced that he did indeed have smallpox as if I had actually seen a 3000-year-old poxvirus" (a *poxvirus* is any virus that can infect humans and other animals, causing diseases such as smallpox, chicken pox, and cowpox) (Hopkins 2012).

Similar detective work has revealed the existence of other infectious diseases early in human history. Mummies like those studied by Hopkins are among the richest sources of

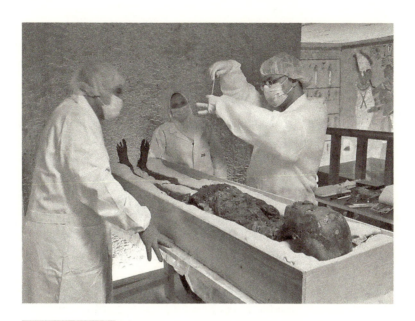

Scientists take DNA samples from the 3,300-year-old mummy of Tutankhamun in Luxor, Egypt, in 2008. The samples indicated that the ancient Egyptian pharaoh had suffered from malaria and a host of other maladies. (AP Photo/Discovery Channel, Barry Iverson)

information because enough of their original bodies remain to permit sophisticated types of modern testing, such as DNA analysis and microanalysis of bone structure and composition. As an example, a research team from the University of Toulouse in France reported in 1998 on the analysis of a 5,400-year-old mummy that appears to have suffered from tuberculosis. Although the team was not able to identify the causative agent that causes tuberculosis (*Mycobacterium tuberculosis*), they were able to collect a segment of DNA from the mummy that is characteristic of that organism (Crubézy et al. 1998). Recent research has been successful in obtaining definitive evidence of the presence of *M. tuberculosis* in a number of Egyptian mummies (see, for example, Zink et al. 2003). Most residents of Christian nations are familiar with references to another infectious disease, leprosy, in the Bible. It is not clear how many of these references actually refer to the modern form of leprosy, now better known as Hansen's disease, and how many to similar, but unrelated diseases (see, for example, "'Leprosy' in the Bible—What Was It?"). In any case modern research suggests that the disease dates back to at least 2000 BCE with the announcement in 2009 of the discovery of a skeleton dating to that period in northwest India (Robbins et al. 2009). Bone structure and composition of the skeleton provided strong indications that the individual had suffered from leprosy during his or her lifetime. Prior to this research, most authorities had accepted the earliest available description of leprosy has having occurred in the Ebers Papyrus, one of the longest medical documents from ancient Egypt, dating to about 1550 BCE (Hulse 1972).

The origin of another infectious disease, malaria, has been the subject of considerable debate and research. Many authorities believe that malaria first appeared in Africa, long before the origin of recorded history, probably by passing across the species barrier from nonhuman animals. Among the earliest mentions of the disease may be those found in Babylonian works, in which Nergal, the god of pestilence and destruction, is sometimes called by humans to rain down his horrors on people by delivering "disease, exhaustion, malaria (?), sleeplessness, worries, and ill health" (Stol 1993, 13). Malaria may also well be the disease to which ancient Chinese and Indians writers refer as far back as 1500 BCE when they describe a potentially fatal feverish condition that arises after heavy rains (which is characteristic of malaria). Indeed, many scholars believe that the so-called king of diseases mentioned in the Indian text, *Atharva Veda*, is probably malaria (Babu 2007, 1). Beyond these older histories, which involve some degree of analysis and interpretation of word meanings, the first clear clinical description of malaria probably dates to the writings of the Greek physician Hippocrates. In his book *On Airs, Waters and Places*, Hippocrates describes a condition he observed frequently in places where there were large deposits of marshy, stagnant water. People living in such areas, he wrote, often suffer from a disease characterized by "large stiff spleens and hard, thin, hot stomachs, while their shoulders, collar-bones, and faces are emaciated." These effects are produced, he taught, by the fact that "their flesh dissolves to feed their spleen" (Winslow 1943, 65; see also Kakkilaya 2012).

The history of infectious diseases is a fascinating and complex field of study. Stories like those above can be repeated for a number of other diseases, including cholera, plague, hepatitis, meningitis, and diphtheria. Over the centuries, information about such diseases has become more reliable, outbreaks have been more clearly recognized, causative agents have been discovered, and treatments and cures have been developed. This story will be resumed within a more recent context in the section on specific diseases presented later in this chapter.

Epidemics in Early Human History

One of the ways in which historians have learned the most about infectious diseases has been in accounts of disease epidemics. An epidemic is an event in which an infectious disease spreads through a community or region, infecting a large section of the people (or other animals) living in that region. (An epidemic that spreads throughout the world is called a *pandemic*.) The disease itself in an epidemic is generally no different in its symptomology than when it affects a single individual. But historians are more likely to take notice of an event in which hundreds or thousands of individuals are killed; they may be more thorough in describing how the disease arrived in an area, how it was spread, the symptoms that individuals showed, the number of people who were sick and died, and the methods that were available to deal with the disease.

Thus, it is hardly surprising that histories of infectious diseases often emphasize particularly noteworthy epidemics. Perhaps the earliest of such widespread epidemics was one that struck Egypt during the 15th dynasty, between about 1650 and

1550 BCE. Experts are uncertain as to the disease involved, with some arguing for influenza (Akhenaten [Amenhotep IV] 2012) and others for the bubonic plague (Kozloff 2006). Probably the most thoroughly studied and best known of the early epidemics was that which swept through Athens between about 430 and 427 BCE. The plague struck Athens in the second year of the Peloponnesian War between the city-state and an army led by the city-state of Sparta. The approaching forces of Sparta had forced most Athenians into the core of the city, behind its gates, increasing the density of population that encourages the development of epidemic conditions. The plague reoccurred on three occasions, first in 430, again in 429, and a third time in the winter of 427–426. As many as a third of the city's residents may have died in the series of epidemics.

No one knows the origin of the epidemic, although some authorities believe that it may have swept up into the European continent from central or northern Africa, carried by both traders and soldiers. There is also no agreement as to the specific disease responsible for the epidemic, with anthrax, bubonic plague, dengue fever, measles, smallpox, typhus, typhoid fever, ebola, and hemorrhagic fever all having their adherents ("The Plague of Athens" 2012). In 1999, however, researchers at the University of Maryland Medical Center announced that they had determined the cause of the epidemic: typhus fever. They used detailed descriptions of symptoms reported by victims of the disease, along with a review of the way the disease spread through the city, to reach their conclusion ("Plague of Athens: Another Medical Mystery Solved at University of Maryland" 2012).

Historically, some epidemics have had profound effects on nations and regions. An example is the so-called Antonine Plague that struck the Roman Empire on a number of occasions between 165 and 180 CE. The epidemic is also known as the Epidemic of Galen for the Roman physician who chronicled the disease. Scholars have been unable to determine the actual disease responsible for the epidemic, although either smallpox or measles appears to be the primary suspect. In any case, the disease swept through the empire, killing an estimated five million people eventually and, at one point, up to 2,000 individuals a day in Rome alone. By some accounts, a quarter of everyone infected by the disease eventually died from it. By all accounts, the epidemic dramatically interrupted the flow of everyday life, essentially ending the recruitment of men for the military, preventing ships from sailing because so many sailors were ill with the disease, causing the death of some of the most important administrators in the empire (including at least two emperors), interrupting the normal planting and harvesting of crops, inspiring the renewal of spiritual and religious movement, and serving as a driving force for a new realization of artistic expression. Many historians suggest that the epidemic was a significant factor in the eventual collapse of the empire in the fifth century (Sabbatini and Fiorino 2009).

Over the centuries, dozens of epidemics have been recorded. Table 1.1 lists some of the most important of those epidemics.

A striking feature of the episodes listed in Table 1.1 is the appearance from time to time of epidemics so widespread that they earn the name of pandemics. Pandemics spread outward from some specific region in which they are endemic across national borders to other countries, regions, and continents. The term *endemic* is used to describe a disease that occurs naturally in some particular region. People who live within that region are accustomed to being stricken by that particular disease from time to time and, as a result, often develop an immunity to the disease that reduces its virulence. An example of the way diseases can spread is found in the appearance of the bubonic plague in Asia, Europe, and North America on a number of occasions between the sixth century and the middle of the 20th century. Experts now recognize three distinct occasions on which the organism that causes the bubonic plague, the bacterium *Yersinia pestis*, swept across broad regions of land infecting and killing tens or hundreds of millions of people. They have worked for decades to determine where the disease came from and how it spread across much of the world.

Table 1.1 Important Epidemics in Human History

Dates	Name	Region	Disease	Estimated Deaths
541–542	Plague of Justinian	Eastern Roman Empire	bubonic plague	25 million
639	Plague of Emmaus	Palestine	bubonic plague	25,000
1338–1351	Black Death	Asia and Europe	bubonic plague	100 million
1485, 1507, 1516, 1529, 1551	English Sweating Sickness	England	unknown	unknown, but relatively small
1617–1619		American colonies	smallpox	unknown
1665–1666	Great Plague of London	England	plague	100,000
1816–1826	First Cholera Pandemic	Asia and Europe	cholera	much greater than 100,000
1829–1851	Second Cholera Pandemic	Asia, Europe, North America	cholera	much greater than 100,000
1847–1848	Typhus Epidemic of 1847	Canada	typhus	more than 20,000
1852–1860	Third Cholera Pandemic	Russia	cholera	1 million
1889–1890	Russian Flu	worldwide	influenza	1 million
1918–1920	1918 Flu Pandemic	worldwide	influenza	75 million
1957–1958	Asian Flu	worldwide	influenza	2 million
1968–1969	Hong Kong Flu	worldwide	influenza	1 million
1974		India	smallpox	15,000

1981–present	HIV/AIDS Pandemic	worldwide	HIV virus	25 million
2002–2003	SARS	Asia	SARS coronavirus	775
2005		Singapore	dengue fever	19
2006		India, Pakistan	dengue fever	more than 100
2008–2009		Zimbabwe	cholera	4,293
2009–2010		West Africa	meningitis	931
2010–present		Hispaniola	cholera	more than 6,500 (as of 2012)
2011		Pakistan	dengue fever	more than 350 (as of 2012)

A plausible explanation, based on recent research, is that the bacterium originated somewhere in China, probably early in human history. It was then transmitted by traders, military excursions, and other mass movements of individuals from its place of origin in China to Constantinople, southern France, Scandinavia, and other "transfer points," from where it spread throughout the Middle East, Europe, and, eventually, to North America. The first such episode, for example, occurred in 541 CE when traders from the Far East are thought to have brought with them to their home port in Constantinople the fleas on which *Y. pestis* live, which were then transferred to humans. The bite of those fleas delivered bubonic plague to the victims, introducing the first phase of the disease to the Eurasian region. Over the next year, the disease is thought to have killed an estimated 40 percent of the city's inhabitants, taking the toll up to 5,000 deaths per day. By the time it disappeared more than a year later, more than 25 million people throughout the world are estimated to have died of the plague (Echenberg 2002; Morelli et al. 2010). This scenario was apparently repeated at least twice more, once beginning in the Middle Ages with the appearance of the bubonic plague in Marseilles in 1347, a plague that was to reappear on the continent a number of times in the next 500 years, and a second time when the disease spread from Hong Kong throughout the world in 1894 (Wade 2010).

As Table 1.1 shows, epidemics and pandemics are hardly a problem of the past. Indeed, one of the most devastating pandemics of all human history, the HIV/AIDS pandemic, rages throughout the world today. The disease, caused by the human immunodeficiency virus (HIV) was first noted in the early 1980s, when it appeared in a small number of men who had sex with other men (MSM) on the two coasts of the United States. Since that time, the disease has spread throughout the world, with arguably its most terrible effects occurring today not only in the United States and other Western nations, but also in every region of the world, most especially sub-Saharan Africa.

Table 1.2   Nations with the Highest Percent of People Infected with HIV, 2009

Nation	Rate of Infection (percent) (estimated)
Swaziland	25.90
Botswana	24.80
Lesotho	23.60
South Africa	17.80
Zimbabwe	14.30
Zambia	13.50
Namibia	13.10
Mozambique	11.50
Malawi	11.00
Uganda	6.50
Kenya	6.30
Tanzania	5.60
Cameroon	5.30
Gabon	5.20
Equatorial Guinea	5.00
Central African Republic	4.70
Nigeria	3.60
Congo, Republic of the	3.40
Chad	3.40
Cote d'Ivoire	3.40
Burundi	3.30
Togo	3.20
Bahamas, The	3.10
South Sudan	3.10
Rwanda	2.90
For comparison:	
United States	0.60
Switzerland	0.40
France	0.40
Canada	0.30
Netherlands	0.20
Israel	0.20
United Kingdom	0.20
China	0.10
Japan	0.10

(*Continued*)

Table 1.2   *(Continued)*

Nation	Rate of Infection (percent) (estimated)
Saudi Arabia	0.01
Afghanistan	0.01
Svalbard	0.00

Source: "Country Comparison: HIV/AIDS—Adult Prevalence Rate." The World Factbook. https://www.cia.gov/library/publications/the-world-factbook/rankorder/2155rank.html.

According to the most recent data available, there are about 34 million people around the world living with HIV/AIDS, of whom 30.1 million are adults, 16.8 million are women, and 3.4 million are children under the age of 15. An estimated 2.7 million people were thought to have been infected by the virus in 2010, of whom 390,000 were children. The World Health Organization (WHO) also estimated that, during 2010, 1.8 million people died of HIV/AIDS, of whom 250,000 were children (HIV/AIDS. Data and Statistics 2012. As Table 1.2 shows, all but one of the 25 nations with the highest percent of individuals infected with HIV are in Africa. In fact, most developed countries rank relatively low on this list with Estonia at number 43, Ukraine at number 44, Russia at number 46, Latvia at number 59, Portugal at number 63, and the United States at number 64 (Country Comparison: HIV/AIDS—Adult Prevalence Rate 2012). As these data suggest, the world's battle with its latest pandemic is very far from over.

The Nature of Infectious Diseases

Perhaps the first question that one might ask about infectious diseases is how tiny organisms like viruses and bacteria can cause such terrible devastation to the human body (and to other animals and plants). No simple answer is available to that question—nor is there room for an adequate answer in a book of this kind—because pathogens act in a variety of ways to interrupt the normal function of an organism's body. Some examples may help understand this process, however.

In a number of cases pathogenic bacteria produce their physiological effects by excreting a toxin, a poisonous substance that interrupts the complex, normal biochemical changes that maintain body function. An example is the toxin that causes tetanus, the bacterium *Clostridium tetani*. *C. tetani* acts on the point where a nerve is attached to the muscle over which it has control. A toxin released by the bacterium has an amplifying effect on the nerve, causing it to stimulate the muscle over and over again. The muscle, in turn, responds repeatedly to that stimulation, resulting in muscle spasms that are characteristic of tetanus. Eventually, a person may go into seizures and may die as a result of the toxin's action.

Different bacteria use different mechanisms when they infect a host organism. For example, the bacterium that causes pertussis (whopping cough), *Bordetella pertussis*, attaches to ciliated cells that normally remove mucus from the throat and other parts of the respiratory system. Once in place, the bacterium then releases toxins that produce a somewhat unusual effect; they stimulate cells in the region where they are attached to produce nitric oxide (NO) gas. That gas, in turn, kills the cilial cells to which bacteria are attached, destroying the body's normal mechanism for eliminating mucus from the respiratory system. Lacking that mechanism, an organism has to cough— and usually cough *hard*—to get rid of the mucus accumulating in their respiratory system; hence the characteristic "whopping" cough associated with pertussis.

Viruses generally use a different form of attack on a host, one that by its very nature is much more dangerous. Viruses are very small particles that are unable to reproduce by themselves. They do so by infecting some other organism—the "host"— and then taking over that organism's reproductive mechanism to make additional copies of itself. The exact method by which they do so varies from virus to virus, but the ultimate result in largely the same in virtually all viral diseases. For example, the human immunodeficiency virus (HIV) first attaches itself to the outer lining of a host cell. It then burrows through that lining and ejects its own genetic material (DNA or RNA) into the host cell. That genetic material travels to the nucleus of the host cell and inserts itself into the DNA of the host cell. When the host cell begins its normal process of reproduction, it tends to "read" the instructions left by the viral particles, rather than its own DNA. Thus, it begins to produce, not copies of itself, but copies of the viral particles. These viral particles then assemble themselves into new complete viruses, burst out of the host cell (destroying the cell in the process), and go elsewhere to find new host cells to infect. The virus causes its damage, then, simply by using host cells to reproduce itself and, in the process, to destroy the host cell. (The reader who is interested in more detail about this topic is referred to Abedon 2012; Fact Sheet—Viruses 2012; Guerrant et al. 1999; Todar 2012.)

Major Infectious Diseases

What are the worst infectious diseases known to humankind? The answer to that question depends to a great extent on the point in history at which one asks the question. It also depends to some degree on the part of the world in which one lives. As one looks back over history, the most serious killers have been smallpox, bubonic plague, cholera, malaria, and HIV/AIDS. That list has changed to a considerable extent today, partly because of the discoveries of antibiotics and other materials for the treatment of these diseases, and partly because of the development of vaccines that protect individuals against diseases. For example, smallpox, once called the king of diseases by some observers, has now been eradicated from earth. The only pathogens capable of causing the disease are stored in two research laboratories in Russia and the United States. Table 1.3 lists the most serious infectious diseases in today's world, based on the number of deaths they cause each year. The data presented in Table 1.3 differ considerably, however, depending on the region of the world in which one lives today. In countries that the WHO has classified as "low-income" countries, 6 of the top 10 most lethal medical conditions are infectious diseases: lower respiratory infections (#1), diarrheal diseases (#2), HIV/AIDS (#3), malaria (#5), tuberculosis (#7), and neonatal infections (#10). By contrast, only four infectious diseases are listed as major killers in "middle-income" countries: lower respiratory infections (#4), diarrheal diseases (#5), HIV/AIDS (#6), and tuberculosis (#8); and only one infectious disease makes the top 10 in "high-income" countries, lower respiratory infections (#5) (The Top 10 Causes of Death 2012).

While "top 10" lists draw attention to some of the worst infectious diseases, the fact remains that many other such diseases still occur throughout the world, causing perhaps fewer numbers of deaths, but still posing major public health problems to a number of local communities and nations. These diseases include such familiar names as dengue fever, hepatitis (in all its forms), influenza, measles, rubella, and yellow fever. Space

Table 1.3 Worst Infectious Diseases Worldwide, 2008

Cause of Death	Diseases Involved	Estimated Number of Deaths (million)	Percent of All Deaths Worldwide
Lower respiratory infections	Primarily, pneumonia and bronchitis	3.46	6.1
Diarrheal diseases	Cholera, enterotoxigenic *Escherichia coli* (ETEC) infection, rotavirus, shigellosis, typhoid	2.46	4.3
HIV/AIDS	Cytomegalovirus infection, *Pneumocystis jiroveci* pneumonia, disseminated *Mycobacterium avium* intracellulare infection, cerebral toxoplasmosis, viral hepatitis, cancers, etc.	1.78	3.1
Tuberculosis	Tuberculosis	1.34	2.4

Source: "The Top 10 Causes of Death." World Health Organization. Fact Sheet No. 310. http://www.who.int/mediacentre/factsheets/fs310/en/index.html.

does not permit a detailed description of the many infectious diseases of concern to public health authorities. The following section will, however, provide a brief introduction to four of these diseases, selected as representative to some extent of dozens of other infectious diseases. Vaccines are available for two of these diseases (smallpox and polio), but not for the other two (dengue fever and hepatitis C).

Smallpox

Smallpox has certainly not taken the largest number of lives in history, but it remains one of the most dreaded of all infectious diseases. The reason for this attitude is that, while the disease has killed millions of people throughout history, it is also characterized by a number of frightening symptoms that have the potential for scarring a person for life. Thus, a person might be spared from death by the disease, but she or he would carry forever the marks of having contracted it.

Medical researchers believe that smallpox first appeared as early as 10000 BCE in central or northeastern Africa. The first credible written evidence of the disease can be traced to records of the Egyptian–Hittite War of about 1350 BCE (Barquet and Domingo 1997). Many historians also trace the earliest evidence for the disease to early in the first millennium BCE, with the discovery of smallpox-like rashes on Egyptian mummies from the period. The number of deaths and illnesses attributed to smallpox over the centuries is stunning. Some scholars estimate that smallpox killed between 300 and 500 million people during the 20th century alone. As late as 1967, WHO had estimated that upward of 15 million people worldwide had contracted the disease, and at least 2 million had died of it (Smallpox 2012).

Smallpox was originally known as *variola*, or *variola vera*, terms derived from the Latin words *varius*, for "spotted," or *varus*, for "pimple." It was given its modern name during the 15th century in Europe to distinguish the disease from another infectious condition, syphilis, also generally known as "the great pox." Two forms of the disease occur, known as variola major and variola minor, differentiated by the seriousness of their effects. Variola major is also the more common form of the disease. Incubation period for variola major ranges from 7 to about 17 days, after which the infected person experiences fever, head and body aches, and a general feeling of malaise. After a few days, small red spots begin to appear in the mouth and on the tongue, which spread across the body. They eventually evolve into red, raised bumps that are characteristic of the disease. The fatality rate from smallpox is about 30 percent. Other complications include encephalitis, infections of the respiratory system and the skin, diseases of the eye and blindness, and swollen joints and arthritis.

Humans have known how to protect individuals from smallpox infection for at least 3,000 years, and probably much longer. The method originally used was called *variolation*. It involved collecting materials from a person who had been infected with smallpox, pus or scabs from the wound, for example, which was then dried and blown into a person's nose and mouth or inserted directly into a cut in the person's skin. Since the material used in the process contained the variola major virus itself, the procedure typically produced relatively large, disfiguring blisters. It was, however, generally successful in protecting the variolated person from developing full-blown smallpox (Fenner et al. 1988, Chapter 6). By the end of the 18th century, medical researchers had learned how to inject material from less virulent variola minor infections (such as those that cause cowpox) through the skin and directly into muscle tissue. This procedure was much safer, with fewer dangerous side effects, and eventually replaced variolation as the procedure of choice in preventing smallpox. Variolation was finally banned in Russia in 1805, in Prussia in 1835, and in Great Britain in 1840 (Fenner et al. 1988, Table 6.1, 247).

Isolating and identifying the causative agent for smallpox was a long and complex process, dating to the late 1880s.

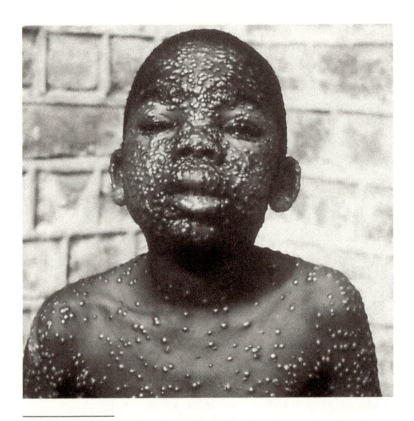

An African child displaying the rash typical of smallpox on his face, chest, and arms, 1970. (Centers for Disease Control)

Pieces of the virus were first unambiguously identified by German researcher Enrique Paschen in 1906, and the virus itself was finally isolated and identified by English bacteriologist J.C.G. Ledingham in 1931. These discoveries made possible the development of vaccines against smallpox, which were then aggressively promoted throughout the world. That effort was so successful that the last recorded case of naturally occurring smallpox was diagnosed in a two-year-old Bangladeshi girl in October 1975. On May 8, 1980, the WHO announced that "the world and all its peoples have won freedom from smallpox" (Pennington 2003, 762).

Poliomyelitis

As with many infectious diseases, there is evidence to suggest that poliomyelitis (more commonly known simply as "polio") has existed among humans since antiquity. The study of Egyptian mummies has found skeletal damage that is consistent with that caused by polio. Drawings and etchings on walls also show individuals who seem to have a condition known as amyotrophy that is characteristic of polio and young children who are walking with a cane (Daniel and Robbins 1997, Chapter 1; Polio 2012). Some authorities believe that the first recorded case of the disease dates to 1773, when the famous Scottish writer Sir Walter Scott was described as having had a high fever that deprived him of the use of his right leg, resulting in his walking with a limp for the rest of his life (Cone 1973, 35).

Although polio has apparently occurred in many parts of the world throughout history, the disease reached epidemic proportions only in the late 19th century, with the first major outbreak having occurred in Vermont in 1894, with a total of 132 cases reported (Merrill and Timmreck 2006, 320–321). After the turn of the century, polio epidemics became common almost every summer, with a few tens of thousands of cases and a few thousand deaths being reported in some years. In 1952, the United States reported the worst numbers in its history, with a record 57,628 cases; 3,145 deaths; and 21,269 individuals permanently paralyzed by the disease (Caplan 2011). Similar outbreaks occurred from time to time in other countries also, including Canada, the United Kingdom, and Sweden.

Polio is transmitted by direct person-to-person contact, through contact with oral or nasal discharges, or through contact with fecal matter from an infected person. Incubation for the disease ranges from 5 to 35 days, with an average of one to two weeks. Initial symptoms include a sore throat, mild fever, headache, vomiting, and general discomfort. The disease progresses into one of two stages, paralytic or nonparalytic, both of which involve damage to the central nervous system. Paralytic polio is characterized by a number of symptoms, most important of which is muscle weakness, which comes on quickly and eventually results in paralysis of one or more parts of the body or the entire body. Nonparalytic polio is accompanied by a number of symptoms, such as mild fever and discomfort and stiffness of the legs, neck, muscles, or other parts of the body. These symptoms pass rather quickly, usually within a few weeks, with no disabling long-term effects.

The causative agent of polio was discovered in 1908 by Austrian physicians and medical researchers Karl Landsteiner and Erwin Popper. The agent was a virus that is now called the poliovirus (Eggers 1999). Discovery of the virus made possible, at least in theory, the development of a vaccine against the disease. A host of technical problems prevented the realization of that hope, however, until the early 1950s, when two vaccines were released at almost the same time. The first vaccine, consisting of dead virus material, was developed by American virologist and medical researcher Jonas Salk. The success of clinical trials on the vaccine was announced in a press conference at the University of Michigan on April 12, 1955. Only five years later, a second polio vaccine, this one consisting of attenuated viral material, was licensed by the Food and Drug Administration (FDA) for use in the United States. The vaccine, developed by American physician and medical researcher Albert Sabin, was administered orally.

The success of the two polio vaccines has been extraordinary. In the United States, the number of polio cases dropped from an average of 35,000 per year between 1935 and 1945 to less than 2,500 cases by 1957, only two years after introduction of the Salk vaccine, and to 61 cases in 1965. The last case of naturally occurring poliomyelitis in the United States was reported in 1979, and the last case resulting from importation of the virus from other countries occurred in 1993. The nation is now free of polio.

The WHO has sponsored an aggressive campaign to repeat that success on a worldwide basis. In 1988, WHO and Rotary International announced the formation of the Polio Global Eradication Initiative, designed to end polio around the world by the year 2013. That program has been very successful. In 1980, WHO had recorded 52,795 cases of polio in 161 countries, a number that dropped to 23,390 in 1990, to 2,971 in 2000, and to 650 in 2011. Although the disease will probably not be completely eradicated by 2013, it has been largely confined to a handful of African and Asian countries, including Pakistan (198 cases in 2011), Chad (132 cases), Democratic Republic of the Congo (93 cases), Afghanistan (80 cases), Nigeria (62 cases), and Côte d'Ivoire (36 cases) (Polio This Week—As of 04 April 2012; WHO Vaccine-Preventable Diseases: Monitoring System. 2010 Global Summary 2012).

Dengue Fever

The first mention of a disease that was probably dengue fever occurred in a medical encyclopedia dating to the Jin Dynasty in China sometime between 265 and 420 CE. The first confirmed epidemics associated with the disease occurred simultaneously in a number of parts of the world in the 1780s. American physician Benjamin Rush is credited with providing the first detailed clinical description of the disease in 1789. Rush called the condition "breakbone fever" because of the intense muscle and joint pain associated with the disease. The modern name is thought to have come from a Swahili phrase *ka-dingo po*, meaning a "cramp-like pain caused by an evil spirit," or from the Spanish word *dengue* which means "careful," referring to the way in which a person with the disease walks (Gubler 2006; Henchal and Putnak 1990; History of Dengue 2012).

Dengue fever is commonly diagnosed on the basis of three characteristic features, the so-called dengue triad: fever, headache, and a characteristic rash that occurs at first as a flat red rash covering the body and later develops into small pimples similar to those associated with measles. The symptoms of dengue fever last only about a week with a fatality rate of less than about 1 percent. Another form of dengue fever, known as dengue hemorrhagic fever is more serious, with the occurrence of hemorrhaging beneath the skin. Dengue hemorrhagic fever is of greatest concern when it is not treated properly, resulting in a death rate that approaches 20 percent.

Dengue fever has become much more common over the past half century. The WHO recorded only 908 cases of the disease worldwide between 1955 and 1959. That number continued to rise over the next five decades until it reached almost a million in the most recent surveys. The disease is characterized by its tendency to occur in epidemics, such as those that struck India (16,517 cases), Indonesia (44,650 cases), Thailand (38,109 cases), and Myanmar (1,655 cases) in 1996 and that swept through Brazil (158,553 cases), Costa Rica (33,470 cases), Honduras (18,591 cases), Peru (5,957 cases), and Venezuela (33,661 cases) in 2005. Epidemiologists now consider dengue fever to be a major public health problem because anywhere from a quarter to a half of the world's population may be at risk for contracting the disease (Dengue—Annual Cases and Deaths by Country (1955–) 2012).

The method of transmission of dengue fever was determined in 1906, when researchers found that mosquitoes belonging to the genus *Aedes*, especially the species *A. aegypti*, transmit a virus between individuals in essentially the same way that yellow fever is transmitted. Scientists have since found that four different viruses are capable of producing dengue fever, and that exposure to one virus does not provide immunity to the other three forms of the virus. Thus, a person can develop dengue fever at least four times by contracting each of the four forms of the disease. This possibility is one reason that developing a vaccine against the disease has thus far been unsuccessful, although research on such a vaccine continues today (Vector-Borne Viral Infections. Dengue Fever 2012).

Hepatitis C

The term *hepatitis* means "inflammation of the liver," a condition that can be caused by both infectious disease and by other conditions (such as excessive alcohol intake). Perhaps the most prominent sign of the disease is jaundice, a yellowish coloration of the skin and the whites of the eyes. Jaundice and hepatitis were first described by the Greek physician Hippocrates in the eighth century CE. Hippocrates also hypothesized, correctly, that at least some forms of the disease he saw could be transmitted from person to person. In 1947, a British medical researcher suggested that two forms of hepatitis occur, which he named infectious hepatitis, or hepatitis A, and serum hepatitis, or hepatitis B (Martin 2003). Three decades later, researchers at the Infectious Disease Section of the National Institutes of Health (NIH) found that some cases of hepatitis could not be associated with either hepatitis A or hepatitis B. They began attributing such cases to a third type of hepatitis, which they originally called non-A non-B hepatitis, or NANBH. That rather clumsy name was retained for only a short while before, in 1989, the disease was renamed hepatitis C (Hepatitis C History 2012).

Four out of five people who are infected with hepatitis C are asymptomatic. The body is unable to "cure itself," however, and the disease tends to become chronic. The chronic state of the disease also tends to be asymptomatic in the vast majority of cases. A person with hepatitis C, then, is not aware that the disease is damaging her or his liver until symptoms of cirrhosis begin to appear. These symptoms include fatigue, loss of appetite, itchy skin, problems with sleeping, retention of water, and mental disturbances such as confusion and hallucinations. Although the most severe conditions associated with hepatitis C occur in fewer than 30 percent of those individuals who are infected, the consequences can be serious, as the most drastic effects of the disease can be treated only by a liver transplant (Hepatitis C. emedicinehealth 2012).

The WHO estimates that 130–170 million people world-wide are chronically infected with hepatitis C. They estimate that the number increases by three to four million annually. About 350,000 people worldwide die each year as a result of cirrhosis of the liver caused by a hepatitis C infection. The countries with the highest rate of the disease are Egypt (22 percent chronic infection rate), Pakistan (4.8 percent), and China (3.2 percent) (Hepatitis C. World Health Organization 2012). The U.S. Centers for Disease Control and Prevention (CDC) has reported that the number of hepatitis C cases in the United States has ranged from about 700 to about 900 cases over the past decade. In 2009, the last year for which data are available, that number was 781, for a rate of 0.3 cases per 100,000 persons. The states with the highest rate of infection were West Virginia (1.7 cases per 100,000), Connecticut (1.5/100,000), and Kentucky (1.5/100,000) (Viral Hepatitis Surveillance. United States 2009).

The virus that causes hepatitis C, now known as the hepac-virus, was discovered in 1989. It is a member of the family *Flaviviridae*, whose other members are responsible for infec-tious diseases such as yellow fever, dengue fever, various forms of encephalitis, and hepatitis G. The genetic structure of the hepacvirus is now well known, although that knowledge has as yet not been successfully translated into a vaccine against the disease. As of mid-2012, a number of vaccines against hepatitis C are in clinical trials (O'Shea 2012). A report in February 2012 by the discoverer of the hepacvirus was hailed by many observers as an important breakthrough in the search for such a vaccine (Hanlon 2012).

The Human Immune System

Perhaps the most remarkable fact about infectious diseases is that they do not kill every organism they attack. From a naive point of view, infectious agents like viruses, bacteria, and fungi have a lot going for them. Over the centuries, they have evolved sophisticated methods of breaking into the human body; attacking cells, tissues, and organs; and causing devastating diseases and death. Indeed, the statistics associated with the great epidemics and pandemics in human history, like those enumerated in Table 1.1, are reminders of how successful disease agents can be in their attacks on humans.

But the sophistication of disease agents is only part of the story. As they have evolved over time to become more and more efficient, so have bodily systems designed to provide protection against foreign invaders, the human immune system. How does the immune system operate to protect the body from infection and damage?

All organisms, ranging from simple bacteria to humans, have some form of immune system. Those immune systems have a dual function, not only to protect an organism against substances that are "not me," but also to adapt in such a way as to recognize modified forms of the original "not me." In humans, that immune system consists of a variety of chemical compounds, cells, tissues, and organs with the ability to recognize a foreign body and then to capture and destroy that body. Any substance that initiates an immune response in the body is known as an *antigen*, a term that comes from German and French words that mean "against" (*anti-*) the "creation" (*-gen*) of something, such as the creation of a disease within the body. Substances that the body produces to combat an antigen are known as *antibodies*.

Primary Immune Response

The first line of defense for humans against invading organisms is the integumentary system, which consists of the skin, nails, and hair. Foreign organisms have a great deal of difficulty breaking into the body through the skin and usually do so only when there is a break in the skin, such as that caused by a cut or a wound. Mucous membranes that line the oral, nasal, and genital cavities are also part of the first line of defense against organisms. Viruses, bacteria, and other microorganisms are trapped in the sticky material that makes up mucous membranes, from which they are then expelled by processes such as sneezing and coughing. Epithelial cells surrounding body openings, like the mouth and nose, also provide defense against invading organisms by releasing enzymes that attack and kill microorganisms.

This first line of defense is not, however, perfect. Foreign organisms can often find a way into the body in spite of the protection offered by skin, mucous membranes, and epithelial cells. It is at that point that the body's immune system takes over, providing a second line of defense against infection. Consider the following scenario.

Roxanne has cut her finger while slicing fruit in the kitchen. That cut in Roxanne's skin provides an opening through which bacteria can enter her body. Assume that these bacteria have never entered Roxanne's body before. Once they have passed through the skin, the bacteria can travel throughout her body by two convenient and complex highways: the bloodstream and the lymph system. These highways also provide the means by which the components of the immune system are able to travel anywhere in the body to battle with bacteria.

The presence of bacteria in Roxanne's body initiates a response known as the *innate immune response*. The innate immune response is genetically determined and present in (almost) every person's body. It is nonspecific in character; that is, it tends to treat all types of foreign invaders in the same way. It does not recognize any difference among bacteria, viruses, pollen, or dust particles. As long as those substances are recognized as "not me," they will trigger a response by the immune system. The primary weapon in the innate immune system is a group of cells called *macrophages* (meaning "big" [*macro-*] "eaters" [*-phages*]). Macrophages are white blood cells that are probably descendants of prokaryotic cells that, many millions of years in the past, became part of eukaryotic organisms and continued to function as prokaryotes. That is, when they see a particle in their vicinity that they recognize as "not me," they approach that particle, engulf and absorb the particle, and then break apart and dissolve the particle. The process by which that occurs is called *phagocytosis*, or "breaking a cell apart by eating." The bacteria that have entered Roxanne's body, then, have a good chance of simply being captured, engulfed, and devoured by macrophages.

But it sometimes happens that a flood of invading microorganisms simply overpowers the innate immune system; macrophages are not able to destroy all of the invading microorganisms. In such cases, a second line of innate immune defense is called into action. The major players in this line of defense are lymphocytes, white blood cells produced in the bone marrow. After they are manufactured, some lymphocytes travel from the bone marrow to the thymus gland, where they are modified so as to function as agents in the immune system. They are then called T-cells ("T" for *thymus*).

The modification in T-cells that takes place in the thymus involves the attachment on their surface of certain characteristic molecular patterns called *pattern recognition receptors*. These receptors have shapes that will fit perfectly into complementary regions on the surface of invading cells, much as a key fits perfectly into a lock. These T-cells are "off-the-shelf" cells that are preconfigured to recognize specific antigens, such as those for a smallpox virus, the *Bacillus anthrax* that causes anthrax, or any other "not me" invading cell.

A second component of the specific defense system is another type of lymphocyte, the B-lymphocyte, or B-cell. B-cells do not leave the bone marrow after they are produced, but, instead, remain there until they have matured and are ready to join the immune system. It is for this reason that they are called B- (for "bone") cells. Only when they have matured do B-cells leave the bone marrow to enter the bloodstream and lymphatic system.

T-cells and B-cells are widely distributed in the bloodstream and lymphatic system at all times, ready to deal with invading "not me" particles. What is it that spurs these cells into action? That process gets under way as soon as macrophages begin their attack on invading microorganisms. As they engulf and digest invading cells, macrophages also "spit out" small pieces of the organisms they have just devoured. These pieces become attached to the surface of a macrophage as a way of identifying the invading particle. It's as if the macrophage has run up a flag on its surface announcing the identity of the invading particles. (This process is called *antigen presentation*.) T-cells with receptor sites on their surface that match those of the invading particles will recognize the "flag" on the macrophage surfaces and be activated to join the battle against those particles. As those T-cells replicate, they differentiate into one of two types: killer T-cells and helper T-cells. As their names suggest killer T-cells search for and destroy cells that have been infected by an invading microorganism. Also, the job of helper T-cells is to notify B-cells that an invasion of foreign bodies has occurred and to activate those cells to take part in the battle against the invaders.

As soon as B-cells have received this news, they begin to differentiate into a somewhat different form known as *plasma cells*. Plasma cells have the ability to secrete specific antibodies that attach to the surface of an invading microorganism, also somewhat similar to planting a flag that will identify the particle. Macrophages and other types of phagocytes (cells that eat other cells) can now recognize these "not me" particles and attack, engulf, and devour them. (A superb detailed visual explanation of the details of the immune response is available at "Cancer and the Immune System," http://www.cancerresearch. org/Resources.aspx?id=586, Figure 3 animation.)

Secondary Immune Response

In most cases, the immune system is successful in repelling an invader. When that happens, certain types of T-cells, called *regulatory T-cells* or *suppressor T-cells*, step in to signal other components of the immune system that the battle is over, thus preventing the system from running amok and continuing its activities endlessly and needlessly. The battle-weary cells then go into "standby" mode and, in most cases, die off within a few days. A few T-cells and B-cells that have remained above the fray, however, survive. These cells carry on their surfaces "memories" of the invader that has just been defeated. These memories consist of molecular fragments that are distinctive codes for corresponding molecular patterns on the surface of the invading molecules. The so-called *memory T-cells* and *memory B-cells* are very long-lived, capable of lasting years of decades in the body without degrading. During this time, they continue to reproduce, vastly increasing their population in the body. Their presence means that a later invasion by the same pathogen will be met by a much more rapid and stronger response by the immune system than was the case with any initial infection. It is for this reason that a person who has contracted an infectious disease early in her or his life is likely to survive later incidents of the disease with fewer and less severe symptoms than with their first experience with the disease.

Vaccination

A person living in the fifth century BCE certainly would not have been familiar with the scientific explanation of the immune system outlined above. Yet he or she might well have been familiar with the fact that individuals who had been exposed to an infectious disease such as smallpox early in their life were likely to survive later episodes of the disease with little or no harm. And they might well have heard of specific treatments that had been developed to make use of that fact, by intentionally exposing children to dangerous diseases early in their lives, with the expectation that doing so would protect them throughout later periods of their life. Such treatments are classified as *vaccinations*, a term about which some background may be necessary.

The Language of Vaccinology

The art and science of providing a person with immunity to one or more infectious diseases is fraught with terminology with which the average person may be only partially familiar. So, here is a brief review of some of those terms. First, there is often confusion among some of the most common terms used in talking about the process by which an individual becomes immune to a disease. The most common of those terms—vaccination, immunization, and inoculation—are sometimes used interchangeably. Differences do exist among these terms, however. In the first place, the term *immunization* refers to any mechanism by which a person becomes immune to a disease. Scientists often speak of two kinds of immunization: active and passive. Active immunization occurs when an individual is exposed to an antigen, as in the extended example above, and her or his body successfully fights off that infection and produces memory cells that help protect against future infections of the same antigen. But active immunization can occur in other ways also, ways that are classified as *artificial active immunization*. In this process, some form of an antigen is introduced into a person's body intentionally to activate that person's immune system against the antigen. This process is generally called *vaccination*, a term first used by the father of modern vaccination technology, Edward Jenner, in 1803. Jenner devised the word because he used infectious material taken from a person with cowpox disease to provide humans with immunity against smallpox, and the Latin word for "cow" is *vacca* (Edward Jenner and the Discovery of Vaccination 2012).

The process by which vaccination occurs most commonly involves the insertion of a special material, called a *vaccine*, into a person's body, usually (but not always) by means of a sharp needle. That process is called an *inoculation*, a procedure that is used with vaccination, but with other kinds of medical procedures also (for more on this point, see Edsall 1964). Vaccines can be classified into a number of categories depending on the material of which they consist. For example, *live vaccines* consist of whole, living pathogens that activate the immune system in essentially the same way a natural infection does. The vaccine developed by Jenner for use against smallpox consisted of live cowpox vaccines. The cowpox virus was sufficiently similar to the smallpox virus to produce antibodies against the more dangerous disease, while producing only mild versions of the much less dangerous cowpox. The advantage of using live vaccines is that they are essentially identical with the mechanism by which infectious diseases occur, so they tend to produce a robust response with long-lived immunity against the disease. The disadvantage, of course, is they may actually cause the disease itself.

One way of overcoming this disadvantage is to treat the pathogen used in a live vaccine in such a way as to reduce its virulence, the degree to which the pathogen can cause the disease. This process is called *attenuation*, and the vaccine produced is called an *attenuated vaccine*. Attenuation can be achieved in a variety of ways. For example, the vaccine developed by Albert Sabin against poliomyelitis was produced by passing the polio virus through a number of steps in which it was exposed to monkey tissue. In the process, the virus "learned" to infect monkey tissue preferentially to human tissue, thus reducing its risk of producing polio in humans when used as a vaccine (Sabin and Boulger 1973). The problem is that not every last polio virus "learned" to prefer monkey tissue to human tissue, and the Sabin vaccine rarely causes polio in children to whom the vaccine was given. That risk is extraordinarily small—about one in a million—but it is not zero. When polio was a relatively common disease (as it was in the middle of the 20th century), a one-in-a-million chance seemed like a reasonable risk to take in vaccinating young children. Now that the incidence of polio has been greatly reduced in the United States and other parts of the world, the number of cases caused by the vaccine (called *vaccine-derive polio*) is of greater concern. In fact, some authorities in 2012 are calling for cessation of the use of the Sabin vaccine in favor of the safer (they say) Salk vaccine, which uses killed viruses (Orent 2012).

A popular alternative to live vaccines, then, is a *killed vaccine*, one in which the causative agent of a disease is present, but inactive. The causative agent for a disease can be killed in a variety of ways, such as heating, the use of chemicals, or exposure to radiation. The Salk vaccine against polio, for example, used viral components that were first heated to a temperature at which the virus could not survive and then treated with formaldehyde. The challenge for someone developing a killed vaccine is to find a way of ensuring that the virus does not survive to cause the disease one is trying to prevent, while, at the same time, ensuring that it retains enough of its live characteristics to activate the human immune system (The Salk Vaccine Trials 2012). Another common variation of the killed vaccine is the *sub-unit vaccine*, which consists of components of a pathogen, such as the coating of viral particles or important proteins from a pathogenic bacterium. The challenge in developing a sub-unit vaccine is to find a component that is sufficiently characteristic of the pathogen to evoke the immune response in a human. Two examples of sub-unit vaccines currently in use include the vaccines against hepatitis B and human papillomavirus (HPV), each of which contains proteins from the viral surface. Such vaccines are desirable if they can evoke the proper immune response because they do not contain enough of the pathogen itself to cause the disease the vaccine is designed to prevent (Making Vaccines: Subunit Vaccine: Hepatitis B 2012).

Another type of vaccine is possible for pathogens that damage cells by the release of a toxin (a poison). That vaccine is made by collecting the toxin and treating it chemically with a water solution of formaldehyde (formalin). The treatment destroys the toxic properties of the toxin, although it does not affect its immunogenic properties (its ability to evoke an immune response). The resulting product is called a *toxoid*. A vaccine consisting of a toxoid can be effective in producing immunity in an individual, while posing a very small risk of infection. Two of the most common toxoid vaccines now in use are those against diphtheria and tetanus.

Conjugate vaccines are a special type of vaccine of special value for young children whose immune systems are not well developed. They are most useful for bacteria whose surface is covered with a coating made of polysaccharides, a complex type of sugar. This coating tends to hide a bacterium's antigens, which consist of proteins or protein segments. When an individual's immune system encounters this type of bacterium, it may not recognize the bacterium's antigens (because they are hidden by the polysaccharide coating) and, as a result, the normal immune response may not be triggered. One way to get around this problem is to create proteins or protein segments that are similar to those found in the bacterium's antigens, and then to attach those units to the polysaccharide coating. The vaccine, then, consists of two parts, the polysaccharide coating and the antigen-like protein portion attached to it. Even a young child's immature immune system is generally able to recognize this configuration and begin to form antibodies against it. The *Haemophilus influenzae* type B (Hib) vaccine is probably the most common example of conjugate vaccines in use today (*Haemophilus influenzae* Type B 2012).

Vaccines are also designated as *monovalent* or *multivalent* (or *polyvalent*) depending on the number of different antigens they contain, one in the former case, and more than one in the latter. (Multivalent vaccines are also called *combination vaccines* or *mixed vaccines*.) Multivalent vaccines have been available since the early 20th century, and two of the vaccines most widely used today, the MMR (measles-mumps-rubella) and DTP (diphtheria-tetanus-pertussis) vaccines are both *trivalent*. That is, each one contains antigens for three different infectious diseases. Immunization can involve the use of three monovalent vaccines (such as one immunization for measles, one for mumps, and one for rubella), or a single trivalent vaccine (a single inoculation of MMR vaccine). Multivalent vaccines can also include antigens for more than one strain of a single disease. In 2007, for example, the GenVec company announced funding for the development of a vaccine against malaria that contains antigens for five different strains of the disease (GenVec Announces Additional Funding for Malaria Vaccine Program from the PATH Malaria Vaccine Initiative 2012). Such a vaccine will, of course, provide a much wide range of protection than a monovalent vaccine that protects against only a single strain of the disease agent. Other multivalent vaccines that are available today include those for polio (3 antigen strains), *Streptococcus pneumonia* (23 strains), and rotavirus (5 strains) (Ellis 1999; Rotavirus Strains 2012).

Medical researchers are always searching for new ways to make vaccines that are more efficacious and safe than existing alternative. One of the most interesting developments in the 21st century has been a practice known as *reverse vaccinology*. The development of a new vaccine traditionally involves the identification of the causative agent, culturing that agent in the laboratory, and then carrying out a series of tests to determine the components of that agent that are most likely to evoke an immune response. This process is complex and time-consuming, and may even be impossible if the causative agent cannot, for example, be cultured in the laboratory. The development of a variety of modern technologies has made possible another approach to vaccine design and development, an approach known as *reverse vaccinology*.

Reverse technology involves the preparation of various gene combinations found in a pathogen and testing them for their ability to evoke an immune response *in silico* (i.e., by means of computer simulation). This method allows a researcher to test a wide variety of possible antigens from a pathogen in a relatively short period of time, producing results that can then be tested in the laboratory (Rappuoli 2001). The first disease with which this approach has been successful is a form of meningitis caused by the bacterium *Neisseria meningitidis* B. No vaccine is currently available for that disease, but reverse vaccinology has provided a number of possible candidates for use in vaccines against the disease. As of 2012, late state clinical trials of new vaccines against the disease have shown strong promise for success (Novartis Phase III Study Shows Meningococcal B Vaccine Candidate Could Be First to Provide Broad Coverage Against Deadly Disease 2012; for future prospects for reverse vaccinology, also see Rappuoli and Aderem 2011). For additional and updated information on other types of experimental vaccines currently under investigation, see "Science News Articles about 'Experimental Vaccine'" at http://esciencenews.com/dictionary/experimental.vaccine.

One remaining feature of vaccines remains to be mentioned: adjuvants. In pharmacology, an adjuvant is any substance that modifies the effect of some drug, usually a vaccine. An example of a nonvaccine adjuvant is caffeine, which has little or no analgesic (pain-killing) effect on its own. But when added to acetaminophen, it enhances the analgesic effect of that drug.

Adjuvants are far more commonly used in vaccines, where they tend to increase the effectiveness of a vaccine. Adjuvants were first discovered in the early days of commercial vaccine production when physicians observed that some batches of a vaccine were more effective in preventing a disease than were other batches. The first guess proposed was that this variation was a result of various levels of contamination in different batches of the vaccine. This hypothesis turned out to be true, but in a somewhat peculiar way. Researchers found out that vaccines in which there was *no* contamination at all were the least efficacious of all batches of vaccine. That is, the presence of some contamination actually improved a vaccine's ability to prevent disease.

Over time, researchers have studied a host of possible "contaminants" to add to vaccines to increase their effectiveness. The most widely used adjuvants today are compounds of aluminum, including alum (hydrated potassium aluminum sulfate), aluminum sulfate, aluminum phosphate, and aluminum hydroxide; calcium phosphate; virosomes (manufactured noninfective fragments of viruses); and preparations containing squalene ($C_{30}H_{50}$), a highly unsaturated hydrocarbon obtained from shark liver oil. Research continues on a number of possible new substances for use as vaccine adjuvants, including the products QS21, a product of the Antigenics company, derived from the soap bark tree (*Quillaja saponaria*), and M59, a product of the Novartis company, that consists of a proprietary mixture of oil in water. The use of adjuvants in vaccines is the subject of serious controversy within the professional and nonprofessional community; it is discussed further in Chapter 2 of this book (see, for example, Adjuvant Index Page 2012; Scheibner 2000/2001).

The History of Vaccination

The origins of vaccination are shrouded in the mists of early human history. Researchers have traced the root of the practice to ancient India or China, although almost nothing is known for certain about its origins. One observer has noted that some of the mystery surrounding the beginnings of the practice are understandable, as some early healers may have wanted to keep their methodology hidden from the common people and, as a result, from historical inquiries many hundreds of years later (Boyston 2012). A number of sources claim that the practice of vaccination dates back to the pre-Christian era, although such claims tend not to cite specific references or to rely on references that are highly questionable. For example, a Smithsonian Institution website on the history of polio vaccination says that "[i]noculation originated in India or China some time before 200 BC," without providing any reference for that claim (History of Vaccines 2012).

Variolation

It is, perhaps, safer to rely on written accounts that describe the practice of vaccination in unequivocal terms for dating the earliest confirmed examples of the procedure. All of these earliest accounts refer to variolation, which, as described earlier in this chapter, is the practice of transferring infectious material from the sores of a person infected with a disease directly to the body of an uninfected person, with the goal of providing immunity to the latter person. A number of variolation methods have been described in the historical record. One of the most common is the process known as *insufflation.* In this process, material taken from a smallpox lesion (either pus or scab) was dried and then inserted into the nose of the uninfected person. This procedure appears to have been used most commonly in China. A second procedure involved the removal of pus from a lesion or, alternatively, the preparation of a solution of ground smallpox scab with water, either of which was then placed into the skin of an uninfected person with a sharp needle. The person conducting the variolation pricked a person's skin with the treated needle in a number of closely spaced sites, a procedure that was still used (in principle, if not in detail) as late as the mid-20th century. In either of these procedures, the inserted infectious material generally produced a mild case of the disease, which then protected the person against more serious, full-blown cases of smallpox. In some cases, however, the process produced the undesired result of engendering the disease itself. Other procedures of inoculating a person against smallpox were also known. For example, children were sometimes dressed in the clothing of other children who had been infected with the disease, with the expectation that this exposure to the disease would prevent its occurrence in the uninfected child (Fenner et al. 1988, Chapter 6).

One of the first written reports of variolation dates to the work of the Chinese physician Yu Mao Kun. In his 1727 book *Ke Jin Jing Fu Ji Ji (Special Golden Mirror and Solutions),* Yu describes how variolation was used widely in many parts of China during the Qing period of the Ming Dynasty (1567–1572) (Flower 2008, 5). A number of writers suggest a much earlier origin of the practice, but rely on less positive historical records for their claims. The early history of immunization in India is as murky as it is for China. Some authorities trace the beginnings of variolation in India to the teachings of Dhanvantari, the physician of the gods and the god of Ayurvedic medicine in the oldest of Hindu traditions recorded in the Vedas and Puranas, the holy writings. According to this tradition, variolation was well known and widely practiced in India at least as early as the fifth century CE (Hindu Culture—Part 2 2012).

More cautious historians rely on written reports that date to about the 18th century. A report by one Robert Coult, a British resident of India writing to a relative in England in 1731, explained how physicians performed variolation. They extracted a small amount of pus from a smallpox lesion on the point of a "pretty large sharp needle" and then made "several punctures in the hollow under the deltoid muscle or sometimes in the forehead, after which they cover the part with a little paste made of boiled rice." Coult went on to say that the practice he was describing had been in use for at least 150 years, and had probably been introduced by a physician by the name of Dununtary, who lived in the small town of Champanagar on the Ganges River. Coult's letter is generally thought to be the first confirmed Western report of variolation practices in India (Marglin 1987).

By the time of Coult's report in 1713, variolation was also being used in other parts of the world, including the Middle East, northern and western Africa, and even parts of Europe. Scholars have been unable to unravel the mechanisms by which the practice (as well as the disease of smallpox itself) migrated from one part of the world to another. Some authorities believe that Arab traders brought both the disease and the practice of variolation from India and, perhaps, China to the Middle East and thence into North Africa. Others argue that the route of transmission went in the other direction, from Africa or, even more likely, from the Middle East, outward into Africa and southern Asia. In any case, reports from all parts of the globe in the mid-18th century confirm that variolation was widely practiced in most known regions of the world (see, for example,

Boyston 2012; Flower 2008, 5–6; Klebs 1913; Marglin 1987; The History of Inoculation and Vaccination for the Prevention and Treatment of Disease 1913).

Methods for preventing infection by smallpox were relatively well known in Europe probably as early as the first part of the 17th century. One of the most common practices used was called "buying the smallpox," in which parents arranged to have their children exposed under controlled conditions to the disease. For example, they might have their children spend a night in the bed of another child who had contracted the disease, or they might purchase a bit of food from a house in which smallpox had recently been present (Burke 1769; Fenner 1988, 254). Of particular interest for the history of immunization is that this practice was apparently common for a long period of time in geographical areas as distinct as Poland, Denmark, Wales, Scotland, England, Algiers, West Africa, and Switzerland, where the practice was even called by the same name (Glynn and Glynn 2005, 47).

In spite of the use of such practices, the introduction of variolation itself is generally credited to the efforts of a single person, Lady Mary Wortley Montagu, in 1721. (This interpretation of the history of variolation in Europe is likely to be somewhat simplistic. See, for example, Buda 2012.) At the time, Lady Wortley Montagu was living in Constantinople with her husband, the English ambassador to the Ottoman Empire. A victim of smallpox herself, Lady Wortley Montagu took a very special interest in the custom she observed in Constantinople of having young children variolated in the fall of every year. She was so impressed with the practice that she had her own son variolated against the disease. She then also wrote long and effusive letters back to England describing the variolation process and encouraging her friends to have their children variolated. Her entreaties were largely met with distrust and indifference by the conservative British medical community, but the general public was eventually won over when Caroline, Princess of Wales (later Queen Caroline), arranged for two public demonstrations of the safety and efficacy of variolation (Case and Chung 1997, 59).

The introduction of variolation to the United States is often also credited to a single event, this one involving the famous American cleric Cotton Mather. In 1706, Mather's parishioners had given him a slave, Onesimus, from North Africa. From Onesimus, Mather learned about the practice of variolation, a procedure for which he saw great promise in the new American colonies. (At about the same time, Mather came across an article about variolation by Dr. Emmanuel Timoni to the British scientific journal, *Philosophical Transactions*. Ironically, Timoni was a physician living in Constantinople at the same time as Lady Wortley Montagu, who also worked diligently to teach European physicians about the process of variolation (see Behbehani 1983). Mather's enthusiasm for variolation was not sufficient to convince the Massachusetts Bay medical community during the smallpox outbreaks that occurred on and off during the first quarter of the 18th century. Not only were questions raised about the safety and efficacy of the procedure but, generally more important, religious leaders preached against using a technique (variolation) that was designed to thwart God's will (presumably to cause illness and death) (Behbehani 1983, 464–466).

From Variolation to Vaccination

During the 18th century, when variolation was gradually winning adherents in England and other parts of the world, another method of vaccination was also in use, although to a far more limited extent. This method was based on the common observation among rural residents that a person who had been exposed to the relatively mild disease known as cowpox was less likely to contract smallpox than were those who had never had such exposure. (The cowpox virus belongs to the same genus as the smallpox virus, but is much less virulent.) In fact, records indicate that a process similar to variolation using materials from cowpox lesions had been used in Great Britain and other European countries during the middle decades of the 18th century. In this procedure, small quantities of pus or scabs from cowpox sources were injected into young children, who then almost invariably became immune to infection by the smallpox virus. In fact, some historians have claimed that individuals from England and Germany, including a Mr. Jensen (about 1770), a Mrs. Sevel (about 1772), and Peter Plett (1791), all in Germany; and Benjamin Jesty (in 1774) and a Mrs. Rendall (about 1782), both in England, had all practiced vaccinations using cowpox (Hammarsten, Tattersall, and Hammarsten 1979; Plett 2006; Vaccination Against Smallpox 2012).

The real breakthrough in this technology occurred in 1796, when English physician Edward Jenner inoculated eight-year-old James Phipps with material taken from a cowpox sore on the hands of milkmaid Sarah Nelmes. After the boy experienced a mild reaction to the procedure, Jenner then injected him with material from a smallpox lesion and found that the boy failed to develop smallpox. Jenner later repeated his experiment on about two dozen more subjects, with similarly satisfactory results with all of them. The primary significance of Jenner's work was that he had found a way of inoculating a person against smallpox without the risk of actually inducing the disease in the patient. Since the person being vaccinated never actually received the smallpox virus, she or he was essentially incapable of developing the disease. Jenner's work was important for another reason also, however. The design of his experiment provided scientific evidence that the procedure actually worked; he demonstrated that patients inoculated with cowpox material did not develop smallpox even when they were given the virus that causes the disease. Medical practitioners no longer had to rely on old wives' tales to have confidence in the new procedure; they had actually data on which to rely. (All of which does not mean that there was not widespread objection to the use of Jenner's technique both within the medical profession and among the general public, a topic of Chapter 2 of this book.) Jenner later gave the name *vaccine* to the material he used in the procedure, after the Latin word *vaca*, for "cow," and the name *vaccination* to the procedure he developed.

News of Jenner's discovery spread rapidly throughout Europe and other parts of the world. Before long, many public health authorities were using his procedure to provide protection against smallpox among large populations. An often-repeated example of the impact made by his discovery is the story of the so-called Balmis Expedition to the New World in 1803. For a number of years, the Spanish colonies in the New World had been wracked by smallpox epidemics for which, of course, there was neither treatment nor any form of prevention. When King Charles IV of Spain heard of Jenner's discovery, he decided to send the new method of vaccination to the New World to reduce the risk of future smallpox epidemics. The method his advisors developed was to recruit 22 orphaned children between the age of 8 and 10 for a voyage to the New World. Two of the children were inoculated with the smallpox vaccine before they left Spain on November 30, 1803. As soon as those two children began to develop the infectious pustules characteristic of cowpox, specimens of the infectious fluid were taken and injected into the arms of two other children on the ship. By means of this method, supplies of the vaccine were always available and could be used to begin vaccinating residents of the New World as soon as the ship reached its destination (Franco-Paredes, Lammoglia, and Santos-Preciado 2005).

Arm-to-arm vaccination proved to be highly successful, but it was accompanied by some serious side effects, primarily the transmission of other infectious diseases, such as hepatitis, leprosy, and syphilis. For example, 44 out of the 63 children who were vaccinated in Rivalta, Italy, in 1861 eventually developed syphilis. A number of those children died of the diseases, and some family members also contracted the disease from the infected children (Fenner et al. 1988, 264–265). These side effects were serious enough that some governmental agencies began to ban the use of arm-to-arm vaccination by the end of the 19th century. In 1898, for example, the British Parliament adopted the Vaccination Act that essentially banned the use of the arm-to-arm procedure (Dudgeon 1963, passim).

Such actions were possible because an alternative method of producing vaccine was available, if not at the time widely used. This method dated to the very early 19th century and involved the inoculation of calves with the cowpox serum. When the calves began to produce the pustules characteristic of the disease, fluid was taken from their lymph system, processed, and used as a vaccine against smallpox. The process involving the production, collection, and purification of calf lymph obtained from inoculated cows has remained the primary method of making smallpox vaccine to the present day. In fact, the only smallpox vaccine currently available in the world was originally produced in the early 1970s. In its current form, a product known as Dryvax, the vaccine is still viable and capable of preventing smallpox. As of 2012, enough doses of the vaccine are available to vaccinate every citizen of the United States against a possible return of the smallpox virus (a second stock of vaccine produced in the 1950s is also still available and still viable) (Smallpox Vaccination and Adverse Events Training Module 2012).

The preceding discussion has focused on smallpox as the classic story of the development of vaccines and vaccination. A similar tale can be told for a number of other infectious diseases. Cholera was another example of an infectious disease that had been infecting human populations for hundreds of years. In 1879, the French chemist and microbiologist Louis Pasteur set out to identify the agent that caused cholera and to develop a method of protection against the disease. He decided to start by studying cholera in chickens, a problem of considerable importance to French farmers at the time. Pasteur injected a group of chickens with the bacteria that cause cholera and found that they became ill, but did not die. He later learned that the bacteria used were less virulent than normal, a fact he blamed on their exposure to oxygen. About a month after this experiment, Pasteur used a fresh batch of chicken cholera bacteria to inject both the original group of chickens, and another group of chickens that had never been inoculated with the bacteria. Again, chickens in the first group became moderately ill, but did not die; but all members of the unvaccinated chickens did die. Pasteur concluded that an infectious agent (the chicken cholera bacteria) that was less virulent than normal (that had become *attenuated*) provided protection against the disease. Pasteur eventually used this information to develop vaccines for a number of animal diseases using a variety of methods to produce attenuated viruses and bacteria. Pasteur's method was also later adapted by other researchers for the development of new vaccines against other diseases. For example, Russian bacteriologist Waldemar Mordecai Wolff Haffkine produced the first vaccine against human cholera in 1892 in a long process, the final step of which involved injecting himself with the experimental vaccine (Bornside 1982; Ilana 1992).

Space does not permit a detailed discussion of the development of other vaccines against infectious diseases. Table 1.4 provides a brief summary of the dates of the first discovery of some of these diseases.

The history of infectious diseases and the vaccines developed for use against them is an exciting and inspiring story of the successes of medical researchers in dramatically reducing the suffering caused by such diseases among humans and other animals. The story has not been one of unalloyed accomplishment about which everyone is entirely pleased, however. From the very moment that vaccines were first conceived and put to use, questions have been raised about both their safety and efficacy. Some of the issues associated with the development and use of vaccines and vaccination procedures are the subject of the next chapter of this book.

Table 1.4   First Discovery of Vaccines

Disease	Year First Developed
Rabies	1885
Tetanus	1890
Typhoid fever	1896
Bubonic plague	1897
Diphtheria	1921
Tuberculosis	1921
Pertussis	1926
Yellow fever	1932
Typhus	1937
Influenza	1945
Polio	1952
Japanese encephalitis	1954
Anthrax	1957
Measles	1963
Mumps	1967
Rubella	1970
Pneumonia (*Streptococcus pneumoniae*)	1977
Meningitis (*Neisseria meningitidis*)	1978
Hepatitis B	1981
Haemophilus influenzae type b (HiB)	1985
Hepatitis A	1992
Lyme disease	1998
Rotavirus	1998
Human papillomavirus	2006

References

Abedon, Stephen T. "Bacterial Mechanisms of Pathogenicity." http://www.mansfield.ohio-state.edu/˜sabedon/biol2060.htm. Accessed on April 9, 2012.

"Adjuvant Index Page." Vaccination Liberation. http://www.vaclib.org/basic/adjuvants.htm. Accessed on April 14, 2012.

"Akhenaten (Amenhotep IV)." Ancient Egypt Online. http://www.ancientegyptonline.co.uk/akhenaten.html. Accessed on April 8, 2012.

Babu, B. V. "History of Malaria Burden." *RMRC News Bulletin* 7, no. 1 (2007): 1–4. http://rmrcorissa.gov.in/news/news.pdf. Accessed on April 8, 2012.

Barquet, Nicolau, and Pere Domingo. "Smallpox: The Triumph over the Most Terrible of the Ministers of Death." *Annals of Internal Medicine* 127, no. 8, part 1 (1997): 635–642.

Behbehani, Abbas M. "The Smallpox Story: Life and Death of an Old Disease." *Microbiological Reviews* 47, no. 4 (1983): 455–509.

Bornside, George H. "Waldemar Haffkine's Cholera Vaccines and the Ferran-Haffkine Priority Dispute." *Journal of the History of Medicine and Allied Sciences* 37, no. 4 (1982): 399–422.

Boyston, A. W. "The Origins of Inoculation." http://www.jameslindlibrary.org/illustrating/articles/the-origins-of-inoculation. Accessed on April 16, 2012.

Buda, Octavian. "Variolation from the Balkans—Through Romanian Territories—to Western Europe, 1678–1802." Pulse Project. http://www.pulse-project.org/node/287. Accessed on April 17, 2012.

Burke, Edmund. *The Annual Register of World Events:A Review of the Year 1769.* London: Longmans, Green, 1769. http://books.google.com/books?id=-29IAAAAYAAJ&pg=RA1-PA83&lpg=RA1-PA83&dq=%22carries+a+few+raisins,+dates,+sugar+plumbs,+or+such+like%22&source=bl&ots=gn30UPiLjg&sig=v2yXKtmt_cw_ZMCKCJ7PGAT0PDo&hl=en&sa=X&ei=Ot-NT4qbAqv-ciQKVvty_CA&sqi=2&ved=0CA8Q6AEwAQ#v=onepage&q=%22carries%20a%20few%20raisins%2C%20dates%2C%20sugar%20plumbs%2C%20or%20such%20like%22&f=false.

Caplan, Arthur. "Vaccination: Facts Alone Do Not Policy Make." *Health Affairs* 30, no. 6 (2011): 1205–1208.

Case, Christine L., and King-Thom Chung. "Montagu and Jenner: The Campaign Against Smallpox." *SIM News* 47, no. 2 (1997): 58–60.

Cone, T. E., Jr. "Was Sir Walter Scott's Lameness Caused by Poliomyelitis?" *Pediatrics* 51, no. 1 (1973): 35.

"Country Comparison :: HIV/AIDS—Adult Prevalence Rate." The World Factbook. https://www.cia.gov/library/publications/the-world-factbook/rankorder/2155rank.html. Accessed on April 9, 2012.

Crubézy E., et al. "Identification of Mycobacterium DNA in an Egyptian Pott's Disease of 5,400 Years Old." *Comptes Rendus de l'Academie des Sciences. Serie III* 321, no. 11 (1998): 941–951.

Daniel, Thomas M., and Frederick C. Robbins, "A History of Poliomyelitis." In Daniel Thomas M., and Frederick C. Robbins, eds. *Polio.* Rochester, NY: University of Rochester Press, 1997.

"Dengue -> Annual Cases and Deaths by Country (1955) ->." World Health Organization. Denguenet. http://apps.who.int/globalatlas/dataQuery/reportData.asp?rptType=1. Accessed on April 18, 2012.

Dudgeon, J. A. "Development of Smallpox Vaccine in England in the Eighteenth and Nineteenth Centuries." *British Medical Journal* 1, no. 5342 (1963): 1367–1372.

Echenberg, Myron. "Pestis Redux: The Initial Years of the Third Bubonic Plague Pandemic, 1894–1901." *Journal of World History* 13, no. 2 (2002): 429–449.

Edsall, Geoffrey. "Smallpox Vaccination vs Inoculation." *The Journal of the American Medical Association* 190, no. 7 (1964): 689–690.

"Edward Jenner and the Discovery of Vaccination." http://library.sc.edu/spcoll/nathist/jenner.html. Accessed on April 13, 2012.

Eggers, Hans J. "Milestones in Early Poliomyelitis Research (1840 to 1949)." *Journal of Virology* 73, no. 6 (1999): 4533–4535.

Ellis, Ronald W. *Combination Vaccines: Development, Clinical Research, and Approval.* Totowa, NJ: Humana Press, 1999.

"Fact Sheet—Viruses." Ecometrex. http://www.ecometrex. com/viruses.htm. Accessed on April 9, 2012.

Fenner, Frank, et al. *Smallpox and Its Eradication.* Geneva: World Health Organization, 1988.

Flower, Darren R. *Bioinformatics of Vaccinology.* New York: Wiley, 2008.

Franco-Paredes, Carlos, Lorena Lammoglia, and José Ignacio Santos-Preciado. "The Spanish Royal Philanthropic Expedition to Bring Smallpox Vaccination to the New World and Asia in the 19th Century." *Clinical Infectious Diseases* 41, no. 9 (2005): 1285–1289.

"GenVec Announces Additional Funding for Malaria Vaccine Program from the PATH Malaria Vaccine Initiative." redOrbit. http://www.redorbit.com/news/health/920712/ genvec_announces_additional_funding_for_malaria_vaccine_ program_from_the/. Accessed on April 14, 2012.

Glynn, Ian, and Jenifer Glynn. *The Life and Death of Smallpox.* London: Profile Books, 2005.

Gubler, D. J. "Dengue/Dengue Haemorrhagic Fever: History and Current Status." *Novartis Foundation Symposium* 277 (2006): 3–16.

Guerrant, Richard L., et al. "How Intestinal Bacteria Cause Disease." *Journal of Infectious Diseases* 179, suppl 2 (1999): S331–S337.

"*Haemophilus influenzae* Type B." http://www.vaclib.org/legal/ MTstate/hib.pdf. Accessed on April 13, 2012.

Hammarsten, J. F., W. Tattersall, and J. E. Hammarsten. "Who Discovered Smallpox Vaccination? Edward Jenner or

Benjamin Jesty?" *Transactions of the American Clinical and Climatological Association* 90 (1979): 44–55.

Hanlon, Jamie. "Vaccine Discovered for Hep C by Michael Houghton Who Discovered HCV in 1989." http://www.natap.org/2012/newsUpdates/022312_01.htm. Accessed on April 12, 2012.

Henchal, Erick, and J. Robert Putnak. "The Dengue Viruses." *Clinical Microbiology Reviews* 3, no. 4 (1990): 376–396.

"Hepatitis C." emedicinehealth. http://www.emedicinehealth.com/hepatitis_c/article_em.htm. Accessed on April 12, 2012.

"Hepatitis C." World Health Organization. http://www.who.int/mediacentre/factsheets/fs164/en/index.html. Accessed on April 12, 2012.

"Hepatitis C History." News Medical. http://www.news-medical.net/health/Hepatitis-C-History.aspx. Accessed on April 12, 2012.

"Hindu Culture—Part 2." A Tribute to Hinduism. http://www.hinduwisdom.info/Hindu_Culture2.htm. Accessed on April 17, 2012.

"History of Dengue." http://www.denguevirusnet.com/history-of-dengue.html. Accessed on April 12, 2012.

"The History of Inoculation and Vaccination for the Prevention and Treatment of Disease." Lecture Memoranda. London: Burroughs Wellcome & Co., 1913. http://archive.org/stream/historyofinocula00burrrich#page/n9/mode/2up. Accessed on January 4, 2013.

"History of Vaccines." Smithsonian Institution. http://americanhistory.si.edu/polio/virusvaccine/history.htm. Accessed on April 17, 2012.

HIV/AIDS. "Data and Statistics." World Health Organization. http://www.who.int/hiv/data/en/. Accessed on April 9, 2012.

Hopkins, Donald R. "Ramses V: Earliest Known Victim?" http://whqlibdoc.who.int/smallpox/WH_5_1980_p22.pdf. Accessed on April 8, 2012.

Hulse, E. V. "Leprosy and Ancient Egypt." *Lancet* 300, no. 7788 (1972): 1024–1025.

Ilana, Löwy. "From Guinea Pigs to Man: The Development of Haffkine's Anticholera Vaccine." *Journal of the History of Medicine and Allied Sciences* 47, no. 3 (1992): 270–309.

Kakkilaya, B. S. "Malaria in Ancient Literature." http://www.malariasite.com/malaria/history_literature.htm. Accessed on April 8, 2012.

Klebs, Arnold C. "The Historic Evolution of Variolation." *The Johns Hopkins Hospital Bulletin* 24, no. 265 (1913): 1–67. http://www.med.yale.edu/library/historical/klebs/pdf%20docs/histvariolation2.pdf. Accessed on January 4, 2013.

Kozloff, Arielle. "Bubonic Plague in the Reign of Amenhotep III?" *KMT* 17, no. 3 (2006): 36–46.

"'Leprosy' in the Bible—What Was It?" WebSpawner.com. http://www.webspawner.com/users/lepbible/. Accessed on April 8, 2012.

"Making Vaccines: Subunit Vaccine: Hepatitis B." http://www.pbs.org/wgbh/nova/bioterror/vacc_hepatitis.html. Accessed on April 13, 2012.

Marglin, Frédérique Apffel. *Smallpox in Two Systems of Knowledge.* Helsinki: UNU-WIDER, 1987.

Martin, N. A. "The Discovery of Viral Hepatitis: A Military Perspective." *Journal of the Royal Army Medical Corps* 149, no.2 (2003): 121–124.

Merrill, Ray M., and Thomas C. Timmreck. *Introduction to Epidemiology*, 4th ed. Sudbury, MA: Jones and Bartlett Publishers, 2006.

Morelli, Giovanna, et al. "*Yersinia Pestis* Genome Sequencing Identifies Patterns of Global Phylogenetic Diversity." *Nature Genetics* 42, no. 12 (2010): 1140–1143.

"Novartis Phase III Study Shows Meningococcal B Vaccine Candidate Could Be First to Provide Broad Coverage Against Deadly Disease." Novartis Global. http://www.novartis.com/newsroom/media-releases/en/2010/1443940.shtml. Accessed on April 14, 2012.

Orent, Wendy. "The Polio Virus Fights Back." http://articles.latimes.com/2011/feb/09/opinion/la-oe-orent-polio-20110209. Accessed on April 13, 2012.

O'Shea, Robert S. "Hepatitis C." Cleveland Clinic. Center for Continuing Education. http://www.clevelandclinicmeded.com/medicalpubs/diseasemanagement/hepatology/hepatitis-C/#bib1. Accessed on April 12, 2012.

Pennington, Hugh. "Smallpox and Bioterrorism." *Bulletin of the World Health Organization* 81, no. 10 (2003): 762–767.

"The Plague of Athens." http://www.ancientgreece.com/essay/v/the_plague_of_athens/. Accessed on April 8, 2012.

"Plague of Athens: Another Medical Mystery Solved at University of Maryland." http://www.umm.edu/news/releases/athens.htm. Accessed on April 8, 2012.

Plett, P. C. "Peter Plett and Other Discoverers of Cowpox Vaccination before Edward Jenner." *Sudhoffs Archives* 90, no. 2 (2006): 219–232. (in German)

"Polio." Online Health Magazine. http://www.allabthealth.com/infections/polio-4090. Accessed on April 11, 2012.

"Polio This Week—As of 04 April 2012." World Health Organization. http://www.polioeradication.org/Dataandmonitoring/Poliothisweek.aspx. Accessed on April 11, 2012.

Rappuoli, Rino. "Reverse Vaccinology, a Genome-based Approach to Vaccine Development." *Vaccine* 19, no. 17–19 (2001): 2688–2691.

Rappuoli, Rino, and Alan Aderem. "A 2020 Vision for Vaccines Against HIV, Tuberculosis and Malaria." *Nature* 473, no. 7348 (2011): 463–469.

Robbins, Gwen, et al. "Ancient Skeletal Evidence for Leprosy in India (2000 B.C.)." *PLoS ONE* 4, no. 5 (2009): e5669, 1–8.

"Rotavirus Strains." Exploring Vaccines. http://explorevac cines.wordpress.com/2011/04/03/rotavirus-strains/. Accessed on April 14, 2012.

Sabbatini, Sergio, and Sirio Fiorino. "The Antonine Plague and the Decline of the Roman Empire." *Le Infezioni in Medicina* 17, no. 4 (2009): 261–275.

Sabin, A. B., and L. R. Boulger. "History of Sabin Attenuated Poliovirus Oral Live Vaccine Strains." *Journal of Biological Standardization* 1, no. 2 (1973): 115–118.

"The Salk Vaccine Trials." http://wps.aw.com/wps/media/ objects/14/15269/projects/ch12_salk/index.html. Accessed on April 13, 2012.

Scheibner, Viera. "Adverse Effects of Adjuvants in Vaccines." *Nexus* 8, no. 1 & 2 (2000/2001). http://www.whale.to/ vaccine/adjuvants.html#ADJUVANTS_. Accessed on January 4, 2013.

"Smallpox." World Health Organization. http://www.who. int/topics/smallpox/en/. Accessed on January 4, 2013.

"Smallpox Vaccination and Adverse Events Training Module." Centers for Disease Control and Prevention. http://www. bt.cdc.gov/training/smallpoxvaccine/reactions/about_vac_ emergency.html. Accessed on April 18, 2012.

Stol, Marten. *Epilepsy in Babylonia.* Gröningen: Styx Publications, 1993.

Todar, Kenneth. "Mechanisms of Bacterial Pathogenicity." http://textbookofbacteriology.net/pathogenesis.html. Accessed on April 9, 2012.

"The Top 10 Causes of Death." World Health Organization. Fact Sheet No. 310. http://www.who.int/mediacentre/factsheets/fs310/en/index.html. Accessed on April 10, 2012.

"Vaccination Against Smallpox." http://www.hubertlerch.com/classes/IH0852/Jenner_Notes.html. Accessed on April 17, 2012.

"Vector-Borne Viral Infections. Dengue Fever." World Health Organization. Initiative for Vaccine Research (IVR). http://www.who.int/vaccine_research/diseases/vector/en/index1.html. Accessed on April 12, 2012.

"Viral Hepatitis Surveillance. United States, 2009." Centers for Disease Control and Prevention. http://www.cdc.gov/hepatitis/Statistics/2009Surveillance/PDFs/2009HepSurveillanceRpt.pdf. Accessed on April 12, 2012.

Wade, Nicholas.. "Europe's Plagues Came From China, Study Finds." *New York Times.* October 31, 2010. http://www.nytimes.com/2010/11/01/health/01plague.html?_r=1&src=me&ref=general. Accessed on January 4, 2013.

World Health Organization. *WHO Vaccine-Preventable Diseases: Monitoring System. 2010 Global Summary.* Geneva: World Health Organization. http://whqlibdoc.who.int/hq/2010/WHO_IVB_2010_eng.pdf. Accessed on April 11, 2012.

Winslow, Charles-Edward Amory. *The Conquest of Epidemic Disease: A Chapter in the History of Ideas.* Princeton, NJ: Princeton University Press, 1943.

Zink, Albert R., et al. "Characterization of *Mycobacterium tuberculosis* Complex DNAs from Egyptian Mummies by Spoligotyping." *Journal of Clinical Microbiology.* 41, no. 1 (2003): 359–367.

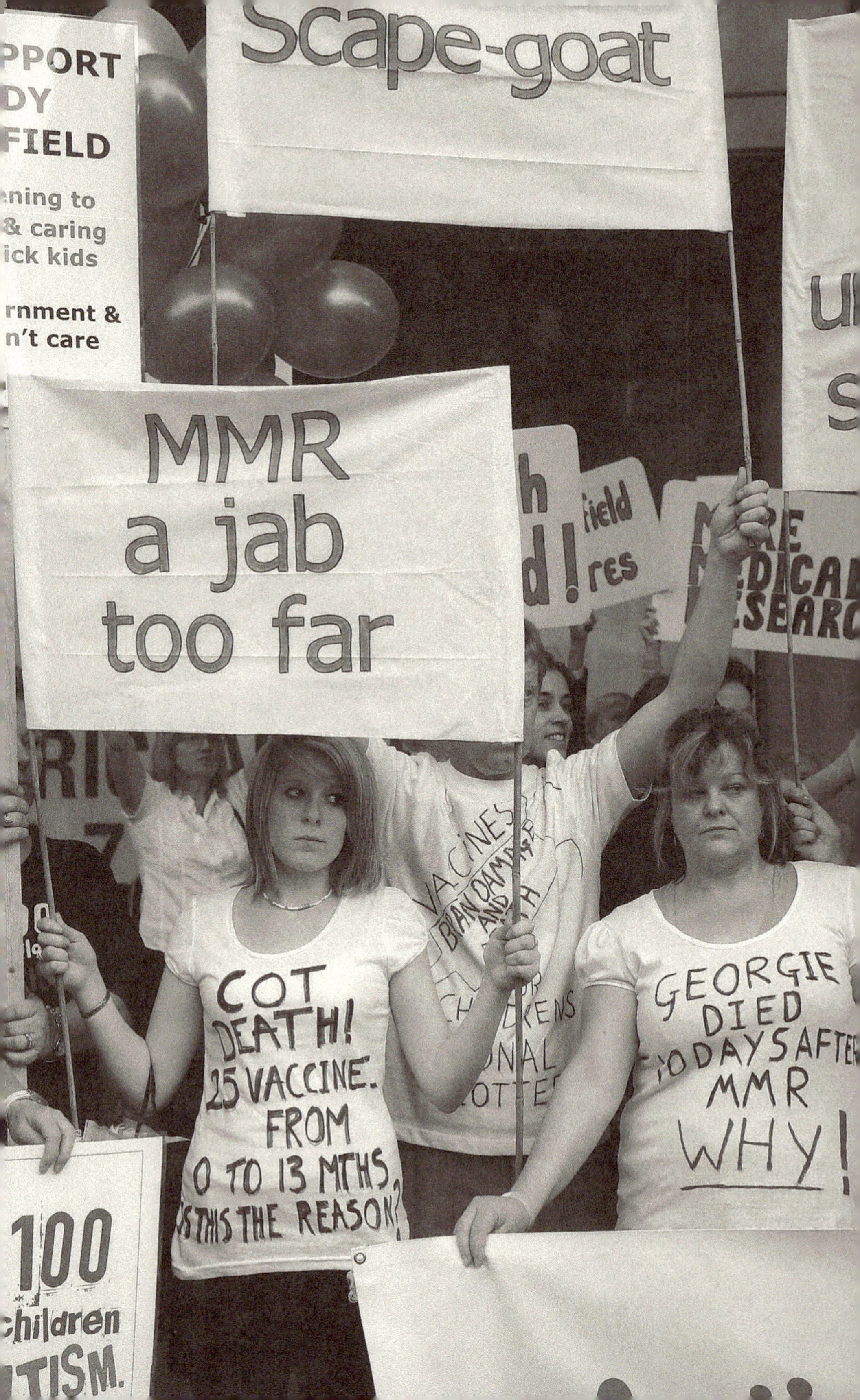
Scape-goat
MMR a jab too far
COT DEATH! 25 VACCINE. FROM 0 TO 13 MTHS IS THIS THE REASON?
GEORGIE
DIED
MMR
WHY!

For a man to infect a family [by vaccination] in the morning with smallpox and to pray to God in the evening against the disease is blasphemy.

Smallpox is "a judgment of God on the sins of the people . . . to avert it is but to provoke him more."

Inoculation is "an encroachment on the prerogatives of Jehovah, whose right it is to wound and smite."

Such were only a few of the judgments offered by religious leaders in the American colonies in the early 1720s against newly established requirements that children be vaccinated against smallpox in the Massachusetts Bay Colony (White 1960, vol. 2, 56). Opponents who offered this view of vaccination also called for the death of Dr. Zabdiel Boylston, a Boston physician, who had aroused their ire by vaccinating his own son against the disease. They called for Boylston's trial, conviction, and execution because of his insistence on "thwarting God's will."

The sentiments expressed here in opposition to vaccination were by no means the first objections to the use of artificial means to prevent the spread of smallpox, nor were they to be the last of such efforts. In fact, questions as to the safety and efficacy of vaccines have been an integral part of the centuries-old

Women picket in support of anti-vaccinationist doctor Andrew Wakefield and his controversial views on a connection between the measles-mumps-rubella (MMR) vaccine and autism. (AP Photo/Sang Tan)

battle to bring smallpox and other infectious diseases under control. This chapter begins with a brief history of such efforts, dating to the earliest known dates to which they can be connected. The chapter continues with a review of the continuing battle being waged against compulsory vaccination in the United States and other countries around the world, as well as the campaign against certain specific mandatory types of vaccination, such as the current controversy over the human papillomavirus and anthrax vaccines.

A Brief History of Opposition to Vaccination

In the centuries before Edward Jenner's discovery of the process of vaccination, the strongest and most common objection to the practice was probably that reflected in the comments with which this chapter opened. Objectors argued that smallpox was not some random event that struck individuals in a haphazard way, but a specific form of punishment ordained by some supernatural being, designed to punish individuals for their sins or to provide some kind of moral lesson. (Humans usually had to decipher that lesson on their own, usually with the help of religious leaders.) Such beliefs were not restricted to any particular religion, but extended to all faiths. For example, efforts by the Egyptian ruler Muhammad Ali in the late 1810s to require vaccination of all children in the country ran into religious teachings that smallpox was sent by God to punish humans, and that vaccinating against the disease was an act of resistance to God's will. Such an act was, of course, in opposition to the teachings of the Koran, and thus not permitted among faithful Muslims (Kuhnke 1990, 114–116).

Religious teachings were by no means the only source of opposition to vaccination. Muhammad Ali's orders for mandatory universal vaccination of children were also resisted because many Egyptians believed that the process represented a way of marking their children. The cowpox scar formed after vaccination was a way, they believed, of identifying them for possible future conscription into military service. Objectors actually had some basis for this concern, as the Egyptian government had previously used tattooing as a method for identifying individuals who were eligible for or who had actually been conscripted into military service. Rural Egyptians, in fact, often referred to the vaccination process as "tatooing smallpox" (Kuhnke 1990, 116–117).

Yet a third objection to vaccination among rural residents in Egypt in particular was the fear that blood from Christians would be mixed with that of Muslims during the inoculation process. Such an event would, of course, also violate the teachings of the Koran, adding yet another reason for people to oppose the newly imposed procedure.

Many opponents of vaccination were gradually convinced over the years, primarily because so many people noticed that their "marked" children were far more likely to survive a smallpox infection than were otherwise similar "unmarked" children. Still, objections against the practice never completely died out over the next few decades (Kuhnke 1990, 115).

A similar reliance on religious teachings as a basis of opposing compulsory vaccination can be found in other countries. In 1888, for example, a group of citizens in the town of Cawnpore, India, presented a petition to local officials objecting to a new program of required vaccination. They pointed out in their petition that a "major portion of the community" believed that smallpox was a "direct expression of the wrath of the Goddess Bhawani or Shitala. It is not a malady that can be cured by medicine," the petition went on, "and any attempt to check its progress will only enrage the Goddess, who is otherwise pacified by prayers and a simple diet" (Bhattacharya, Harrison, and Worboys 2005, 64).

As in Egypt, the objections to vaccination in India were not entirely religious. For example, residents in the town of Unnao, India, presented a petition similar to the one from Cawnpore a year later. The main objection in the Unnao petition was that bodily fluids from two different castes might be mixed during the procedure, an act that would clearly violate the country's strong system of separating individuals of different castes (Bhattacharya, Harrison, and Worboys 2005, 65). This concern was based on the fact that the most common method of vaccination in India at the time involved the use of a lower-caste child who had become infected with smallpox. That child was taken from place to place and used as a source of smallpox fluid for the vaccination of other children, of whatever caste. The risk for upper-caste families, then, was that their children would become contaminated by contact with a lower-caste child (Arnold 1988, 55; see also Brimnes 2004).

As the practice of vaccination became more popular in Europe, it almost immediately encountered strong opposition from both the medical community and the general public. Not only was religion a strong factor in the condemnation of the practice, but so was the viewpoint of a very large number of scientists and medical experts interested in the problems of smallpox treatment and prevention. As an example, a conference of the International Anti-Vaccination League was held in Paris in December 1880, at which representatives from Belgium, France, the Netherlands, Switzerland, the United Kingdom, the United States, and the Kingdom of Württemberg met to discuss issues surrounding the use of vaccination for the prevention of smallpox. At the completion of the conference, the league's executive committee issued a report that contained a statement of nine conclusions as to why the practice of vaccination should be suppressed. The last of those conclusions was:

> In view of the confusion of opinion which prevails in every medical assembly amongst the so-called authorities, whenever the subject of Vaccination is discussed, it is unwise, impolitic, unjust and tyrannical to enforce Vaccination; that such enforcement retards all improvement in the treatment, and all discoveries for the prevention of small-pox; and that all Compulsory Legislation

with regard to Vaccination ought to be repealed. (Tebb 1884, 62)

The English Vaccination Laws

Opposition to vaccination in Great Britain reached a peak during the second half of the 19th century, largely as a result of a series of laws enacted by the British Parliament with regard to the practice. The first of those laws, adopted in 1840, banned the practice of variolation because, the Parliament decided, variolation was always more dangerous for a person than was vaccination. Demonstrating that it still supported the concept of vaccination, however, the Parliament also included in the law a provision that assigned to the Poor Law Commission the responsibility for providing free vaccinations for all children whose parents requested the service (Brunton 2008; Wolfe and

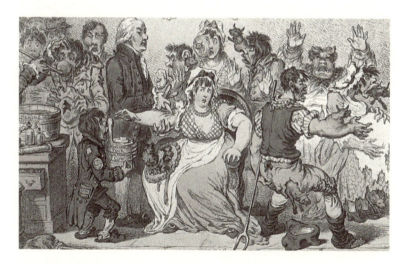

Anti-Vaccine Society cartoon by James Gillray, 1802. Entitled "The Cow-Pock or the Wonderful Effects of the New Inoculation," the etching mocked Edward Jenner's efforts at inoculation using the cowpox virus, suggesting the transformation of patients into cows. Despite controversy, support of vaccination was strong in the early part of the 19th century. (Library of Congress)

Sharp 2002). In 1853, Parliament passed a second vaccination act, dramatically changing the government's policies toward the practice. It introduced a provision *requiring* all children under the age of four months to be vaccinated against smallpox. The act also put into place a system by which all new births were to be registered with the government, parents were to be notified of the vaccination requirement, and fines were to be assessed against parents who did not comply with the law. The 1853 law is of historic significance because it established in Great Britain for the first time the principle that public health concerns (the spread of smallpox) trumped individual rights concerns (the right of parents to refuse vaccination). That controversy has remained at the core of the anti-vaccination sentiment that has permeated countries around the world for the past 150 years (Durbach 2000; Wolfe and Sharp 2002).

Reaction to the 1853 act was rapid and sometimes violent. Riots broke out in a number of cities and towns, including Ipswich, Henley, and Mitford. Throughout the nation, large numbers of parents simply refused to follow the law and were arrested, fined, rearrested, and re-fined for (often repeated) violations of the law (Williamson 1984). Opponents of the law also began to organize against its provisions. Those organizations ranged in size from small, local committees against vaccination to national organizations like the Anti-Vaccination League, founded in London in 1853. Arguably the most important of the local groups was the Leicester Anti-Vaccination League which, according to one historian, "came to have an influence out of all proportion to its size," to a considerable extent because the city itself was a hotbed of resistance to the law of 1853 (Ross 1967-68, 38). As an example, one resident in the city was arrested a total of 25 times for continually refusing to allow her children to be vaccinated (Howard 2003). The city is perhaps best known in this regard for a mammoth protest march held in March of 1885 when an estimated 80,000–100,000 citizens took to the streets demonstrating against compulsory vaccination (History of Anti-Vaccination

Movements 2012). The anti-vaccination leagues not only planned and carried out local protest demonstrations and other acts of civil disobedience, but also published newsletter, wrote and distributed tracts against vaccination, and lobbied members of parliament to change the 1853 law.

If the goal of the anti-vaccination leagues was to get Parliament to change its mind about compulsory vaccination, they were unsuccessful. Parliament continued to pass additional, stricter versions of the 1853 law in 1867, 1871, 1873, and 1885. In one regard, these laws made vaccination more palatable by offering modest payments to parents who had their children vaccinated, but also more restrictive as stiffer penalties were applied for those who did not permit vaccinations. More broadly, however, the new laws expanded the range of vaccination requirements and increased the severity of penalties for noncompliance. The 1867 revision, for example, extended the age for mandatory vaccination of children to 14 and allowed penalties for noncompliance to accumulate against an individual or family.

These stronger laws only engendered stronger responses from those who opposed mandatory vaccination. After adoption of the 1867 law, opponents of vaccination began to speak more openly and more clearly about the issue of compulsory vaccination as an attack on civil liberties. At a time when individual freedoms were becoming a more important principle within the body politic in England (and elsewhere across Europe), this charge of interference with one's right to make one's own choices resounded broadly across the general population. No sooner was the 1867 act passed by the Parliament than another large national organization, the Anti-Compulsory Vaccination League, was formed in London to protest against the act in particular and mandatory vaccination in general. The organization's announced goal was "[t]he entire repeal of the Vaccination Acts; the disestablishment and disendowment of the practice of vaccination; and the abolition of all regulations in regard to vaccination as conditions of employment in the

Army, Navy, and in all State departments, or of admission to Educational or other Institutions" (Hawden 1902). The league also began to publish a number of publications on the subject of mandatory vaccination, including the journals *Anti-Vaccinator*, *National Anti-Compulsory Vaccination Reporter*, and the *Vaccination Inquirer*, as well as occasional papers such as "The Story of a Great Delusion," "Vaccination a Delusion," "Exit Dr. Jenner," "Why Vaccinate?" and "The Protest of an Anti-Vaccinist" (Hawden 1902).

Among the Vaccination Act revisions, perhaps the most significant was the one passed in 1898. That act contained two new major provisions. The first provision was a ban on arm-to-arm (human lymph) vaccination, leaving only vaccination by calf lymph as a permitted method of treatment. The second provision was a so-called conscience clause, which allowed individuals opposed to vaccination to indicate that opposition and to request a certificate of exemption for their children. In order to carry out this provision of the law, local vaccination boards were authorized to set up and administer vaccination programs for each community (The Vaccination Act, 1898). The conscience clause that permitted parents to "opt out" of vaccination for their children revealed the breadth and depth of opposition to vaccination in Great Britain at the time. In the year following passage of the act, about 600 communities chose the required vaccination boards by general election. Of that, at least a fifth were elected on the basis of a pledge to *not* enforce the new legislation (Address by Miss Lily Loat 2012). And by the end of 1898, more than 200,000 certificates of exemption had been granted throughout the country (Durbach 2002).

After adoption of the 1898 act, anti-vaccinationists continued to press their demands for a reduction in compulsory vaccinations, arguing that the process through which an individual had to go to get an exemption was too complex and time-consuming. They finally achieved their objective in the British elections of 1906 in which a new government was installed. One outspoken anti-vaccinationist claimed that more than 300 of those who had been elected to Parliament in the 1906 election had pledged in advance to repeal or modify the 1898 law (Address by Miss Lily Loat 2012). And one of the first acts by the new Parliament was, in fact, an effort to water down provisions in the 1898 bill. The main change was the elimination of the provision to which anti-vaccinationists had objected by which vaccination exemptions were granted by appeal to a local board. In its place was a new provision by which parents could simply file an affidavit stating their objection to having their children vaccinated at any time within four months following the birth of a child. As a result of the 1907 provisions, vaccination rates in Great Britain continued to fall precipitously over following decades, with about 75 percent of all children having been vaccinated in the years immediately following adoption of the act, and only a 34 percent vaccination rate by 1939. Compulsory vaccination against smallpox was finally abandoned entirely with the creation of the National Health Service in 1948 (Baxby 1999; Durbach 2002).

Anti-Vaccinationism in the United States

The introduction of variolation to the United States by Cotton Mather, as described in the opening of this chapter, brought with it many of the concerns and complaints about the practice from citizens who thought the practice was violating the wishes of God, on the one hand, or were concerned about deliberating infecting individuals with a deadly disease, on the other. Nonetheless, the practice of variolation did spread through the young colonies and, as a consequence, resulted in significant decreases in morbidity and mortality due to the disease during much of the 18th century. This success did not last long, however, in quieting the concerns of many citizens, and by the end of the century, a number of colonies had passed laws prohibiting the practice of variolation within their borders (Behbehani 1983, 466).

Objections against vaccination in the United States reached a high point in 1879 when William Tebb, leader of the anti-vaccination movement in Great Britain, arrived in the United States to inspire Americans in the campaign against vaccination. Largely as a result of his visit, supporters founded the Anti-Vaccination Society of America (primarily a local organization based in Terre Haute, Indiana, in spite of its name), followed soon afterward by creation of the New England Anti-Compulsory Vaccination League, in 1882, and the Anti-Vaccination League of New York City, in 1885 (The Anti-Vaccination Society of America 2012). The American anti-vaccination movement spread rapidly from the East Coast across the nation, bringing challenges to existing compulsory vaccination laws throughout the country. It was eventually successful in having such laws repealed in a number of states, including California, Illinois, Indiana, Minnesota, Utah, West Virginia, and Wisconsin (Wolfe and Sharp 2002). One of the movement's striking "successes" occurred in Milwaukee, Wisconsin, in 1894–1895 when it managed to close down a vaccination program in that city by calling on fears among citizens of immigrants and foreigners, with whom the disease was often associated (Leavitt 1976).

One of the leaders of the anti-vaccinationist movements in the United States in the early 20th century was John Pitcairn, who had immigrated to the United States while he was still a teenager. Pitcairn made his fortune in a variety of industrial fields, including oil development, railroads, and steel manufacturing. He was also a founder of the Pittsburgh Plate and Glass Company (now PPG). After retiring from business, he became a philanthropist and activist for a variety of social causes. One of those causes was the anti-vaccinationist movement to which he came, partly because of his strong religious background in the Swedenborgian Church and his commitment to the principles of homeopathic medicine, but more because of his belief that compulsory vaccination laws were an improper invasion by government into the private lives of individual citizens (Colgrove 2005).

Pitcairn's interest in the vaccination question appeared to have been spurred in about 1906 when members of his church decided to refuse vaccination during a smallpox epidemic in their community. He soon joined with fellow industrialist and philanthropist Charles M. Higgins to form the Anti-Vaccination League of America in Philadelphia. He became a spokesman for the movement and was in wide demand as a speaker on the subject, especially in his home state of Pennsylvania. He is perhaps best known for a speech he gave in March 1907 to the Committee on Public Health and Sanitation of the Pennsylvania General Assembly, in which he criticized the practice of mandatory vaccination. In that speech, he asked

Shall the citizen have the freedom to decide for himself and his children, whether he will submit to vaccination; or shall he be forced to bow his head to a medical dogma that has been utterly rejected by many eminent medical men? . . . Shall we witness unmoved the establishment by . . . government of a practice that deprives us of freedom in matters of *medical* faith? (Pitcairn 2012b)

Pitcairn is also best known for an article he wrote for the *Ladies Home Journal* in May 1910 entitled "The Fallacy of Vaccination," later published as a very popular pamphlet. The article continues to be cited by opponents of vaccination in the early 21st century (Pitcairn 2012a). In 1911, Pitcairn was appointed to the Pennsylvania State Vaccination Commission which, by law, was required to include two anti-vaccinationists.

An important turning point in the American anti-vaccinationist movement occurred in 1902. In an effort to combat an outbreak of smallpox in the city of Cambridge, Massachusetts, the board of health issued an order requiring all citizens to be vaccinated against the disease. One Henning Jacobson chose to ignore that order and refused to be vaccinated. His argument was a classical individual's freedom stand, arguing that the government had no right to tell him how to live his life or what to do with his body. Jacobson was tried in the local court, found guilty, and fined $5. He refused to accept that judgment, however, and appealed the court's decision, eventually all the way to the United States Supreme Court. In 1905, the Court ruled in favor of the state in the case of *Jacobson v. Massachusetts*. The Court began by acknowledging that, in a democracy, personal freedom was an ultimate right and privilege. It said that

> There is, of course, a sphere within which the individual may assert the supremacy of his own will and rightfully dispute the authority of any human government, especially of any free government existing under a written constitution, to interfere with the exercise of that will. (*Jacobson v. Massachusetts* 2012)

Nonetheless, the Court went on, there are circumstances under which personal freedom and liberty is not absolute (the classic argument that a person cannot shout "fire" in a crowded theater). It then went on to point out that

> it is equally true that, in every well ordered society charged with the duty of conserving the safety of its members the rights of the individual in respect of his liberty may at times, under the pressure of great dangers, be subjected to such restraint, to be enforced by reasonable regulations, as the safety of the general public may demand. (*Jacobson v. Massachusetts* 2012)

Jacobson's guilt was confirmed, and he was ordered to pay the $5 fine (Gostin 2005).

Jacobson v. Massachusetts is generally recognized as the standard on which U.S. vaccination law, and, indeed, public health law in general, has been based ever since the 1905 decision. The Court reaffirmed its position on the legality of mandatory vaccination laws in 1922 in the case of *Zucht v. King*. That case involved a complaint against mandatory vaccination laws established by the city of San Antonio, Texas. In a brief decision, the Court reiterated the fact that

> Long before this suit was instituted, *Jacobson v. Massachusetts*, 197 U.S. 11, had settled that it is within the police power of a state to provide for compulsory vaccination. That case and others had also settled that a state may, consistently with the federal Constitution, delegate to a municipality authority to determine under what conditions health regulations shall become operative. *** And still others had settled that the municipality may vest in its officials broad discretion in matters affecting the application and enforcement of a health law. *** A long line of decisions by this Court had also settled that, in the exercise of the police power, reasonable classification may be freely applied, and that regulation is not violative of the equal protection clause merely because it is not all-embracing. (*** = citations deleted)

The Court thus concluded that

> these ordinances confer not arbitrary power, but only that broad discretion required for the protection of the public health. (*Zucht v. King* 2012)

Jacobson v. Massachusetts had a deep and widespread impact on the anti-vaccinationist movement in the United States. Prior to that ruling, the movement had been somewhat disorganized, functioning largely on a local or regional level. Within three years of the Court's decision, however, the first truly national anti-vaccination society, the Anti-Vaccination League of America, was founded. Reflecting the movement's past history, the League announced that it was a "national confederation" of local associations organized to oppose vaccination. In response to the Court's pronouncement, the League declared that it based its campaign on true Constitutional principles. It said that

> We have repudiated religious tyranny; we have rejected political tyranny; shall we now submit to medical tyranny? (As quoted in "Toward a Twenty-first-century," *Jacobson v. Massachusetts* 2008, 1823)

Opponents of vaccination also began to establish other national organizations to battle compulsory laws. These organizations included the Citizens Medical Reference Bureau, founded in New York City in 1919; the American Medical Liberty League, established in 1918; the National League for Medical Freedom, founded in 1910; and the Constitutional Liberty League of America, an offshoot of the National League for Medical Freedom. Most of these organizations were rather short-lived, achieving only a modest influence on vaccination practices in most cities and states (Colgrove 2005, *passim*; Whorton 2004, 278–279).

As their names suggest, most of these organizations based their objections to vaccination not only on potential (and, they believed, widespread) adverse effects of the procedure, but also on the rights of individuals in a free society to choose the medical practices to which they would be exposed. (This theme remains a vital component not only of the continuing debate over compulsory vaccination in 21st-century America, but also of the ongoing debate over the extent and limitations of medical coverage in the United States engendered by the passage of the Patient Protection and Affordable Care Act of 2010.) But objections to compulsory vaccination also came from another source, which remains a powerful force against the practice in modern-day society: nontraditional healers, such as chiropractors, homeopaths, holistic practitioners, and naturopaths.

The late 19th and early 20th centuries saw the rise of a number of new systems of healing outside the general category of allopathy, or traditional method. These systems included chiropractic, the diagnosis and manipulation of the spine and joints to cure disease; homeopathy, the use of small amounts of substances known to produce disease in otherwise healthy people; and naturopathy, treatment of medical disorders by adjustment of diet and the use of techniques such as hydrotherapy, heat, and massage. The concept of injecting individuals with admittedly harmful products, such as cowpox or poliovirus, would appear to be fundamentally incompatible with such approaches to healing by chiropractic, naturopathic, or homeopathic techniques. And some founders of these disciplines did make rather clear statements about their objections to the use of vaccination to prevent infectious diseases. For example, the founder of chiropractic medicine, David D. Palmer, wrote that

> It is the very height of absurdity to strive to 'protect' any person from smallpox or any other malady by inoculating them with a filthy animal poison. . . . No one will ever pollute the blood of any member of my family unless he cares to walk over my dead body to perform such an operation. (Busse, Morgan, and Campbell 2005)

Palmer's son, Batlett Joshua, repeated this view in a 1909 statement when he expressed the philosophy behind the treatment of smallpox by chiropractic techniques.

> Chiropractors have found in every disease that is supposed to be contagious, a cause in the spine. In the spinal column we will find a subluxation that corresponds to every type of disease. If we had one hundred cases of small-pox, I can prove to you where, in one, you will find a subluxation and you will find the same condition in the other ninety-nine. I adjust one and return his functions to normal and you could do the same with the other ninety-nine. (Busse, Morgan, and Campbell 2005)

A significant fraction of present-day chiropractors subscribe to this approach to the treatment of infectious diseases and vaccination, as will be discussed in more detail below.

A similar view about vaccination was expressed by Benedict Lust, who brought the study of naturopathy to the United States from Europe. Lust wrote in his 1918 book, *Universal Directory of Naturopathy*,

> The contemporary fashion of healing disease is that of serums, inoculations and vaccines, which, instead of being an improvement on the fake medicines of former ages are of no value in the cure of disease, but on the contrary introduce lesions into the human body of the most distressing and deadly import. . . . Who would be fool enough to swallow the putrid pus and corruption scraped from the foulest sores of smallpox that has been implanted in the body of a calf? (Atwood and Barrett 2012)

As late as 1968, naturopaths in the United States were continuing to make this argument, suggesting that a mild case of smallpox was not necessarily a bad thing, in that it might "cleanse the body" of more serious diseases, such as tuberculosis and syphilis. In a report submitted to the Department of Health, Education, and Welfare, the National Association of Naturopathic Physicians submitted as evidence of their principles of practice a standard 1948 textbook in the field, which noted that "[n]aturopaths do not believe in artificial immunization" (Spitler 1948, 214 and 271, as cited in HEW Report on Naturopathy [1968] 2012).

Homeopaths have traditionally held similar views about vaccination. Arguably at the extreme edge of these views is a hypothesis proposed by the renowned homeopath James Compton Burnett. In his 1884 book, *Vaccinosis and Its Cure by Thuja*, Burnett argued not only that vaccination was useless in curing smallpox, but that it actually engendered a new type of infection, which he called *vaccinosis*. Symptoms of the disease included acne, pimples, neuralgia, cephalalgia (head pain), paresis (muscular weakness), and sties in the eyes (Burnett 1884, 12, 57). The purpose of Burnett's book was to demonstrate that this condition could be treated by using the herb *Thuja occidentalis*. At least some remnants of this philosophy remain among naturopaths today (see, for example, Tyler 2012).

At this point, it may be appropriate to indicate that Great Britain and the United States were by no means the only countries in the world affected by an anti-vaccinationist sentiment. A somewhat less well-known movement swept through Brazil at the beginning of the 20th century. The movement was engendered by an outbreak of smallpox and a number of other infectious diseases in Rio de Janeiro in 1904. In an effort to bring the outbreak under control, the government adopted a law requiring mandatory vaccination of all citizens. The so-called Law of Mandatory Vaccine allowed health teams, accompanied by the police, to enter private homes and forcibly, if necessary, vaccinate all residents found there. When informed of the law, citizens began rioting, looting shops, turning over and burning trams, tearing up tram tracks, and attacking government buildings. The event, now known as Revolta da Vacina (The Vaccine Revolt), has been called the most terrible riot of the Republic. It involved tens of thousands of citizens that left 30 people dead and more than 100 wounded. The city government held out against the protest movement; however, vaccinations continued, and the smallpox epidemic eventually ebbed (The Revolt of the Vaccine 2012; also see Meade 1989; Nachman 1977).

Vaccination Laws in the United States

State and local governments in the American colonies were well aware of the advances in vaccination practices and policies. One of the earliest expressions of colonial concerns on the topic dates to 1792 when the Virginia state legislature adopted an omnibus bill covering many aspects of smallpox infections and inoculations. The bill imposed heavy fines ($3,000 per incident) for intentionally transmitting the disease, while also acknowledging and establishing regulations for inoculations as a method of preventing smallpox (A Collection of All Such Acts of the General Assembly of Virginia of a Public and Permanent Nature as Are Now in Force 1803, 200).

As smallpox continued to wreck devastation throughout the colonies, additional laws were proposed and adopted. As early as 1802, Massachusetts had made a formal statement recommending (but not requiring) that all school age children be vaccinated against smallpox. This policy was adopted largely as a result of the urging of Dr. Benjamin Waterhouse. Two decades later, the first legal requirement for the vaccination of schoolchildren was adopted by the city of Boston in 1827, followed by a similar statewide requirement by Massachusetts in 1855. Similar policies and requirements were soon adopted by states across the country, including New York (1862), Connecticut (1872), Indiana (1881), Illinois (1882), Wisconsin (1882), Arkansas (1882), Virginia (1882), California (1888), Iowa (1889), and Pennsylvania (1895), as well as a number of cities and towns (Hodge and Gostin 2012, 28).

Today, all 50 states require children to be immunized against certain infectious diseases before they are allowed to enter schools. These state laws are very much alike in that they generally assign responsibility for listing the diseases against which students have to be immunized and the provisions under which those immunizations are to occur. The laws are somewhat different in the many details involved in assigning such responsibilities. As an example, the current law dealing with immunization in Michigan was passed in 1978 and has been updated and amended many times since then. The amended law says that the state Department of Public Health "shall maintain a list of reportable diseases, infections, and disabilities that designates and classifies communicable, serious communicable, chronic, or noncommunicable diseases, infections, and disabilities. The department shall review and revise the list under this subsection at least annually," and that the department shall also "[e]stablish procedures for control of diseases and infections, including, but not limited to, immunization and environmental controls" (Public Health Code 2012, Section 333.5111). In a recent amendment to the original law, the Michigan legislature included a provision by which children could be exempt from immunization, providing that parents (or their legal substitutes) provided an official certificate of exemption (Public Health Code 2012, Section 333.9208).

Exemption certificates are now common in U.S. state laws. Every state, with the exception of Mississippi and West Virginia, allow a child to be exempted from the school immunization requirement for religious reasons, and 20 states also allow children to be exempted for "philosophical" reasons, objections to immunization that fall outside the realm of religious beliefs. For example, the state of Washington provides that "Any child shall be exempt in whole or in part from the immunization measures required by [the state immunization law] upon the presentation of any one or more of the certifications required by this section, on a form prescribed by the department of health." The three types of exemption certificates permitted are those that are

> . . . signed by a healthcare practitioner that a particular vaccine required by rule of the state board of health is, in his or her judgment, not advisable for the child" [i.e., that the immunization would pose a risk to the child's health];
> . . . signed by any parent or legal guardian of the child or any adult in loco parentis to the child that the religious beliefs of the signator are contrary to the required immunization measures" [i.e.,, a religious objection]; or
> . . . signed by any parent or legal guardian of the child or any adult in loco parentis to the child that the signator has either a philosophical or personal objection to the immunization of the child [that is, a philosophical

objection]. (Immunization Program—Exemptions 2012; for more detail, also see States with Religious and Philosophical Exemptions from School Immunization Requirements 2012)

The list of diseases against which children must be immunized varies somewhat from state to state, but generally corresponds to the recommendations of the U.S. Centers for Disease Control and Prevention (CDC). Those diseases are *Haemophilus influenzae* type b (Hib), diphtheria, hepatitis A, hepatitis B, influenza, measles, mumps, pertussis (whooping cough), pneumococcal disease, polio, rubella (German measles), tetanus (lockjaw), rotavirus, and varicella (chickenpox). Vaccines have recently become available also for other diseases that, for the most part, tend to be mentioned less commonly in state laws. One of those diseases is meningitis, for which a vaccine has been available since the 1970s, but for which no state requirement was established until the late 1990s. Currently, 37 states have some type of meningitis vaccination requirement, most commonly for secondary- or college-level students. As with other types of immunizations, students may opt out of meningitis immunizations for medical, religious, or philosophical reasons in some states.

The other infectious disease for which a vaccine now exists is human papillomavirus (HPV) disease. The vaccine for this disease became available in 2009. Thus far, no state has added the HPV vaccine to its list of required immunizations, although the majority of states have taken some type of action to promote or encourage its use. As of 2012, twenty states have adopted bills that educate parents and children about the benefits of HPV vaccination and/or provided funds for a voluntary HPV immunization program (HPV Vaccine 2012).

Laws dealing with immunization of specific subpopulations of U.S. citizens and visitors also exist. The largest such subpopulations is adults, for whom there are no required immunizations at either the state or federal level. (The CDC does, however, recommend certain types of immunizations for adults; see 2012 Adult Immunization Schedule 2012.) Another large subpopulation for whom immunization requirements exist is members of the military. Entering members of the military services are required to have immunizations for the following infectious diseases: adenovirus, types 4 and 7; cholera; hepatitis A and B; influenza; Japanese encephalitis; measles; meningococcal disease; mumps; plague; polio; rabies; rubella; tetanus-diphtheria; typhoid; varicella; and yellow fever. Current members of the military are also required to keep their immunizations up to date (Immunizations and Chemoprophylaxis 2012; for more detail on U.S. immunization laws, see Immunization and Vaccination Laws in the U.S. 2012).

Vaccination Laws Worldwide

As one might expect, immunization laws vary widely from country to country around the world. The World Health Organization (WHO) maintains a very useful database of immunization requirements worldwide that lists the antigens to which a citizen is required to be vaccinated, the recommended vaccination schedule, and regions of the country in which requirements may vary. The database allows a person to select any country in the world and any one of a number of antigens to find the specific legal requirements for immunization in any part of the world. According to the most recent version of that database, the most common vaccines required worldwide are those against tuberculosis (the Bacille Calmette Guérin vaccine; 172 countries); polio (the oral polio vaccine; 154 countries); measles, mumps, and rubella (117 countries); hepatitis B (115 countries); diphtheria, tetanus, and pertussis (102 countries); and influenza (76 countries) (these numbers may vary since different countries may express their requirements in somewhat different vaccination formulations) (Vaccine Schedule Selection Form 2012).

The number of immunizations required also varies widely around the world. The nation that requires immunization against the largest number of antigens is Italy, with 27 different types of immunizations required for children ranging in age from 3 months to 15 years. The countries with the least stringent immunization requirements are those in Africa and Asia, including Equatorial Africa, Ethiopia, Mauritania, Tanzania, (five antigens each); and Bangladesh, Eritrea, Mali, Mozambique, Myanmar, Pakistan, Somalia, Timor-Leste, Uzbekistan, and Zambia (six antigens each). The great majority of nations in Africa require immunization against fewer than 10 antigens, while those in developed nations tend to require immunization against a dozen or more antigens (Vaccine Schedule Selection Form 2012).

Finally, immunization laws are also an important consideration for people moving from one country to another, either as visitors or as migrants. Every nation has specific provisions for the kinds of immunizations a person needs to have in order to enter the country on a temporary or permanent basis. As of late 2012, immunizations required of immigrants to the United States are for mumps, measles, rubella, polio, tetanus and diphtheria, pertussis, *haemophilus influenzae* type b (Hib), hepatitis A, hepatitis B, rotavirus, meningococcal disease, varicella, pneumococcal disease, and seasonal influenza (New Vaccination Criteria for U.S. Immigration 2012).

Vaccination Epidemics

In addition to the very strong religious opposition offered to the practice of variolation and vaccination described above, many individuals and organizations expressed concern about both procedures on the basis of their safety and efficacy. Especially in the case of variolation, critics pointed out that individuals being inoculated were receiving the very substance that caused smallpox in the first place. Rather than reducing the risk of their contracting the disease, they claimed, variolation was likely to *increase* their chance of becoming ill. A similar, although obviously not identical, argument was used against the practice of vaccination, in which cowpox materials were purportedly used to protect against smallpox. As an example, a modern website claims that one of the worst epidemics in the world's history, the Spanish influenza of 1918, was caused by compulsory vaccination of U.S. soldiers against the disease. "That was the first war in which all the known vaccines were forced on all the servicemen," this blogger writes. "This mishmash of poison drugs and putrid protein of which the vaccines were composed, caused such widespread disease and death among the soldiers that it was the common talk of the day, that more of our men were being killed by medical shots than by enemy shots from guns" (Peterson 2012).

In fact, this argument had a sound basis, because, throughout history, variolation and vaccination have both resulted in the outbreak of diseases they were designed to prevent. Although critics would argue that such outbreaks highlight the fallacy of the theoretical basis on which variolation and vaccination are based, most such events can be traced to more mundane (although certainly no less tragic) explanations. One of the classic stories in the history of vaccination in this regard occurred in 1802 in Massachusetts. Dr. Benjamin Waterhouse, one of the earliest converts to Jenner's method of vaccination, attempted to corner the market on smallpox vaccine in order to guarantee his own financial success in using the procedure. In desperation, other doctors who also wanted to use Jenner's system of vaccination were forced to look for other sources of the vaccines. One such source was pus taken from the infected arm of a British soldier who was thought to have been vaccinated against the diseases. As it turned out, the infection was not from a smallpox vaccination (which the solider had not had), but from a smallpox infection itself. When the vaccine prepared from the soldier's infection was used to inoculate a number of residents of Marblehead, Massachusetts, 68 of the vaccinated developed the disease itself and eventually died of it (Behbehani 1983, 480).

Reports of outbreaks of infectious diseases *caused* by vaccines intended to prevent those very diseases were common during the first century following Jenner's development of the vaccination procedure. That such would be the case is hardly surprising. Little was known about the importance of sterile techniques in preparing any type of medical product, including vaccines, so contamination was a constant and serious problem in maintaining a successful record for vaccination. Recognition of this problem in the United States led to the passage of the Vaccine Act of 1813. That act was inspired to a considerable extent by problems such as the one described in the preceding lines, in which individual physicians attempted to obtain smallpox vaccine by whatever means possible, often resulting in the use of contaminated products. The 1813 act was intended to ensure that American citizens would have access to adequate amounts of pure vaccine at no cost to themselves (the federal government paid for the vaccine and for shipping it to consumers). That act remained in force for less than a decade. It was repealed in 1822 when Congress decided that control over vaccination issues could better be handled by the individual states (Griffin 2009, 536; Singla 2012).

Individual states were relatively uninterested in taking on the task of dealing with vaccinations, in general, or of regulating vaccines, in particular. In fact, it was not until 1855 that Massachusetts became the first state to pass a law mandating that children be vaccinated in order to attend public schools. It was even much later (1894) that New York City decided to establish standards for the potency and purity of diphtheria vaccines, which were then largely being imported from Germany (Government Regulation 2012). By that time, the U.S. Congress was about ready to become involved once more in the regulation of vaccines. In 1902, it passed the Biologics Act, which charged the Hygienic Laboratory (predecessor to the National Institutes of Health) with the task of regulating the production of vaccines and antitoxins. The act was passed in response to two vaccine-related tragedies of the preceding year when 13 children in St. Louis and 9 children in Camden, New Jersey, died as a result of being vaccinated with contaminated diphtheria and smallpox vaccines, respectively (*Science and the*

Regulation of Biological Products: From a Rich History to a Challenging Future [2002]).

Over the past century, then, the U.S. government has closely and, to a large extent, effectively monitored the safety and efficacy of vaccines in the United States, as has been the case in all developed countries of the world. In spite of this impressive track record, outbreaks of infectious diseases have continued, events that anti-vaccinationists have often taken as additional evidence of the inherent lack of safety involved in the process of vaccination. In addition to blanket condemnations of the safety of vaccines, anti-vaccinationists have also appointed to specific events, such as the following as reasons for concern about mandatory vaccination policies.

Kyoto, Japan: 1948

In November 1948, public health officials in Kyoto, Japan, became concerned when a number of cases of diphtheria were reported in the city. Since children in the city at the time were routinely being vaccinated against the disease, they had no ready explanation for the mini-epidemic. Later investigations found that the Osaka Red Cross Research Institute had produced four batches of diphtheria toxoid, but sterilized only two of them. When the vaccine was sent to Tokyo for assay, the two good batches, purely by chance, were selected for testing, and the whole shipment was approved. Eventually, more than 600 children in Kyoto who received the vaccine became ill. Of that, 99 were hospitalized and 68 eventually died of the disease (Nishimura 2008).

Complications Resulting from DTP Vaccinations: Mid-1970s

By the mid-1970s, many children throughout the world were being routinely vaccinated with a trivalent vaccine against diphtheria, tetanus, and pertussis (the DTP vaccine). Some medical authorities expressed concern, however, about possible serious adverse events associated with the use of the vaccine. In 1974, three researchers at the Great Ormond Street Hospital for Sick Children in London published a paper suggesting that 36 children had experienced serious neurological damage as a result of being inoculated with the DTP vaccine. They suggested that in many cases, the problem may not have been with the vaccine, but with idiosyncratic characteristics of the children that predisposed them to harm from it (Kulenkampff, Schwartzman, and Wilson 1974).

This research report engendered a great deal of debate among public health officials, parents, government officials, medical researchers, and other interested stakeholders. A significant decrease in vaccination rates with DTP prompted a number of researchers to try to pin down the cause(s) for the London findings. These efforts were inspired to a considerable degree and then carefully monitored by a group of parents whose children had suffered adverse reactions as a result of being vaccinated with the DTP vaccine, a group called the Association of Parents of Vaccine Damaged Children (APVDC). One researcher, Gordon Stewart, eventually came to the conclusion that DTP vaccination was contraindicated among children with certain predisposing factors, such as existing neurological abnormalities. Other studies contradicted Stewart's findings and suggested that there was no common explanation for the range of adverse events reported with use of the DTP vaccine (Stewart 1986).

Polio: 1955

The first polio vaccine, an inactivated poliovirus vaccine, was approved for use in the United States by the U.S. Food and Drug Administration (FDA) on April 12, 1955. Only two weeks later, reports began to come in that a number of children who had been vaccinated with the new vaccine had come down with polio. By April 27, 260 individuals had been diagnosed with the disease, about a third of whom had received the vaccine and two-thirds who had been in close contact with someone who had been contacted. The U.S. Laboratory of Biologics Controls asked the manufacturer of that vaccine, Cutter Laboratories, to recall all stock of the vaccine, which the company did. Further investigation revealed that two batches of the vaccine had not been properly sterilized and carried low levels of live virus. All vaccinations with the new vaccine were immediately halted and not renewed until the fall of 1955 (Offit 2007).

Rotavirus: 1999

Rotavirus is the leading cause of severe acute diarrhea among children under the age of five throughout the world. It is thought to cause nearly half a million deaths of young children annually throughout the world. The disease is somewhat less common in the United States. In the early 2000s, it was the causative agent for more than 2.7 million cases of rotavirus gastroenteritis, 60,000 hospitalizations, and about 40 deaths annually in the United States. In August 1998, the U.S. FDA licensed a new vaccine for use against the disease, a vaccine called RotaShield. The vaccine was in use for only slightly more than a year when Wyeth Lederle, manufacturer of the vaccine, voluntarily withdrew it from the market. The reason for the decision was that the vaccine was suspected of causing a small number of cases of intussusception, an obstruction of the bowel that can cause serious problems in young children. Eventually, evidence suggested that the event occurred about once in every 5,000 instances of vaccination. After RotaShield was withdrawn from the market, research on the vaccine continued, and the FDA licensed two new products, RotaTeq in 2006, and Rotarix in 2008 (Rotavirus Vaccine (RotaShield®) and Intussusception 2012). This incident is an event in which a clear connection between the use of a vaccine and a specific adverse effect has been demonstrated.

In 2012, a special committee on the U.S. Institute of Medicine reported on an exhaustive study designed to determine the cases in which and the extent to which vaccines may have been or are responsible for a variety of medical conditions. The medical conditions chosen by the committee to study were those that had been reported to the National Vaccine Injury Compensation Program, whether those claims had been approved or not. The committee reviewed more than 1,000 research studies on which to base its conclusions. The major thrust of those conclusions was that

> Vaccines are not free from side effects, or "adverse effects," but most are very rare or very mild. Importantly, some adverse health problems following a vaccine may be due to coincidence and are not caused by the vaccine. (Adverse Effects of Vaccines: Evidence and Causality 2012; for the full report, see Stratton et al. 2012)

As comments in the rest of this chapter will demonstrate, that conclusion does not conform with the opinions of many people in the United States and around the world who are still convinced of the reality of many harmful effects of vaccines.

The Legal Status of Vaccination

As discussed above, Great Britain adopted a series of vaccination laws throughout the second half of the 19th century and into the 20th century. It was by no means the only nation, however to take such actions. One of the earliest laws passed concerning vaccination was one adopted in 1806, in Piombino and Lucca, part of the Napoleonic Principalities, now Italy. This law required that anyone with smallpox be quarantined in their home, which is surrounded by armed guards. Anyone not reporting a case of the smallpox or attempting to flee the territory was assessed a substantial fine. As a result of these regulations, "every child [was soon being] inoculated within two months after its birth" (Varieties, Literary and Philosophical 1808, 61). A number of other countries adopted some form of compulsory vaccination at about the same time: Bavaria (1807), Denmark

(1810), Norway (1811), Russia (1812), Sweden (1816), and Hanover (1821) (Hopkins 2002, 86). These laws were not always well enforced, and the impact on local rates of morbidity and mortality due to the disease was sometimes minimal. As a result, new laws requiring revaccination or laws instituting new vaccination requirements began to appear toward the middle of the century, and again in the 1870s.

Especially noteworthy among these laws was the one promulgated in 1874 in Germany by Kaiser Wilhelm I. The law mandated that every child who had not already had smallpox or who was medically not a candidate for vaccination be inoculated against the disease within her or his first year of life (Vaccination Law of April 8th 1874 2012). Public health authorities noted the apparent success of the Kaiser's proclamation. A 1907 report by the Medical Society of the State of Pennsylvania, for example, noted that the mortality rate from smallpox dropped dramatically in Prussia between 1874 and 1886, and by 1897, "there were but five deaths from this disease in the entire German Empire with a population of 54,000,000." By contrast, Prussia's next-door neighbor, Austria, experienced no such decline in smallpox death. Its mortality rate ranged between 39.28 and 94.79 per 100,000 of population between 1872 and 1884, compared to a mortality rate of 1.91 per 100,000 in Prussia during the same period (as quoted in Government Regulation 2012).

Modern Anti-Vaccinationism

In the last century, vaccines have saved more lives than any other health intervention. The World Health Organization estimates that every year, more than two million deaths are prevented worldwide due to immunization.

Immunization is an important, cost-effective and successful public health intervention. It effectively prevents disease, improves the health of Canadians, and reduces pressures on our health care system.

Vaccines have led to the eradication of smallpox, the near eradication of polio, and the control of other diseases, including polio and whooping cough, which once maimed or killed in large numbers. (Immunization: The Most Successful Public Health Measure 2012)

This powerful endorsement of vaccination by the Public Health Agency of Canada is typical of the support that immunization programs have among public health authorities worldwide. Indeed, the vast majority of the conventional medical community appears to have no hesitation in recommending mandatory vaccination schedules for young children and, in some cases, adults, against a number of infectious diseases. Yet, that position is certainly not held universally. As has been true throughout history, a substantial number of individuals and organizations believe that mandatory vaccinations (and, in many cases, even voluntary vaccinations) are not only useless to the health of individuals and the general public, but also actually harmful to personal and public health.

Modern anti-vaccinationists have adduced a very extensive array of arguments against the inoculation of children, in particular, and all animals, in general. Interestingly enough, many of those arguments reflect opinions that were first expressed more than 150 years ago, and have continued to hold sway with some portion of the population ever since (see, for example, Wolfe and Sharp 2002, Box A). Among the most common of those arguments are the following.

Vaccines Cause Illness

[T]he venom of the vaccinator may work in the veins of the victims for years and years, crippling, blinding, causing limbs or features to rot off, and entailing hopeless disfigurements and disabilities in comparison to which that medical bugbear—the pitting of small-pox—is but an insignificant trifle. (Mrs. Hume-Rothery 1880, 8)

Not only do vaccines not work, they actually cause diseases. . . . Published studies from reputable journals have
linked vaccines to causing AIDS, autism, cancer, diabetes,
hearing/vision loss, hepatitis B, mumps, measles, polio
and rubella. . . . We have a national policy that supports
the murder of completely innocent infants. (Nagel 2012)

These two commentaries were written 130 years apart, but
they express a very common view, namely that vaccines may
not only not *prevent* disease, they may actually *cause* disease.
This argument appears over and over again in modern anti-
vaccinationist writings to an extent that cannot adequately be
reviewed in this book. As an example, one anti-vaccinationist
website offers links to scientific reports linking vaccination with
more than 150 different diseases and medical conditions ranging from abortion, allergies, apnea, and appetite disorders to
encephalitis, eczema, epilepsy, and Fanconi anemia to shaken
baby syndrome, singles, sinusitis, and skin disorders (Vaccine
Disease 2012). A sample of the claims that have been made
linking vaccines with disease may suffice:

- Childhood vaccinations against a variety of infectious diseases may be responsible for the recent surge in the number of cases of type 1 and type 2 diabetes. "Lab research
  has confirmed that pertussis vaccine can cause diabetes
  in mice," "[o]ne virus, the rubella virus, has already been
  shown to be associated with diabetes," and "mumps disease
  has been strongly associated with the development of Type
  1 diabetes." (Juvenile Diabetes and Vaccination: New Evidence for a Connection 2012)

- Vaccines cause damage to both the body and the brain
  that are not readily noticeable either by an individual who
  has been immunized or by medical specialists. This damage causes a variety of central nervous system effects, some
  of which mimic the effects of a stroke: "ALL vaccines are

causing immediate and delayed, acute and chronic, waxing and waning, impairments to blood flow, throughout the brain and body. This IS causing us all to become chronically ill, sick, and causing brain damages along a continuum of clinically silent to death. This is causing ischemic 'strokes'." (Aufderheide 2012)

- Two large classes of disease, autoimmune disease and cancer, are caused by vaccines, because the viruses used in those vaccines causes tissues to become inflamed, and that inflammation is invariably the first stage in the development of these two classes of disease. "The act of inoculating viruses into the body, bypassing secretory IgA (as explained in my documents at www.drcarley.com) causes corruption of the immune system leading to ALL autoimmune diseases and cancer." ([untitled website] 2012)

- The inflammatory effects of vaccine may also be responsible for the increasing number of cases of Alzheimer's disease now being seen in many countries. "Theoretical data on the inflammatory nature of vaccines, especially in the large numbers given to children at an early age while their nerves are developing response patterns for future life, means that they cannot be ruled out as one main factor that primes the Alzheimer's pump." (Richards 2012)

- "Conclusive evidence" now exists that swine flu vaccine causes permanent neurological damage. On the basis of this "evidence," the government of Finland in 2011 agreed to pay "lifetime medical care" for 79 children who developed narcolepsy as a direct result of having been given the swine flu vaccination. (Adams 2012a)

- National governments around the world know that vaccines can cause disease, and they promote vaccination as a way of causing death and reducing population problems around the world. "Vaccines harm countless millions of children each year in ways that are usually never linked to vaccines (mild mental retardation, suppressed immune

function, learning disabilities, etc.) . . . every world government already knows that vaccines are murder. They know
vaccines kill and maim children." (Adams 2012a)

- A possible explanation as to how vaccines cause health
problems is based on the fact that white blood cells are
large cells, and vaccination increases the number of white
blood cells to the point that the clog blood vessels, causing
inflammation, mini-strokes, and ischemia. "Dr. Andrew
Moulden has actual proof that every single vaccine is dangerous to the body and does eventually cause Autism and
death. He found out that when the body is injected viruses
and adjuvants, your immune system goes in hyper-drive
and creates an overload of white cells in the blood stream."
(Don't Take H1N1 Vaccine this Fall!! [Proof That All Vaccines Cause Damage] 2012)

- Exposure to vaccines may produce not only physical symptoms, but also a wide range of psychological, mental, and
emotional disorders. For example, it may be that vaccines
administered to very young children may affect their growing nervous systems, producing results that may not be apparent for years or decades. Some researchers believe that
these effects may manifest themselves in the form of anti-
social behavior, sexual abnormalities, or violent behavior.
"[T]he sociopathic personality which has emerged on a
mass scale in recent decades—and which is responsible for
a disproportionate amount of crime and social violence—
is causally linked to the childhood vaccination programs.
In other words, vaccination causes encephalitis which in
turn leads to these post-encephalitic states and conditions."
(Coulter 2012)

In addition to hypotheses of the types listed here, some observers are more constrained in their views on the connection
between vaccines and medical and health issues, arguing for
a limited relationship between, perhaps, one specific vaccine
and one specific health issue. For example, one researcher has

suggested the possibility that HIV/AIDS disease originated in humans when the hepatitis B vaccine was first being tested in the late 1970s and early 1980s. He suggests that contamination of the vaccine by monkey viruses may have lead to a new form of the virus that crossed the species boundary into humans. He further warns that continued use of the now-approved hepatitis B vaccine may pose a threat to countless young children who are routinely immunized with the vaccine around the world (Cantwell 2012; for a detailed discussion of other putative vaccine-disease links, see Misconceptions about Immunization 2012).

The Vaccine-Autism Link

Probably the most active debate about a link between vaccination and disease in recent history erupted in the late 1990s, when British gastroenterologist Andrew Wakefield published a paper in the prestigious British medical journal *The Lancet* claiming to have found "a genuinely new syndrome," which he called *autistic enterocolitis*. The syndrome was characterized by a combination of autism-like symptoms and various gastrointestinal disorders in young children, all of whom had been vaccinated with the MMR vaccine. Wakefield suggested that the condition might have been caused by the vaccine. He hypothesized that the three components of the trivalent MMR vaccine might have "overloaded" the children's immune systems, producing the observed gastrointestinal disorders (MMR Research Timeline 2012).

The MMR vaccine was first introduced to the United Kingdom in 1988 and had rapidly become widely popular as a form of protection against measles, mumps, and rubella. By 1995, more than 90 percent of British children were being immunized with the MMR vaccine (MMR Timeline 2012). By the turn of the century, two contrasting trends had developed as a result of Wakefield's research. On the one hand, he and a handful of colleagues continued to argue for a correlation between vaccination and the development of autism-related symptoms and gastrointestinal disorders. For example, Wakefield and a colleague, John O'Leary, director of pathology at Coombe Women's Hospital in Dublin, appeared before the U.S. Congress with evidence that 24 of 25 children with autism who had been tested had traces of measles virus in their guts. This evidence, O'Leary said, provided "compelling evidence" of a link between the MMR vaccine and autism (MMR Research Timeline 2012).

On the other hand, members of the mass media picked up on at least the suggestion in Wakefield's research that vaccinations might be responsible for the rapid increase in autism cases seen at the end of the 20th century. Later research on this episode pointed to a "media frenzy" that pushed the putative connection between vaccines and autism far beyond the level that scientific research had provided. As a result, very large numbers of the parents of autistic children, the general population, and even the medical community began to assume that the autism-vaccine link had essentially been proved (Moore 2006).

Wakefield's research had some very practical consequences for public health practices in Great Britain, the United States, and other countries. In the first place, his hypothesis about the relationship of vaccines and autism was responsible, most experts agree, for a decrease in the rate of MMR vaccinations (and that of other types of vaccinations as well) throughout the world. Those rates fell in some countries from more than 90 percent to about 70 percent. In many countries, rates have not fully returned to their pre-Wakefield levels as of 2012 (Alazraki 2012).

In addition, thousands of parents in the United States and many other countries began to file suit to collect damages for children with autism who had, they believed, contracted the condition as a consequence of being vaccinated. The first such suit was filed in April 1994 in Great Britain against the manufacturers of the MMR vaccine by attorney Richard Barr on behalf of parents of more than 1,000 autistic children. That suit was later withdrawn when supporters of the claim released that they had insufficient evidence to go forward (Fitzpatrick 2012). In the United States, more than 5,000 similar cases were also brought by parents of autistic children in the Office of Special Masters of the U.S. Court of Federal Claims, generally known as the Vaccine Court. These cases were eventually consolidated into three test cases, all of which were decided in favor of the defendants (Rope 2012).

At the same time that these two opposing waves were in motion, a third process was under way, the normal process by which scientific investigators attempt to verify and validate new claims, such as those being made by Wakefield and O'Leary. Only a month after Wakefield's original announcement, for example, the British Medical Research Council issued an announcement that no evidence existed to support the association between vaccination and autism or gastrointestinal disorders. A month later, a group of Finnish researchers reported on a 14-year study in which they found no cause-and-effect relationship between the MMR vaccine and either autism or gastrointestinal problems. And less than a year later, additional research from the hospital at which Wakefield was employed found no such relationship (MMR Timeline 2012). Whatever the general public and the media believed, by the early years of the 21st century, virtually no medical scientist of repute subscribed to Wakefield's autism-vaccine link.

The beginning of the end of this story occurred in February 2004, when investigative reporter Brian Deer of the *Sunday Times* revealed that Wakefield had, for two years prior to his 1998 paper, been receiving fees amount to more than £450,000 from attorneys planning to bring suit against vaccine manufacturers. He had apparently also applied for a patent for a new measles vaccine that would have been in competition with vaccines available from the companies that would have been defendants in that suit. Finally, Wakefield's own research appears to have violated some essential regulations and policies regarding experimentation with human subjects (Andrew Wakefield

2012; Deer 2011). A month later, 10 of the 11 coauthors of Wakefield's original paper withdrew their support for the paper (the other coauthor could not be reached for comment). They said in a letter to *The Lancet* that

> We wish to make it clear that in this paper no causal link was established between MMR vaccine and autism as the data were insufficient. However, the possibility of such a link was raised and consequent events have had major implications for public health. In view of this, we consider now is the appropriate time that we should together formally retract the interpretation placed upon these findings in the paper, according to precedent. (Murch et al. 2004, 750)

Wakefield's original paper was finally fully retracted by the editors of *The Lancet* in 2010, and he was removed from the British medical register in the same year, preventing him from practicing medicine in the United Kingdom (Editors of *The Lancet* 2010, 445; Triggle 2010). In spite of this rejection of Wakefield's original findings and interpretations, he still has the support of a number of organizations and individuals. As of May 2012, more than two dozen organizations and more than 4,000 individuals had signed an online petition indicating that they still believed in Wakefield's original contentions about the possible connection between vaccines and autism (We Support Dr. Andrew Wakefield 2012).

Vaccines and Gulf War Syndrome

Gulf War Syndrome (GWS) is a term used to describe a medical condition characterized by a combination of symptoms that include fatigue, skin rashes, diarrhea, muscle pain, and cognitive problems. The condition occurred among military personnel, primarily from the United States, who served in the 1991 Gulf War against Iraq. A wide number of possible causes have been suggested for the condition, although none has been unambiguously agreed upon by the medical profession. (Recently, the number of possible causative agents appears to have been reduced to three factors: chemical nerve agents, pesticides, and pyridostigmine bromide pills [Hodges 2012].) Among a number of anti-vaccinationists, however, a lingering suspicion remains that vaccinations may be one possible cause of GWS.

For example, one observer, Dr. Russell Blaylock, suggests that vaccines may trigger an effect in the brain called the "bystander effect," in which excess quantities of the vaccine destroy healthy cells in the brain as well as the foreign toxin introduced in the vaccine. He suggests that injecting too many vaccines within too short a period of time may produce this kind of effect, producing the symptoms that are associated with GWS. Dr. Blaylock claims that studies on the safety of vaccines focus only on short periods of time after immunization, and not on long-term effects, like those observed with GMS. He points out that there are "a growing number of scientific studies that are demonstrating serious dangers in our present vaccine policy, including altered brain development, seizures and a loss of brain cell connections called synapses," consequences of which pediatricians and family practice physicians are "completely unaware" (Blaylock 2012).

A number of observers have suggested that the use of an illegal adjuvant, squalene, in an experimental anthrax vaccine was responsible for GWS symptoms. They point out that some vaccines used during the Gulf War had not gone through adequate testing, and that, as a result, some of those vaccines had unexpected and devastating side effects on military personnel on whom they were used. They point to a number of studies conducted during and after the war that suggested a strong link between the vaccines used during the Gulf War and the high number of GWS cases observed after the war was concluded. This relationship was explored in detail in a 2004 book by journalist Gary Matsumoto, *Vaccine A: The Covert Government Experiment That's Killing Our Soldiers and Why GI's Are Only the First Victims*. According to one reviewer, Matsumoto admits that he "cannot state with 100 percent certainty that any of the individual cases he investigated so impressively are linked to anthrax vaccinations required of military servicemen and servicewomen." But, "[t]he circumstantial evidence is so massive, however, that it is persuasive. Experienced journalists, and lawyers, know that circumstantial evidence is as good as direct evidence if its quality is high and enough of it exists" (*Vaccine A: The Covert Government Experiment That's Killing Our Soldiers and Why GI's Are Only the First Victims* 2012).

In contrast to the claims made by anti-vaccinationists, the U.S. government has come to the conclusion that vaccines were not a factor in the development of GWS among veterans of that war. In what was probably the most comprehensive government study on GWS, researchers concluded that, while a number of methodological issues remained unresolved, "Gulf War epidemiologic studies have not identified any individual vaccine, including the anthrax vaccine, to be a prominent risk factor for Gulf War illness" (Research Advisory Committee on Gulf War Veterans' Illnesses 2008, 126).

Vaccines Do Not Work

Another very common argument made by anti-vaccinationists is that mandatory vaccinations should be discontinued because the very purpose for which they are designed, reducing the rate of infectious diseases, is not achieved. This argument claims essentially that the incidence and prevalence of infectious diseases has decreased over the past century, not because vaccinations have been so successful, but because of other factors, the most important of which is the general improvement of public health practices in virtually every part of the world. One of the most compelling presentations of this viewpoint can be found in a series of more than two dozen graphs prepared by Raymond Obomsawin, who claims to have a doctoral degree in health science and human ecology (Biographical Sketch of: Raymond Obomsawin 2012; but also see Friedlander 2012 for an opposing interpretation of these graphs). These graphs show, in general, the incidence (number of newly reported cases annually) of a number of infectious diseases from some early date (such as 1850, 1880, or 1913) to some years after the introduction of a vaccine for each disease. The graphs show, without exception, that the incidence of an infectious disease has dropped precipitously prior to the date the vaccine was introduced, and only modestly after that time. The last set of graphs purport to show the effectiveness of a vaccine in reducing the risk for an infectious disease.

These graphs indicate, for example, that the influenza vaccine is "0% effective" for children under the age of two with "little or no effectiveness" for elderly individuals living in communities in group homes and the Bacillus Calmette-Guérin (BCG) vaccine for tuberculosis is "0% effective" for those who have received two doses of the vaccine. They also suggest that among children who come down with mumps in one 2006 Iowa study, 92 percent had been vaccinated against the disease, and only eight percent had not. Similar studies show that 86 percent of the children in a 2001 Oregon study who developed chickenpox had been vaccinated against the disease, and 14 percent had not, and 90 percent of those vaccinated against pertussis in a 1993 Ohio study contracted the disease, while only 10 percent of those not vaccinated did so (Obomsawin 2012).

Another example of this view is that provided by a blogger who claims to have a background in "astronomy, physics, human physiology, microbiology, genetics, anthropology and human psychology," as well as "nutrition and holistic health." He writes that he had previously offered a $10,000 reward to anyone who could provide scientific evidence that the H1N1 vaccine is both "safe and effective." No one ever took him up on that offer, he points out, simply because flu shots *"simply don't work* [emphasis in the original] on 99 out of 100 people (and that's being generous to the vaccine industry . . .)." The basic point the blogger makes is that it would have not been possible for anyone to take him up on his original claim because no scientific evidence exists on the efficacy of vaccines. He concludes that "vaccine pushers often insist it's unethical to test whether their vaccines really work. You just have to 'take it on faith' that vaccines are universally good for everybody" (Adams 2012b).

Some medical specialists hold views that are the same as or similar to those expressed by this blogger. For example, Dr. Philip Incao is a physician with a medical degree from the Albert Einstein College of Medicine in New York City. He claims to be one of the few practitioners of anthroposophic medicine in the United States, a form of holistic medicine. Incao has written and spoken about the general ineffectiveness of vaccines. For example, he testified in 1999 before the Health Committee of the Ohio House of Representatives with regard to compulsory vaccination for hepatitis B in the state. Incao based his objections to pending legislation to a large extent on his belief that there was insufficient scientific evidence that the vaccine (or any vaccine) had been adequately tested for safety and efficacy. At one point in his testimony, he noted that

The best way to determine the risk-benefit profile of any vaccination is well known and in theory is quite simple: Take a group of vaccinated children and compare them with a matched group of unvaccinated children. If the groups are well-matched and large enough and the length of time the children are observed following vaccination long enough, then such a study is deemed the "gold standard" of vaccine research because its data is as accurate a reflection as medical research is capable of achieving of how vaccinations are actually affecting our nation's children.

Incredible as it sounds, such a common-sense controlled study comparing vaccinated to unvaccinated children has never been done in America for any vaccination. (Emphasis in original; Dr. Incao's Hepatitis B Vaccination Testimony in Ohio 2012)

Big Business and Big Government

Again, a voice from the past:

> An Englishman's house is no longer his own. Under
> favour of the odious Vaccination Acts a poor man's house
> may be entered by the emissaries of the Medical Star
> Chamber, to ascertain whether his children have been
> blood-poisoned according to law. . . . Parents are fined
> and imprisoned for refusing to submit their children to
> what they regard and justly regard, as the deadly risk of
> receiving into their infant veins corrupt matter, laden
> with who knows what horrible taints of foul disease?
> (Mrs. Hume-Rothery 1871, 2)

Many anti-vaccinationists of the 19th century, like Mrs. Hume-Rothery, believed that vaccination was a grand scheme of the formal medical profession to take control of the lives—or at least, the health—of their children. Some of their 21st-century descendants hold similar views, with the inclusion, in many cases, of Big Government as a coconspirator with Big Business in the process of "selling" vaccination to the general public and, sometimes, the medical community.

The basic argument in this regard is that vaccines may or may not be effective and they may or may not be safe. (Anti-vaccinationists tend to say they are neither.) The bottom line, however, is that governments have conspired with large pharmaceutical corporations to impose massive programs of mandatory vaccination (currently in the United States, 69 doses of 16 different vaccines) to ensure that those companies make very large profits. The implied position of both industry and government, then, is that it really doesn't make much difference whether vaccines are efficacious and safe or not, as long as they can be sold in huge quantities.

Observers of the pharmaceutical industry may disagree as to how long such a situation has existed. A number of observers point out that vaccine production has historically been one of the least profitable functions of most pharmaceutical companies. For this reason, the number of such companies producing vaccines plummeted during the last decade of the 20th century and the first decade of the 21st century (Cohen 2002; Offit 2005). Many anti-vaccinationists dispute that argument. They believe that the imposition of ever more extensive vaccination schedules by government has been carried out to a considerable extent in order to ensure high profits for pharmaceutical companies. The theme of one book on the topic is that "vaccination is big business and big money for doctors, for the drug companies and for the government" (What Do You Really Know about Vaccines? 2012). Programs for the development and production of vaccines against the H1N1 virus in 2009 and against seasonal influenza vaccines have come under special scrutiny by anti-vaccinationists. As one critic has written:

> The pharmaceutical industry, with public health officials and the mainstream media acting as a mass marketing team, is about to pull off the biggest profiteering scheme in the history of the world. The swine flu hoax, perpetrated on a global level, will generate unheard of profits from a non-existent pandemic. (Pringle 2012)

Critics often quote representatives of the pharmaceutical industry to reinforce the point they are making. An example of this practice is a statement made by Bruce Carlson, a spokesperson at Kalorama, a company that follows developments in the pharmaceutical industry. A number of anti-vaccinationists quoted Carlson in 2009 when he observed that "[t]he vaccine market is booming. It's an enormous growth area for pharmaceuticals at a time when other areas are not doing so well." The reason for that boom, according to many critics, was not a concern for improved public health, but a "manufactured" public health crisis, the H1N1 (swine flu) scare of that year (Gallander and Stadelmann 2012).

Concerns about the role of "big business" in the promotion of mandatory vaccination schedules is often linked with concerns about the role of "big government" in aiding and abetting such programs. The theme is that both government and industry profit from expanded vaccination programs, industry because of the profits it makes and government because of the greater control it has over the lives of individual citizens. Some critics see mandatory vaccination schedules as simply the first step of a process in which the federal government will eventually take over all health decisions once made by individuals. One anti-vaccinationist highlights the "unhealthy" connection between big business and big government in a pamphlet warning about the health and political risks of the swine flu vaccine. He writes that

> nobody is allowed to offer alternatives for preventing swine flu. Government medical bureaucrats are the sole source of official information, and they're getting their marching orders from Big Pharma, while you pick up the bill! (Blaylock 2012)

Those who are concerned about the "big business"–"big government" connection often point to the fact that individuals responsible for making and carrying out government policy on vaccination schedules commonly have substantial financial interests in the pharmaceutical industry, usually because they hold stock in pharmaceutical companies. One commentator on the topic, for example, has pointed out that

> [c]onflicts of interest are the norm in the vaccine industry. Members and Chairs of the FDA and CDC vaccine advisory committees own stock in drug companies that make vaccines; individuals on both advisory committees own patents for vaccines under consideration or affected by the decisions these committees make. The CDC grants conflict-of-interest waivers to every member of their

advisory committee a year at a time, allowing full participation in the discussions leading up to a vote by every member whether or not they have a financial stake in the decision. (Phillips 2012)

Alternatives to Vaccination

A point frequently made by anti-vaccinationists is that, even if one acknowledges differences of opinion about the safety and efficacy of vaccines, the fact is that a number of alternatives are available to immunization that are known to be at least as safe and efficacious, if not much safer and more effective, than are commercially produced vaccines. For example, nutritionists sometimes argue that the best way to avoid infectious diseases is to eat a sensible diet that strengthens a person's immune system naturally. Such a diet would avoid saturated fats, processed sugar, certain types of medicines such as decongestants and antihistamines, and antibiotics (under most circumstances) (Neustaeder 2012).

Another alternative to traditional forms of vaccination is a homeopathic program called homeoprophylaxis (HP). As would be expected of a homeopathic procedure, HP involves giving a young child very low doses of the material that causes the infectious disease against which one wishes to provide prevention. One suggested schedule, for example, has a child receiving doses of Pertussin (which contains the bacterium that causes whooping cough) at one and two months of age, doses of Pneumococcinum (which contains the bacterium that causes pneumonia) at three and four months of age, doses of *Lathyrus sativus* (a legume that protects against neurodegenerative conditions) at five and six months of age, and so on. No more than one material at a time is ever given to avoid "overloading" the immune system and reducing the effectiveness of the treatment (Vaccine Free: Homeopathic Alternatives to Vaccination 2012). In the broadest sense, HP is similar to vaccination in that substances are introduced into the body to stimulate the immune system, although the method of preparation and manner of administration is very different for the two procedures. A conventional vaccine, for example, consists of live (attenuated) or dead pathogens suspended in a mixture that may contain other substances potentially harmful to an animal body. The mixture is administered by an injection ("shot") that may be painful and traumatic for a person. By contrast, the active ingredient in HP is a very small amount of pathogen compounded into a sugar pill that is easily swallowed without causing upset to a patient. Although a number of individuals have chosen to use HP instead of conventional vaccination, there appears to be little or no scientific evidence that HP actually produces immunity against the diseases for which it is used (see, for example, Crislip 2012; Homeopathy Plus [Complaint No 2011/05/004] 2012).

Another possible alternative to early childhood vaccination is not really an alternative, but instead a suggestion to delay some immunizations until an individual's immune system is better able to withstand the stress placed on it by vaccines. One writer, for example, has recommended delaying the tetanus vaccine until a child begins to walk, the rubella vaccine until an individual reaches child-bearing age, and the hepatitis B vaccine until an individual is likely to become sexually active. She also suggests the possibility of skipping some vaccinations entirely because the diseases against which they protect are so rare in the United States, so mild in their effects (chickenpox), or so easily avoided by quarantine (mumps) (McCormick 2012). This suggestion is based on a concept known as *herd immunity*, the theory that vaccinating a large fraction of a population against a disease greatly reduces the risk that the disease will be transmitted throughout the population. That is, as the number of individuals immune to a disease increases, the chances that the disease will be passed on to nonvaccinated individuals becomes less and less (for a technical description of herd immunity, see Herd Immunity and Vaccination 2012.).

A number of anti-vaccinationists have argued that a host of natural methods are available for use in place of immunizations. One website, for example, recommends "cleanliness and proper sanitation," "breast feeding," "proper nutrition (i.e., unrefined vegan diet)," "hydrotherapy," "colloidal silver minerals," and "herbs" (Many Say "No" to Vaccinations 2012). Colloidal silver is a finely divided form of the metal suspended in a water solution that is administered orally. Proponents of the substances claim that it has been shown to be toxic to more than 600 disease agents, and, thus, can be used in place of almost any vaccine. Testimonials to the treatment frequently come with detailed descriptions as to how one can easily prepare the product in her or his own home (see, for example, Colloidal Silver v/s the Flu Vaccine 2012).

Too Aggressive Vaccination Schedules

A concern mentioned above that runs through many criticisms of the traditional vaccination schedule in most countries is that young children receive too many different vaccines within too short a period of time. The schedule most often recommended in the United States, for example, calls for a baby to receive 26 shots containing 14 different antigens before the age of two, often receiving five shots at once. A schedule this intense, say some anti-vaccinationists, tends to "overwhelm" a young child's immune system, causing more damage than good to the child's body. This view of vaccination is sometimes described as the "too many too soon" movement. It appears to have been especially popular among a few celebrities who have experienced disastrous vaccination events in their personal lives. These individuals tend to point out that they do not oppose the concept of vaccination in and of itself, although they do think the vaccination schedule should be less condensed. At a "Green Our Vaccines" rally in 2008, for example, actor Jim Carrey said that his goal was not to "destroy the vaccine program," but to call for "balance and moderation" in vaccination schedules. He pointed out that children are not "bottomless pits that you endlessly pour substances into" (Brady and Dahle 2012).

A number of physicians have taken advantage of this concern about vaccination schedules to design alternative schedules that reduce the number of vaccines given in early childhood and/or spread out the time between vaccinations. One example is a schedule devised by pediatrician Robert W. Sears. As with other "too many too soon" spokespersons, Sears insists that he is not an anti-vaccinationist; he acknowledges the value of vaccines in protecting a child's health, but believes that the risk of adverse side effects can be reduced by stretching out the length of time during which children receive their shots. Children never receive more than two shots at a time on this schedule, and vaccinations are spread out over five to six years, rather than the 24 months in a traditional vaccination schedule. Sears also has proposed a "selective" vaccination schedule in which some less important vaccines are not given at all during childhood. No scientific evidence is available on the relative merits of traditional, alternative, and selective vaccination schedules, so parents generally must choose one or another option based on their own information and feelings, in consultation with their pediatrician (What Is the Alternative Vaccine Schedule? 2012).

A number of research studies have been conducted, however, on the general theory that "too much too soon" is harmful to children's health. One such study, reported in 2010, examined difference in neuropsychological traits between three groups of children, aged 7 to 10 years, one of which consisted of children who had received the traditional vaccination schedule recommended by the CDC, one of which made up of children who received a more lengthy ("delayed") schedule, and one of which consisted of children who had had no vaccinations of any kind. The researchers discovered that the "traditional" group performed better than either of the two other groups on 12 measures and were no different statistically from those groups on two other measures. They concluded that "[t]imely vaccination during infancy has no adverse effect on neuropsychological outcomes 7 to 10 years later. These data may reassure parents who are concerned that children receive too many vaccines too soon" (Smith and Wood 2010, 1134).

Threats from Thimerosal and Adjuvants

One of the very old arguments posed by anti-vaccinationists against the use of vaccines with young children is the potential harm posed by preservatives and adjuvants used in the vaccines. (See Chapter 1 for a discussion of adjuvants in vaccines.) This argument notes that even if pure vaccines themselves were safe for use, the addition of preservatives and adjuvants to increase their potency introduces an additional factor that may pose a threat to children's health. Preservatives are added to vaccines to kill pathogens that may be present in the vaccine that have the capacity to cause diseases, including those diseases for which the vaccine is itself intended. Historically, the preservative that has received the greatest amount of attention is a mercury-containing organic compound whose chemical name is ethyl (2-mercaptobenzoato-(2-)-O,S)e mercurate(1-) sodium, but that is much better known as thiomersal, or thimerosal. Thimerosal has been widely used since the 1930s in a wide variety of antiseptic and antifungal substances, perhaps the best known of which has been sold under the trade name of Merthiolate.

Thimerosal has also been used as a preservative in vaccines. In fact, until fairly recently, it was the most widely used of all vaccine preservatives. Over the past few decades, however, concerns have been raised about possible mercury toxicity posed by the use of thimerosal in vaccines. Critics of vaccination have argued that the use of thimerosal has been responsible for a large number of neurological disorders in young children (see, for example, Dangers of Vaccines Mercury and Thimerosal 2012). In response to these concerns, pharmaceutical manufacturers and the U.S. FDA have worked to reduce or eliminate the amount of thimerosal in vaccines. Today, the compound is absent from 25 of the 30 vaccines routinely recommended for childhood vaccinations and is present in very low or trace amounts in the remaining five vaccines (Vaccines, Blood & Biologics 2012). Because of this change, critics of vaccination tend to raise concerns about the risks posed by thimerosal in vaccines to a lesser degree than has been the case in the past.

Such is not the case with adjuvants, however. Anti-vaccinationists still tend to worry about the health risks posed by compounds added to vaccines to increase their potency. The two adjuvants most commonly mentioned in this regard are compounds of aluminum and an unsaturated hydrocarbon obtained primarily from shark oil, called squalene.

Aluminum Compounds

In the popular literature, the compounds of aluminum used as adjuvants in vaccines are commonly lumped together and called simply "aluminum." That term is, of course, incorrect, because aluminum is a metallic element that is never used as an adjuvant. It appears in vaccines only in the form of compounds such as aluminum hydroxide or aluminum sulfate. Scientists have known since 1886 that compounds of aluminum are neurotoxins, that is, capable of causing damage to brain cells. This fact was first discovered when physicians noted that members of the Prussian army who had had limbs amputated and then covered with pastes made of aluminum compounds were prone to develop nervous system disorders. Little laboratory research was done on the problem, however, until the early 1970s, when research on rabbits showed that aluminum was responsible for observable changes in brain cell structure and function (Mahdi et al. 2006, 19). In the last quarter of the 20th century, extensive research was conducted on a number of problems related to the toxic effects of aluminum, including many studies on the possible relationship of the use of aluminum in everyday life (such as aluminum cookware) and

Alzheimer's disease. Generally speaking, no strong correlation between aluminum and neurological disease in humans has been found, and those neurotoxic effects that have been observed are still largely unexplained (Toxicological Profile for Aluminum 2008).

Whatever the scientific evidence may say, many anti-vaccinationists are convinced that the use of aluminum compounds as vaccine adjuvants poses a serious risk to the health of young children. One prominent anti-vaccinationist, for example, has written that aluminum compounds may be even more dangerous to harmful to the developing brains of young children than thimerosal. He suggests that aluminum compounds "may even exceed the toxicity of mercury in the human body," reaching levels 14.7 to 49 times greater than that recommended by the FDA (Dr. Mercola 2012b).

Some vaccine critics have pointed to recent research that claims to demonstrate the mechanism by which aluminum produces its neurotoxic effects and that confirms the view that aluminum compounds are a far greater risk for young children than the medical profession has previously been willing to admit. The authors of an oft-cited paper in this regard begin by noting that although the neurotoxic effects of aluminum are well known, as well as its effects as a stimulator of the immune system, "it is somewhat surprising to find that in spite of over 80 years of use, the safety of Al adjuvants continues to rest on assumptions rather than scientific evidence" (Tomljenovic and Shaw 2012, 223). They then describe the biochemical mechanisms by which aluminum appears to exert its effects on the nervous and immune systems before reaching their conclusions about the safety of vaccines that contain aluminum compounds. They say in that regard that children should not be regarded as "small adults" since their unique physiology makes them more susceptible to toxins than are adults. Vaccine makers appear to have disregarded this fact because most vaccines contain levels higher than those generally recognized as safe for humans. They suggest that "a more rigorous evaluation of potential vaccine-related adverse health impacts in pediatric populations than what has been provided to date is urgently needed" (Tomljenovic and Shaw 2012, 228; for further examples of concerns about aluminum adjuvants, also see Aluminum 2012; Merchent 2012; Mercola 2012a).

Given the widespread use of aluminum compounds in vaccines, it is probably not surprising that many public health experts are convinced of their safety. The National Network for Immunization Information, for example, points out that aluminum compounds have been used in vaccines for more than 75 years, and that serious side effects are rare. The service points to a recent review article about aluminum adjuvants that "found no evidence that aluminum salts cause any serious or long-lasting adverse events" (Aluminum Adjuvants in Vaccines 2012). The Vaccine Education Center at the Children's Hospital of Philadelphia offers a similar overview. It notes that aluminum adjuvants have been "used for decades and have been given to over a billion people without problem" (Hot Topics: Aluminum 2012). And the FDA points to a 2011 study on the safety of aluminum adjuvants that concludes that the risk to infants during the first year of life is "extremely low" and that "the benefits of aluminum-containing vaccines administered during the first year of life outweigh any theoretical concerns about the potential effect of aluminum on infants" (Study Reports Aluminum in Vaccines Poses Extremely Low Risk to Infants 2012).

Squalene

Concerns about the presence of squalene in vaccines were discussed above in a review of GWS. More recently, anti-vaccinationists have been worried also about the use of squalene in other vaccines, especially those against the H1N1 virus and other forms of influenza. This concern rests on the assumption that squalene is associated with the same diseases in humans as have been observed in experimental animals, such as rats and mice. Investigative reporter Gary Matsumoto, for example, has suggested that vaccine researchers intentionally added squalene to a new vaccine, fully aware of the potential damage it could cause to humans who were given the vaccine. The list of potential diseases included multiple sclerosis, myelitis, Guillain-Barré syndrome, uveitis, neurodermatitis circumscripta and disseminata, amyloidosis, lupus erythematosus, dermatomyositis, scleroderma, chronic pericarditis, Raynaud's disease, rheumatoid arthritis, rheumatoid myositis, and acute glomerulonephritis (Matsumoto 2004, 50). All of these diseases are autoimmune conditions, initiated when the human immune system is challenged with squalene.

The determination by researchers that squalene was not responsible for GWS complications did not completely silence critics of squalene's use as an adjuvant in other vaccines. During the development of vaccines against H1N1 in 2009, for example, U.S. government officials indicated that squalene would not be used as an adjuvant for the new vaccines being developed, although anti-vaccinationists were convinced that such would not be the case. One critic of vaccines in general, Joseph Mercola, warned that fewer than 100 children were likely to die in an H1N1 flu epidemic in the United States, while 75 million children were being at risk of autoimmune diseases as a result of using squalene-containing vaccines. He opined that

> there can be no argument that unnecessary mass injection of millions of children with a vaccine containing an adjuvant known to cause a host of debilitating autoimmune diseases is a reckless, dangerous plan. (Mercola 2012c; also see Newborg 2012; Squalene—A History of Vaccine Development and the Newest Adjuvant 2012)

Most public health authorities hold somewhat different views toward the use of squalene as vaccine adjuvant. WHO, for example, has written in answer to the question, "Are squalene-containing vaccines safe?" that

Over 22 million doses of squalene-containing flu vaccine have been administered. The absence of significant vaccine-related adverse events following this number of doses suggests that squalene in vaccines has no significant risk. (Global Advisory Committee on Vaccine Safety 2012)

In its review of the status of squalene as an adjuvant, the FDA declared that the compound is "naturally occurring and safe" (AVIP–Questions and Answers 2012).

Old Wine in New Bottles

As noted above, one of the features of modern anti-vaccinationist teachings is their close connection with messages from the distant past. Although very much milder than was once the case, many religious leaders today continue to object to the practice of vaccination for a variety of reasons. For example, the Roman Catholic Church encourages its members to avoid vaccines that may have been made using cell lines taken from aborted fetuses (Vaccines Prepared from Cells Derived from Aborted Human Fetuses: A Statement of the Catholic Medical Association 2012). And a number of fundamentalist Protestant churches continue to teach that disease is a form of punishment delivered by God that humans must accept rather than fight against. Or, at most, they should restrict their concerns about infectious diseases to prayers that they will be spared from such punishments (Some Outbreaks of Vaccine-Preventable Disease in Groups with Religious or Philosophical Exemptions to Vaccination 2012). Some observers suggest that the increase in the number of preventable infectious diseases over the past few decades reflect to some extent these religious concerns, which are concretely expressed in a rising number of religious exemptions granted to people who hold such beliefs (see, for example, Omer et al. 2009).

Religious opposition to vaccination is not restricted to Christian sects. There is also concern, for example, within the

Muslim world about the health, political, social, and other risks of immunization. For example, Muslim fundamentalist objections have been one of the main reasons for the failure of polio eradication efforts in countries such as Afghanistan, Nigeria, and Pakistan. At least one of the reasons for this opposition is the fear among radical Islamists that immunization may be a method for the sterilization of Muslim children (Warraich 2012).

Just as concerns about vaccination among some religious groups have lingered over the decades, so has the objection by many alternative medical practitioners, including homeopaths, naturopaths, and chiropractors. Some of these concerns have been noted earlier in this chapter. Studies of practicing chiropractors and chiropractic students suggest that members of the profession still have serious doubts about the efficacy of vaccination in preventing infectious diseases. For example, a 2006 survey of 166 chiropractors in Kansas found that 42.7 percent agreed that immunizations were effective in preventing infectious diseases, and 27.7 percent thought that vaccines were safe, even when administered properly and appropriately (Holman and Nyberg 2012). A 2002 study of 467 chiropractic students throughout Canada found that the number of individuals who agreed with vaccination dropped from 60.7 percent in their first year of study to 39.5 percent in their last year of study. Researchers concluded that this decrease in support for immunization was a result of "informal sources of vaccine information, such as the chiropractic literature and informal talks," rather than formal lectures which, in general, were supportive of vaccination practices (Busse et al. 2002, 1531).

The Human Papillomavirus Vaccine

In addition to raising questions about the practice of vaccination in general, anti-vaccinationists sometimes dispute the need, safety, and efficacy of specific vaccines. Such was the case with the vaccine against anthrax developed for use during the

Gulf War, discussed earlier in this chapter. Another example of this type of conflict developed in the early 21st century with the development of a vaccine against HPV.

HPV is the causative agent for a number of infections that develop in the mouth, throat, and genital area. The virus exists in more than 150 different forms, about 40 of which are responsible for sexually transmitted infections, such as genital warts. As unpleasant and painful as these infections may be, they are only the precursors of far more serious diseases. HPV is now thought to be the cause of nearly 75 percent of all cases of cervical cancer, 70 percent of all cases of vaginal cancer, and 50 percent of all cases of vulvar cancer in women, as well as 85 percent of all cancer of anal cancer in men and women (Huynh 2012). These diseases are serious health problems, with cervical cancer causing more than 4,000 deaths annually in the United States, and accounting for the third largest number of cancer cases among women worldwide each year (HPV and Cancer 2012).

In 2006, the U.S. FDA approved a new vaccine, Gardasil®, for use against the HPV virus. The vaccine had been in development for more than 20 years and had undergone extensive testing in experimental animals and humans. The FDA concluded that the vaccine was both safe and effective for human use. In January 2007, the FDA went one step further, adding the HPV vaccine to its list of recommended routine childhood immunizations. The schedule recommended by the FDA was three doses for all girls aged 11–12, although the FDA pointed out that girls as young as nine could also benefit from the vaccine. The FDA also recommended so-called catch up shots for older girls and women who had not yet had the vaccine. In 2009, the FDA also approved a second vaccine against HPV called Cervarix®.

The availability of these vaccines has prompted a number of individuals and organizations to call for mandatory vaccination against HPV among young girls and boys. Their argument is that such vaccinations will reduce the health risks faced later in life by both men and women and will, therefore, reduce health costs for individuals and governments. For example, Melinda Wharton, deputy director of the Center for Disease Control and Prevention's National Center for Immunization and Respiratory Diseases, has said that "far too few U.S. girls are getting the HPV vaccine, a vaccine we know that can protect them against cervical cancer. . . . We've got in our possession a very powerful tool, a vaccine that prevents cancer. . . . If we all take actions to protect girls starting today, we'll have generations of women who will never be diagnosed with cervical cancer and that would be a great outcome to have" (NIS Teen Briefing 2012).

As of 2012, nearly all of the states have considered laws requiring mandatory HPV vaccination for young girls entering school or for state-funded education programs about the vaccine. Thus far, only one state, Texas, has adopted such a law, and that too only briefly. In 2006, Governor Rick Perry issued an executive order requiring that young girls be vaccinated for HPV before entering school. The state legislature quickly overturned that order, however, so that, as of 2012, no state has yet adopted mandatory HPV vaccination (HPV Vaccine 2012).

Objections to mandatory HPV vaccination go beyond the traditional arguments against vaccinations in general. They often focus on the fact that HPV is a sexually transmitted virus, and that protecting young women and men against the virus is only likely to increase the likelihood of their becoming sexually promiscuous at an early age. In any case, groups objecting to mandatory HPV vaccination believe that decisions involving a child's potential sexual activity are strictly within the domain of parental and family actions and are no business of the government (Position Statement: HPV Vaccine 2012). An example of this viewpoint can be found in a position paper released by the Catholic Medical Association in January 2007. That paper noted that

Given the importance of parental involvement for raising children, and particularly in forming their children in chastity, it would be counterproductive to override their ethical objections and negate their authority on this issue. (Catholic Medical Association Position Paper on HPV Immunization 2012)

Where to from Here?

In some respects, the objection of anti-vaccinationists to mandatory immunization may seem like the flailing of a small, perhaps uninformed, minority against a successful, entrenched, and dominant worldwide public health profession. Certainly there is virtually no objection or opposition to mandatory vaccination against most infectious diseases within that profession today. The procedure is supported by virtually every relevant public health entity, including, to name but a few organizations, the American Academy of Pediatrics, American Academy of Family Physicians, American Academy of Physician Assistants, American College Health Association, American Medical Association, Association of State and Territorial Health Officials, National Association of County and City Health Officials, National Association of Pediatric Nurse Practitioners, Pharmaceutical Research and Manufacturers of America, Society for Adolescent Health and Medicine, U.S. Centers for Disease Control and Prevention, Department of Health of the United Kingdom, Canadian National Advisory Committee on Immunization, National Immunization Council and Child Health Program of Mexico, and the World Health Organization.

An example of the view of most public health authorities is that expressed recently by Dr. Martin Myers, Executive Director of the National Network for Immunization Information: "there is in fact no credible 'controversy' about the safety or effectiveness of the currently US licensed childhood vaccines," he wrote to this author. "Rather, some uninformed and misinformed individuals have articulated scientifically unsubstantiated claims about vaccines" (Myers 2012). Indeed, some leaders of the public health profession have decided that it may be best simply to ignore the arguments of the anti-vaccinationists and to proceed with established programs of mandatory vaccination in all settings in which they are appropriate.

Still, the anti-vaccinationists apparently refuse to be silenced, making their case strong enough that large numbers of parents have chosen to opt out of mandatory vaccination programs wherever that option is available. Those parents do not appear to be convinced by or concerned about the rise in infectious disease rates wherever that practice has become more widely popular. This argument has been going on for as long as immunizations have been available, in one form or another, and it would be optimistic to suggest that they are likely to disappear within any of our lifetimes.

References

"2012 Adult Immunization Schedule." Centers for Disease Control and Prevention. http://www.cdc.gov/vaccines/recs/schedules/adult-schedule.htm. Accessed on April 23, 2012.

Adams, Mike. "Conclusive Link Now Admitted: Swine Flu Vaccine Causes Chronic Nervous System Disorders." 2012a. http://www.naturalnews.com/033816_swine_flu_vaccines_neurological_disorders.html. Accessed on April 24, 2012.

Adams, Mike. "Evidence-based Vaccinations: A Scientific Look at the Missing Science Behind Flu Season Vaccines." 2012b. http://www.naturalnews.com/029641_vaccines_junk_science.html. Accessed on April 25, 2012.

"Address by Miss Lily Loat." http://www.sparks-of-light.org/loat-early%20fight%201926.html. Accessed on April 20, 2012.

"Adverse Effects of Vaccines: Evidence and Causality." http://www.iom.edu/~/media/Files/Report%20Files/2011/Adverse-Effects-of-Vaccines-Evidence-and-Causality/Vaccine-report-brief-FINAL.pdf. Accessed on April 22, 2012.

Alazraki, Melly. "The Autism Vaccine Fraud: Dr. Wakefield's Costly Lie to Society." Daily Finance. http://www.dailyfinance.com/2011/01/12/autism-vaccine-fraud-wakefield-cost-money-deaths/. Accessed on April 25, 2012.

"Aluminum." Vaccine Risk Awareness Network. http://vran.org/about-vaccines/vaccine-ingredients/aluminum/. Accessed on April 27, 2012.

"Aluminum Adjuvants in Vaccines." National Network for Immunization Information. http://www.immunizationinfo.org/issues/vaccine-components/aluminum-adjuvants-vaccines. Accessed on April 27, 2012.

"Aluminum Hydroxide." World Association for Vaccine Education. "Andrew Wakefield, M.D." The Skeptic's Dictionary. http://www.skepdic.com/wakefield.html. Accessed on April 25, 2012.

"The Anti-Vaccination Society of America." The History of Vaccines. http://www.historyofvaccines.org/content/blog/anti-vaccination-society-america-correspondence. Accessed on April 21, 2012.

Arnold, David. *Imperial Medicine and Indigenous Societies.* Manchester: University of Manchester Press, 1988.

Atwood, Kimball C., and Stephen Barrett. "Naturopathic Opposition to Immunization." http://www.quackwatch.com/01QuackeryRelatedTopics/Naturopathy/immu.html. Accessed on April 21, 2012.

Aufderheide, Jeffrey John. "Vaccinations Are Causing Impaired Blood Flow (Ischemia), Chronic Illness, Disease and Death for Us All." Vactruth.com. http://vactruth.com/

2009/08/03/vaccinations-are-causing-impaired-blood-flow-ischemia-chronic-illness-disease-and-death-for-us-all-hp/. Accessed on April 24, 2012.

"AVIP–Questions and Answers." [U.S. Food and Drug Ad ministration]. http://www.fda.gov/ohrms/dockets/dockets/80n0208/80n-0208-c000037–15–01-vol151.pdf. Accessed on April 27, 2012.

Baxby, Derrick. "The End of Smallpox." *History Today* 49, no. 3 (1999): 14–16.

Behbehani, Abbas M. "The Smallpox Story: Life and Death of an Old Disease." *Microbiological Reviews* 47, no. 4 (1983): 455–509.

Bhattacharya, Sanjoy, Mark Harrison, and Michael Worboys. *Fractured States: Smallpox, Public Health and Vaccination Policy in British India 1800–1947.* New Delhi: Orient Longman, 2005.

"Biographical Sketch Of: Raymond Obomsawin." http://www.whale.to/v/obomsawin.html. Accessed on April 25, 2012.

Blaylock, Russell L. "Beware Swine Flu Vaccination." *The Blaylock Wellness Report.* http://w3.newsmax.com/blay lock/62b.cfm. Accessed on April 26, 2012.

Blaylock, Russell L.. "Vaccinations: The Hidden Danger." *The Blaylock Wellness Report* 1, no. 1 (2004). http://files.meetup.com/195767/blaylock_Vaccinations_1.pdf. Accessed on January 5, 2013.

Brady, Jonann, and Stephanie Dahle. "Celeb Couple to Lead 'Green Vaccine' Rally." ABC News. http://abcnews.go.com/GMA/OnCall/story?id=4987758#.T5m6Zqs7U1I. Accessed on April 26, 2012.

Brimnes, Niels. "Variolation, Vaccination and Popular Resis-tance in Early Colonial South India." *Medical History* 48, no. 2 (2004): 199–228.

Brunton, Deborah. *The Politics of Vaccination: Practice and Policy in England, Wales, Ireland, and Scotland, 1800–1874.* Rochester, NY: University of Rochester Press, 2008.

Burnett, James Compton. *Vaccinosis and Its Cure by Thuja.* London: The Homeopathic Publishing Company, 1884. http://www.archive.org/stream/vaccinosisandit00burngoog/ vaccinosisandit00burngoog_djvu.txt. Accessed on April 21, 2012.

Busse, Jason W., Lon Morgan, and James B. Campbell. "Chiropractic Antivaccination Arguments." *Journal of Manipulative and Physiological Therapeutics* 28, no. 5 (2005): 367–373.

Busse, Jason W., et al. "Attitudes toward Vaccination: A Survey of Canadian Chiropractic Students." *Canadian Medical Association Journal* 166, no. 12 (2002): 1531–1534.

Cantwell, Alan, Jr. "Are Vaccines Causing More Disease than They Are Curing?" New Dawn Magazine. http://www. newdawnmagazine.com/Articles/Vaccine_Genocide.html. Accessed on April 24, 2012.

"Catholic Medical Association Position Paper on HPV Immunization." Catholic Medical Association. http://www. cathmed.org/assets/files/Position%20Paper%20on%20 HPV%20Immunization.pdf. Accessed on April 28, 2012.

Cohen, Jon. "U.S. Vaccine Supply Falls Seriously Short." *Science* 295, no. 5562 (2002): 1998–2001.

Colgrove, James. "Science in a Democracy: The Contested Status of Vaccination in the Progressive Era and the 1920s." *Isis* 96, no. 2 (2005): 167–191.

A Collection of All Such Acts of the General Assembly of Virginia of a Public and Permanent Nature as Are Now in Force. Richmond: Samuel Pleasants, Jun., and Henry Pace, 1803. http://books.google.com/books?id=mxREAAAAY AAJ&pg=PA200&lpg=PA200&dq=virginia+smallpox+in oculation+1792&source=bl&ots=NAiwoAvMkg&sig=0

vRk_mHUdQWUf_ePaZoG9iSo9gs&hl=en&sa=X&ei=JZ
GVT7i2NLTViAKWgI3oDw&ved=0CE8Q6AEwBw#v=o
nepage&q&f=false. Accessed on April 23, 2012.

"Colloidal Silver v/s the Flu Vaccine." http://colloidalsilverse-
crets.blogspot.com/2008/04/colloidal-silver-vs-flu-vaccine.
html. Accessed on April 26, 2012.

Coulter, Harris L. "Vaccination and Social Violence." http://
www.whale.to/vaccines/coulter5.html. Accessed on April
24, 2012.

Crislip, Mark. "Homeopathic Vaccines." http://www.science
basedmedicine.org/index.php/homeopathic-vaccines/. Accessed on May 12, 2012.

"Dangers of Vaccines Mercury and Thimerosal." WANT-
TOKNOW.INFO. http://www.wanttoknow.info/060215v
accinesmercurydangers. Accessed on April 27, 2012.

Deer, Brian. "How the Case Against the MMR Vaccine Was
Fixed." *British Medical Journal* 3421, no. (2011): c5347.
http://www.bmj.com/content/342/bmj.c5347.full. Accessed on April 25, 2012.

"Don't Take H1N1 Vaccine this Fall!! (Proof That All Vaccines
Cause Damage)." Godlike Productions. http://www.god
likeproductions.com/forum1/message875052/pg1. Accessed
on April 24, 2012.

"Dr. Incao's Hepatitis B Vaccination Testimony in Ohio."
http://www.goodlight.net/vacexpert/ohio.htm. Accessed on
April 25, 2012.

Dr. Mercola. "The Neurological Poison So Common Your
Doctor Probably Pushes It." 2012a. 2http://articles.mer
cola.com/sites/articles/archive/2012/04/11/vaccination-
impact-on-childrens-health.aspx. Accessed on April 27,
2012.

Dr. Mercola. "New Revelation: The Neurotoxin Far Worse
than Mercury . . ." 2012b. 3 http://articles.mercola.com/
sites/articles/archive/2011/09/21/

could-this-be-the-most-dangerous-aspect-of-vaccines.aspx. Accessed on April 27, 2012.

Dr. Mercola. "Squalene: The Swine Flu Vaccine's Dirty Little Secret Exposed." 2012c. 4http://articles.mercola.com/sites/ articles/archive/2009/08/04/squalene-the-swine-flu-vac cines-dirty-little-secret-exposed.aspx. Accessed on April 27, 2012.

Durbach, Nadja. " 'They Might As Well Brand Us': Working-Class Resistance to Compulsory Vaccination in Victorian England." *Social History of Medicine* 13, no. 1 (2000): 45–63.

Durbach, Nadja. "Class, Gender, and the Conscientious Objector to Vaccination, 1898–1907." *Journal of British Studies* 41, no. 1 (2002): 58–83.

Editors of The Lancet. "Retraction—Ileal-Lymphoid-Nodular Hyperplasia, Non-Specific Colitis, and Pervasive Developmental Disorder in Children." *The Lancet* 375, no. 9713 (2010): 445.

Fitzpatrick, Michael. "Medicine on Trial." Spiked Health. http://www.spiked-online.com/articles/00000006E019. htm. Accessed on April 25, 2012.

Friedlander, Ed. "The Anti-Immunization Activists: A Pattern of Deception." http://www.pathguy.com/antiimmu.htm. Accessed on April 25, 2012.

Gallander, Benj, and Ben Stadelmann. "Big Pharma has H1N1 Fever." http://www.contratheheard.com/cth/contra guys/091127.html. Accessed on April 26, 2012.

Global Advisory Committee on Vaccine Safety. "Squalene-based Adjuvants in Vaccines." http://www.who.int/vaccine_ safety/topics/adjuvants/squalene/questions_and_answers/ en/. Accessed on April 27, 2012.

Gostin, Lawrence O. "*Jacobson v Massachusetts* at 100 Years: Police Power and Civil Liberties in Tension." *American Journal of Public Health* 95, no. 4 (2005): 576–581.

"Government Regulation." History of Vaccines. http://www. historyofvaccines.org/content/articles/government-regula tion. Accessed on April 22, 2012.

Griffin, John P. *Textbook of Pharmaceutical Medicine,* 6th ed. New York: John Wiley and Sons, 2009.

Hawden, W. R. "Vaccination Absurdities and Contradictions." 1902. http://www.vaclib.org/books/archive1/hadwen/ab surd.htm. Accessed on April 20, 2012.

"Herd Immunity and Vaccination." Supercourse. http://www. pitt.edu/˜super1/lecture/lec1181/index.htm. Accessed on May 12, 2012.

"HEW Report on Naturopathy (1968)." http://www.quack watch.com/01QuackeryRelatedTopics/Naturopathy/hew. html. Accessed on April 21, 2012.

"History of Anti-Vaccination Movements." The History of Vaccines. http://www.historyofvaccines.org/content/articles/ history-anti-vaccination-movements#Source 2. Accessed on April 19, 2012.

Hodge, James G., and Lawrence O. Gostin. "School Vaccina- tion Requirements: Historical, Social, and Legal Perspec- tives." http://www.publichealthlaw.net/Research/PDF/vac- cine.pdf. Accessed on April 23, 2012.

Hodges, Kyle. "Researchers Narrow Gulf War Syndrome Causes." http://www.army.mil/article/21654/researchers- narrow-gulf-war-syndrome-causes/. Accessed on April 25, 2012.

Holman, S., and S. Nyberg. "Attitudes and Beliefs Toward Routine Vaccination: A Survey of Kansas Chiropractors." http://soar.wichita.edu/dspace/bitstream/handle/10057/ 817/grasp0643.pdf?sequence=1. Accessed on April 28, 2012.

"Homeopathy Plus (Complaint No 2011/05/004)." http:// www.tga.gov.au/industry/advertising-reg9–2011–05–004- homeopathy-plus.htm. Accessed on May 12, 2012.

Hopkins, Donald R. *The Greatest Killer: Smallpox in History, with a New Introduction.* Chicago: University of Chicago Press, 2002.

"Hot Topics: Aluminum." The Children's Hospital of Philadelphia. http://www.chop.edu/service/vaccine-education-center/hot-topics/aluminum.html. Accessed on April 27, 2012.

Howard, Colin R. "The Impact on Public Health of the 19th Century Anti-vaccination Movement." *Microbiology Today* 305 (2003): 22–23.

"HPV and Cancer." National Cancer Institute. http://www.cancer.gov/cancertopics/factsheet/Risk/HPV. Accessed on April 28, 2012.

"HPV Vaccine." National Conference of States Legislatures. http://www.ncsl.org/issues-research/health/hpv-vaccine-state-legislation-and-statutes.aspx. Accessed on April 23, 2012.

Mrs. Hume-Rothery. *Women and Doctors, or Medical Despotism in England.* Manchester: Abel Heywood & Son, 1871.

Mrs. Hume-Rothery. *What Small-Pox & Vaccination and the Vaccination Acts Really Are,* 2nd ed. Leicester, England: E. Lamb, 1880. [Reprinted from the *National Anti-Compulsory Vaccination Reporter*]. http://archive.org/stream/what smallpoxvacc587hume#page/n0/mode/2up. Accessed on January 5, 2013.

Huynh, Harmony Phuong. "Gardasil Continues to Stir Heavy Controversy." *USCience Review.* http://www-scf.usc.edu/~uscience/gardasil_vaccine.html. Accessed on April 28, 2012.

"Immunization: The Most Successful Public Health Measure." Public Health Agency of Canada. http://www.phac-aspc.gc.ca/im/measure-intervention-eng.php. Accessed on April 23, 2012.

"Immunization and Vaccination Laws in the U.S." Lawyers. com. http://health-care.lawyers.com/Immunization-and-Vaccination-Laws-in-the-US.html. Accessed on April 24, 2012.

"Immunization Program—Exemptions." http://apps.leg. wa.gov/RCW/default.aspx?cite=28A.210.090. Accessed on April 23, 2012.

"Immunizations and Chemoprophylaxis." Air Force Joint Instruction 48–110, etc. http://www.operationalmedicine. org/ed2/Instructions/AirForce/48011000.pdf. Accessed on April 23, 2012.

"*Jacobson v. Massachusetts.* 197 U.S. 11 (1905)." http://su preme.justia.com/cases/federal/us/197/11/case.html. Accessed on April 21, 2012.

"Juvenile Diabetes and Vaccination: New Evidence for a Connection." National Vaccine Information Center. http:// www.nvic.org/vaccines-and-diseases/Diabetes/juveniledia betes.aspx. Accessed on April 23, 2012.

Kuhnke, LaVerne. *Lives at Risk: Public Health in Nineteenth-Century Egypt.* Berkeley, CA: University of California Press, 1990.

Kulenkampff, M., J. S. Schwartzman, and J. Wilson. "Neurological Complications of Pertussis Inoculation." *Archives of Disease in Childhood* 48, no. 10 (1974): 46–49.

Leavitt, Judith Walzer. "Politics and Public Health: Smallpox in Milwaukee, 1894–1895." *Bulletin of the History of Medicine* 50, no. 4 (1976): 553–568.

Mahdi, Abbas Ali, et al. "Aluminium Mediated Oxidative Stress: Possible Relationship to Cognitive Impairment of Alzheimer's Type." *Annals of Neurosciences* 13, no. 1 (2006): 19–24.

"Many Say 'No' to Vaccinations." http://www.gilead.net/vac cinations.html. Accessed on April 26, 2012.

Matsumoto, Gary. *Vaccine A: The Covert Government Experiment That's Killing Our Soldiers and Why GI's Are Only the First Victims.* New York: Basic Books, 2004.

McCormick, Samantha. "Vaccine Skepticism: Adverse Effects and Alternatives." http://www.gentlebirth.org/archives/immnza1.html. Accessed on April 26, 2012.

Meade, Teresa. " 'Living Worse and Costing More': Resistance and Riot in Rio de Janeiro, 1890–1917." *Journal of Latin American Studies* 21, no. 1–2 (1989): 241–266.

Merchent, Tenna. "Aluminum-hydroxide in Vaccines Causes Serious Health Problems." http://www.proliberty.com/observer/20071206.htm. Accessed on April 27, 2012.

"Misconceptions about Immunization." http://www.quackwatch.com/03HealthPromotion/immu/immu00.html. Accessed on April 26, 2012.

"MMR Research Timeline." *BBC News.* http://news.bbc.co.uk/2/hi/health/1808956.stm. Accessed on April 24, 2012.

"MMR Timeline." *The Guardian.* http://www.guardian.co.uk/society/2010/jan/28/mmr-doctor-timeline. Accessed on April 24, 2012.

Moore, Andrew. "Bad Science in the Headlines." *EMBO Reports* 7, no. 12 (2006): 1193–1196.

Murch, Simon H., et al. "Retraction of an Interpretation." *The Lancet* 363, no. 9411 (2004): 750.

Myers, Martin. Personal communication to author, May 3, 2012.

Nachman, Robert G. "Positivism and Revolution in Brazil's First Republic: The 1904 Revolt." *The Americas* 34, no. 1 (1977): 20–39.

Nagel, Rami. "Vaccines Exposed: A Hidden Crime Against Our Children." http://www.naturalnews.com/022400.html. Accessed on April 23, 2012.

Neustaeder, Randall. "What Are the Alternatives to Vaccination?" http://www.healthychild.com/vaccine-choices/what-are-the-alternatives-to-vaccination/. Accessed on April 26, 2012.

"New Vaccination Criteria for U.S. Immigration." Centers for Disease Control and Prevention. http://www.cdc.gov/im-migrantrefugeehealth/laws-regs/vaccination-immigration/revised-vaccination-immigration-faq.html#whatvaccines. Accessed on April 23, 2012.

Newborg, Herb. "Swine Flu Scare: It's All about the Adjuvant." http://www.infowars.com/swine-flu-scare-its-all-about-the-adjuvant/. Accessed on April 27, 2012.

"NIS Teen Briefing." Centers for Disease Control and Prevention. http://www.cdc.gov/media/releases/2011/t0825_nis_teenbriefing.html. Accessed on April 28, 2012.

Nishimura, Sey. "Promoting Health During the American Occupation of Japan The Public Health Section, Kyoto Military Government Team, 1945–1949." *American Journal of Public Health* 98, no. 3(2008): 424–434.

Obomsawin, Raymond. "Immunization Graphs: Natural Infectious Disease Declines; Immunization Effectiveness; and Immunization Dangers." December 2009. http://genesgreenbook.com/resources/obamsawin/Immunization-Graphs-RO2009.pdf. Accessed on April 25, 2012.

Offit, Paul A. "Why Are Pharmaceutical Companies Gradually Abandoning Vaccines?" *Health Affairs* 24, no. 3 (2005): 622–630.

Offit, Paul A. *The Cutter Incident: How America's First Polio Vaccine Led to the Growing Vaccine Crisis.* New Haven, CT: Yale University Press, 2007.

Omer, Saad B., et al. "Vaccine Refusal, Mandatory Immunization, and the Risks of Vaccine-Preventable Diseases." *New England Journal of Medicine* 360, no. 19 (2009): 1981–1988.

Peterson, Barbara. "The 1918 Influenza Epidemic was a Vaccine-caused Disease." http://spktruth2power.wordpress.com/2009/07/11/the-1918-influenza-epidemic-was-a-vaccine-caused-disease/. Accessed on April 22, 2012.

Phillips, Alan. "Dispelling Vaccination Myths: An Introduction to the Contradictions Between Medical Science and Immunization Policy." http://www.whale.to/v/phillips.html. Accessed on April 26, 2012.

Pitcairn, John. "The Fallacy of Vaccination." http://www.wellwithin1.com/pitcairn.htm. Accessed on April 20, 2012a.

Pitcairn, John. "Vaccination." http://books.google.com/books?id=sTtos1wiIvkC&pg=PA1&lpg=PA1&dq=john+pitcairn+vaccination&hl=en#v=onepage&q=john%20pitcairn%20vaccination&f=false. Accessed on April 20, 2012b.

"Position Statement: HPV Vaccine." http://www.focusonthefamily.com/topicinfo/Position_Statement-Human_Papillomavirus_Vaccine.pdf. Accessed on April 28, 2012.

Pringle, Evelyn. "Swine Flu Vaccine is Big Business for Pharmaceuticals." http://www.ktradionetwork.com/health/swine-flu-vaccine-is-big-business-for-pharmaceuticals/. Accessed on April 26, 2012.

"Public Health Code." (State of Michigan). http://www.legislature.mi.gov/(S(3r0rdp2shfmq2srgox40xyi5))/mileg.aspx?page=GetObject&objectname=mcl-333-5111. Accessed on January 4, 2013.

Research Advisory Committee on Gulf War Veterans' Illnesses. Gulf War Illness and the Health of Gulf War Veterans. Washington, DC: Government Printing Office, 2008.

Richards, Byron J. "Are Vaccinations Causing Early Alzheimer's?" http://www.wellnessresources.com/health/articles/are_vaccinations_causing_early_onset_alzheimers_disease/. Accessed on April 24, 2012.

Rope, Kate. "The End of the Autism/vaccine Debate? *CNN Health*. http://www.cnn.com/2010/HEALTH/09/07/p. autism.vaccine.debate/index.html. Accessed on April 24, 2012.

Ross, Dale L. "Leicester and the Anti-Vaccination Movement, 1853-1889." *Leicestershire Archaeological and Historical Society* 436 (1967–68.): 35–44. http://www.le.ac.uk/lahs/downloads/RossPagesfromvolumeXLIIIsm-7.pdf. Accessed on January 4, 2013.

"Rotavirus Vaccine (RotaShield®) and Intussusception." Centers for Disease Control and Prevention. http://www.cdc.gov/vaccines/vpd-vac/rotavirus/vac-rotashield-historical.htm. Accessed on April 22, 2012.

Science and the Regulation of Biological Products: From a Rich History to a Challenging Future. Rockville, MD: Center for Biologics Evaluation and Research, [2002].

Singla, Rohit K. "Missed Opportunities: The Vaccine Act of 1813." http://leda.law.harvard.edu/leda/data/229/rsingla.pdf. Accessed on April 22, 2012.

Smith, Michael J., and Charles R. Wood. "On-time Vaccine Receipt in the First Year Does Not Adversely Affect Neuropsychological Outcomes." *Pediatrics* 125, no. 6 (2010): 1134–1141.

"Some Outbreaks of Vaccine-preventable Disease in Groups with Religious or Philosophical Exemptions to Vaccination." CHILD, Inc. http://childrenshealthcare.org/?page_id=200. Accessed on April 28, 2012.

Spitler, Harry Riley. *Basic Naturopathy: A Textbook*. [n.p]: American Naturopathic Association, Inc., 1948.

"Squalene—A History of Vaccine Development and the Newest Adjuvant." 12160 Social Network. http://12160.info/profiles/blogs/squalene-a-history-of-vaccine. Accessed on April 27, 2012.

"States with Religious and Philosophical Exemptions from School Immunization Requirements." National Conference of State Legislatures. http://www.ncsl.org/issues-research/health/school-immunization-exemption-state-laws.aspx. Accessed on April 23, 2012.

Stewart, G. T. "The Law Tries to Decide Whether Whooping Cough Vaccine Causes Brain Damage: Professor Gordon Stewart Gives Evidence." *British Medical Journal* 293, no. 6540 7(1986): 203–204.

Stratton, Kathleen R., et al., eds. *Adverse Effects of Vaccines: Evidence and Causality.* Washington, DC: National Academies Press, 2012.

"Study Reports Aluminum in Vaccines Poses Extremely Low Risk to Infants." U.S. Food and Drug Administration. http://www.fda.gov/BiologicsBloodVaccines/ScienceResearch/ucm284520.htm. Accessed on April 27, 2012.

Tebb, William. *Compulsory Vaccination in England: With Incidental References to Foreign States.* London: E.W. Allen, 1884.

Tomljenovic, Lucija, and Christopher Shaw. "Mechanisms of Aluminum Adjuvant Toxicity and Autoimmunity in Pediatric Populations." *Lupus* 21, no. 2 (2012): 223–230.

[anonymous]. "Toward a Twenty-first-century Jacobson v. Massachusetts." *Harvard Law Review* 121, no. 7 (2008): 1822–1841.

Toxicological Profile for Aluminum. Atlanta, GA: Agency for Toxic Substances and Disease Registry, September 2008.

Triggle, Nick. "MMR Doctor Struck from Register." 2010. http://news.bbc.co.uk/2/hi/health/8695267.stm. Accessed on April 25, 2012.

Tyler, Gina. "Vaccinosis—What Parents Need to Know." http://hpathy.com/homeopathy-papers/vaccinosis-what-parents-need-to-know/. Accessed on April 21, 2012.

[untitled website]. http://www.drcarley.com/. Accessed on April 24, 2012.

"The Vaccination Act, 1898." *British Medical Journal* 2, no. 1974 (18988): 1351–1354.

"Vaccination Law of April 8th 1874." http://archive.org/stream/vaccinationlawa00germgoog#page/n3/mode/2up. Accessed on April 23, 2012.

"Vaccine A: The Covert Government Experiment That's Killing Our Soldiers and Why GI's Are Only the First Victims." http://www.whale.to/a/matsumoto.html. Accessed on April 25, 2012.

"Vaccine Disease." http://www.whale.to/vaccines/diseases.html. Accessed on April 23, 2012.

"Vaccine Free: Homeopathic Alternatives to Vaccination." http://vaccinefree.wordpress.com/homeopathicvaccine/. Accessed on April 26, 2012.

"Vaccine Schedule Selection Form." World Health Organization. http://apps.who.int/immunization_monitoring/en/globalsummary/ScheduleResult.cfm. Accessed on April 23, 2012.

"Vaccines, Blood & Biologics." U.S. Food and Drug Administration. http://www.fda.gov/biologicsbloodvaccines/safety availability/vaccinesafety/ucm096228.htm#t1. Accessed on April 27, 2012.

"Vaccines Prepared from Cells Derived from Aborted Human Fetuses: A Statement of the Catholic Medical Association." http://www.cogforlife.org/cmastatement.pdf. Accessed on April 28, 2012.

"Varieties, Literary and Philosophical." *The Universal Magazine* 9 (January–June 1808). http://books.google.com/books?id=530EAAAAQAAJ&pg=PA61&lpg=PA61&dq=piombino+lucca+vaccination+laws&source=bl&ots=q2QRcxcC_x&sig=bv0pHDd2sroiPW6S-dZQbFwKMeQ&hl=en&sa=X&ei=eYSVT5bIEOaIiALju4H9Dw&ved=0CEEQ6AEwB

Q#v=onepage&q=piombino%20lucca%20vaccination%20
laws&f=false.

Warraich, Haider J. "Religious Opposition to Polio Vaccination." *Emerging Infectious Diseases* [Internet journal]. http://
wwwnc.cdc.gov/eid/article/15/6/09-0087_article.htm

"We Support Dr. Andrew Wakefield." http://www.wesupport
andywakefield.com/. Accessed on April 25, 2012.

"What Do You Really Know about Vaccines?" http://www.
immunitionltd.com/book/vaccination-is-not-immuniza
tion.htm. Accessed on April 26, 2012.

"What Is the Alternative Vaccine Schedule?" WebMD. http://
children.webmd.com/vaccines/features/robert-sears-alterna
tive-vaccine-schedule. Accessed on April 26, 2012.

White, Andrew Dickson. *A History of the Warfare of Science
with Theology,* 2 vols. New York: Dover Publications, 1960.
[Reprint of the original 1896 edition]

Whorton, James C. "From Cultism to CAM: Alternative
Medicine in the Twentieth Century." In Johnston, Robert
D., ed. *The Politics of Healing: Histories of Alternative Medi-
cine in Twentieth-Century North America.* London:
Routledge Press, 2004.

Williamson, Stanley. "One Hundred Years Ago. Anti-
Vaccination Leagues." *Archives of Disease in Childhood* 59,
no. 12 (1984): 1195–1196.

Zucht v King. "260 U.S. 174 (1922)." http://supreme.justia.
com/cases/federal/us/260/174/case.html. Accessed on
April 21, 2012.

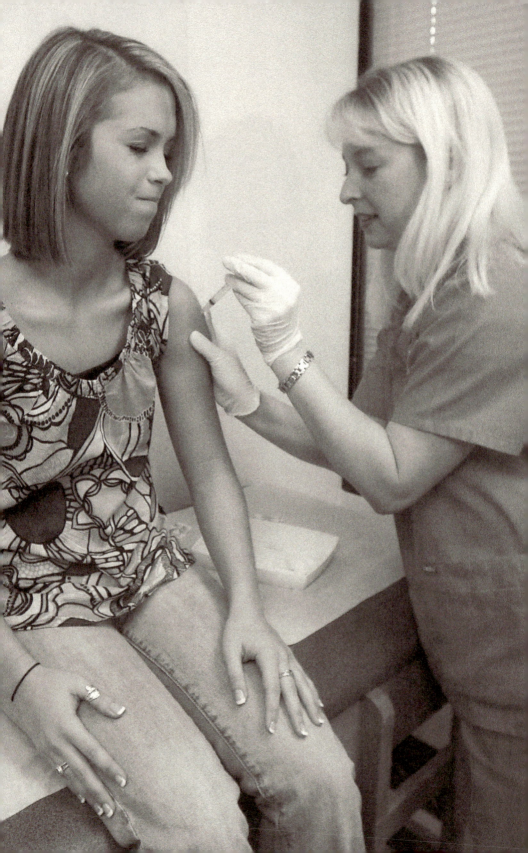

Virtually from the moment that the process of vaccination was invented, critics have raised questions about the safety and efficacy of the procedure. They have imagined side effects that ranged from the scientifically possible, such as an increased risk for developing the disease against which one is being vaccinated, to the absurd, such as the fear that vaccinated children would grow miniature cows on their arms (from the cowpox vaccine). At the same time, many people have long been convinced of the enormous medical benefits that vaccination can offer both to the individuals and the general society. They point out that many diseases that once ravaged human society have now been greatly reduced as a threat to human health, or even completely eradicated. This chapter presents some papers dealing with one or the other of these positions and with other aspects of vaccination of interest to the general public.

HPV VACCINE FOR ALL
Bob Roehr

Everyone should get the quadrivalent HPV vaccine (Gardasil, manufactured by Merck) regardless of gender or age.

An 18-year-old in Georgia receives her third and final application of the HPV vaccine in 2007. (AP Photo/John Amis)

The reason is that we have only proven the tip of the iceberg of how it can protect us by reducing rates of cervical and anal cancers. There are many scientific reasons to believe that it can provide a much broader range of health benefits, but unfortunately the clinical trials to prove them would have to be very large, long, and expensive; they probably never will be done.

Start with the obvious: The human papillomavirus (HPV) vaccine initially was approved only for use in young women. Never before or since has a vaccine been so limited.

Why? Because approval by the U.S. Food and Drug Administration (FDA) is based upon the data submitted to it. Pharmaceutical companies decided that preventing cervical cancer was the most important reason to create a HPV vaccine—it was also the fastest and cheapest way to prove that a vaccine worked. So they built clinical trials around the high cancer-risk HPV types 16 and 18, and HPV types 5 and 11 that cause warts that are less likely to become cancerous. They only looked at the question in young women.

Men are fortunate in that they have a much lower risk of developing HPV-related cancers, but they are the primary vehicle through which the virus is transmitted to women. Researchers knew that vaccinating men as well as women would be the most effective way to break the cycle of new transmission of the virus for everyone.

Proving that would require a very large, long, and expensive clinical trial and there was still the risk that the FDA might not approve that use because the men did not benefit directly, while taking on an infinitesimally small risk associated with any vaccination.

Men do develop HPV-related anal cancers. The virus can be transmitted by fingers (their own or another person's) or even catch a ride in sweat flowing from their genital regions or that of their partners.

Researchers decided that the easiest population to study whether or not the vaccine protected against developing anal warts was young gay men. It was a difficult trial to conduct but it eventually proved that the vaccine protected against anal cancers in men. The FDA expanded the label indication to include young men as well as young women.

HPV Diseases

The HPV is a remarkably diverse family with more than a hundred distinct types and additional variations within types. Each grows in its own very specific ecological niche on the human body, be it between your fingers but not your toes, the mucosal tissue of your throat and penis but not the skin on your calf, or in your bladder, etc.

Some people have an immune system that can fight off one type of HPV but not another, so we all have many different types of HPV living on us. The types and numbers of those viruses is like the population of a country, they grow in number and change in diversity over time.

Sometimes the virus seizes control of the DNA in a patch of skin cells, causing it to grow warty formations rather than normal tissue. And sometimes those warts can become cancerous and even kill, if they are allowed to grow unchecked.

Oropharyngeal cancers, located in the back of the mouth and into the throat, are one of the most rapidly growing categories of cancer in the United States. Most of that increase has been attributed to HPV infection. It predominately strikes young white men in their 30s.

Why is this happening? Researchers attribute it to a combination of biology and patterns of sexual activity. HPV is a localized infection; it doesn't spread inside the body. But the antibodies to the virus are systemic; that means the first site of exposure is likely to become infected, but the antibodies generated by that infection will protect other parts of the body from becoming infected later on.

Is the HPV vaccine likely to protect against oral and penile cancers? Again, all biological logic points to the fact that it will, but the difficulty and cost of conducting the medical studies to conclusively prove that fact means they probably never will be done.

Other Benefits

Traditional vaccines are most effective at revving up one's immune system to prevent an initial infection from occurring. That is why clinical trials were conducted in young women and men, while they were still relatively unexposed to HPV types. This is the tip of the iceberg of what we know for sure about HPV vaccine protection. Other areas of benefit remain hidden below the water line.

A person's immune system declines with age. It is likely that many warts and cancers that appear as a person grows older are the result of an exposure to HPV that occurred years earlier. An active immune system holds the infection in check, but as the immune function declines, the virus becomes more active and visible signs of the infection emerge.

One of the hot new trends in medicine is to use vaccines as therapy, particularly for treating cancer. The concept is that even after one is infected, it might make sense to stimulate the immune system to make a better response, and perhaps even clear the infection.

Another factor likely in play is cross-protection. A vaccine stimulates the immune system to make antibodies that exactly fit the targeted virus. Cross-protection is when that same antibody can also bind to and neutralize other somewhat similar viruses, though perhaps not as well or efficiently as it binds to the targeted virus.

Given how closely related many of the other HPV viruses are, it is no surprise that some of the antibodies generated by the quadrivalent vaccine have shown some cross-protection against other HPV types in the laboratory. It is logical to assume that some of this also occurs in the human body, but it would be difficult and expensive to show that with a clinical trial.

All of this has led me to believe that persons of all ages might benefit from the quadrivalent HPV vaccine. But I can't prove it.

Further Reading

Kahn et al. "Vaccine-Type Human Papillomavirus and Evidence of Herd Protection after Vaccination Introduction." *Pediatrics* 1320, no. 2 (August 2012): e249–e256.

Bob Roehr is a biomedical journalist based in Washington, DC. He writes regularly for the British Medical Journal *and the American Association for the Advancement of Science.*

HPV VACCINE MANDATES: LITTLE BENEFIT, REAL HARM
Diane M. Harper

The World Health Organization states, "There is no such thing as a 'perfect' vaccine which protects everyone who receives it AND is entirely safe for everyone."

With today's technology, cervical cancer is not completely preventable by any combination of screening and/or vaccination. It is the balance of the good that HPV vaccines can do for a small portion of the population, weighed against the costs, harms, and risks to the millions of masses that is the basis of this debate. HPV vaccines are a wonderful option to have for those who value the level of benefit that preventing abnormal Pap tests and their subsequent treatment entails. But HPV vaccines are not a substitute for regular Pap screening and if used that way will result in an increase in the number of women with cervical cancer.

Should states require that young girls receive the HPV vaccine?

No. It is a silly use of public funding resources that could be better spent on sexual education classes. HPV infection is a very common skin-to-skin infection, 95 percent of which never goes on to cause cancer. Hundreds of millions of women are infected with HPV, but only a fraction of a small portion develops cervical cancer. Even for those women whose HPV infections do not clear and do progress to CIN 3, the recognized cervical cancer precursor, only one in five (20%) with CIN 3 will develop cervical cancer over 5 years, and only two in five (40%) with CIN 3 will develop cervical cancer over 30 years. Pap screening for all women 21 years and older will detect almost all of the CIN 3 disease that a woman might have. Once it is detected, the CIN 3 disease is easy to treat in the doctor's office, with 100 percent success. The most important health-care advice a woman can take is to get her Pap smears regularly done throughout her lifetime.

No. One HPV vaccine, Gardasil, has been shown to last for five years. Cervarix, the other HPV vaccine, has been shown to last for 9.4 years. If given to a young girl at 12 years of age, there is no indication that she will be protected for her lifetime. She has a real risk of HPV exposure throughout her entire lifetime, not just for five years. Population health models show that if the HPV vaccine does not last for at least 15 years, no cancers can ever be prevented; women will just get the cancers at a later time in life after the vaccine has worn off.

No. Among girls younger than 11 years, 7–15 percent already have high-risk HPV infections due to sexual abuse or other types of HPV skin-to-skin transmission. Gardasil clearly does not work in those who have already had HPV infections. These girls are better served by routine Pap smear examinations beginning when they are 21 years of age or if they have any symptoms. They are only appropriately identified by their primary care physician, not by a surrogate mandatory vaccine provider.

No. The HPV vaccine, Gardasil, has over 20,000 reports to the CDC of side effects happening after girls have received it. Eight percent of these reports are considered serious, requiring hospitalization, visits to the emergency room, or resulting in death. The Guillain Barré syndrome has been documented and confirmed after Gardasil injection. Twenty-six girls have been awarded money from the National Vaccine Injury Compensation Program for their injury from Gardasil. Many girls and their parents would rather their daughter be screened with Pap tests her entire life than take the risk that Gardasil will cause her damage or paralysis for the rest of her life.

No. If a girl should happen to be pregnant when she receives Gardasil, there is no reassurance that her baby will develop normally. Many regulatory bodies such as the FDA in the United States and others throughout the world are carefully watching the reports of the babies born to mothers who received Gardasil while pregnant.

No. HPV vaccines are an option, not a necessity. The purpose of having the option of HPV vaccination is to offer women the opportunity to have less chance of an abnormal Pap test. With Gardasil, the chances of an abnormal Pap test are reduced by 17 percent and the chances of needing treatment for a CIN 3 lesion are reduced by 45 percent. With Cervarix, the chances of an abnormal Pap test are reduced by 27 percent and the chances of needing treatment for a CIN 3 lesion are reduced by 90 percent.

No. Gardasil only protects against two of the HPV types that can cause cervical cancer (HPV16, 18). Cervarix only protects against seven of the HPV types that can cause cervical cancer (HPV16, 18, 31, 33, 45, 51, 52). There are 14 HPV types that can cause cervical cancer. Only Pap testing can detect the changes in the cells that all 14 HPV types can cause.

No. There is even less evidence that all boys should be vaccinated with Gardasil. The major concern is that the protective antibodies wear off in two of five (40%) boys after only two years! Vaccinating boys will do very little to protect them long-term from HPV and even less to protect girls from HPV. Boys are best served by circumcision and by careful teaching of the nine steps of appropriate condom use in sexual education classes.

No. Mandating HPV vaccination for the prevention of genital warts as a reason to assault young girls with three painful shots is clearly misguided. While genital warts are not pretty, it is rare that they will kill you, and common that they will go away with treatment. For every one girl that has a genital wart, there are 23 women with abnormal Pap tests. For every one boy that has a genital wart, there are 23 women with abnormal Pap tests. Clearly there are far more people with abnormal Pap tests than with genital warts, and the prevention of abnormal Pap tests should be considered a greater good in considering the benefits of HPV vaccination.

No. While speculation, hypotheses, and assumptions abound about prevention against other cancers associated with HPV, prophylactic HPV vaccines have not prevented any anal cancers in any studies to date.

No. Gardasil requires three shots at specific time intervals to be effective. Cervarix, on the other hand, is effective in just one dose. In the United States at this time, over half of the $3.5 billion spent on Gardasil shots are wasted. Either girls get only one or two shots, or they fail to get the three shots on time. Mandating HPV vaccination only increases the profit for Merck and its shareholders when state health monies could be used to a better population good.

No, HPV vaccination should not be mandatory. It is simply silly for states to require that young girls receive the HPV vaccine. HPV vaccination is an option that requires much discussion about the benefits versus harms of all means of cervical cancer prevention. That discussion should be had on an individual basis just as the decision whether or not to vaccinate should be made by each individual and not by the state.

Diane M. Harper, MD, MPH, MS, Professor of Medicine, Director of Gynecologic Cancer Prevention Research Group, and Director of the Center of Excellence for Women's Health at University of Missouri-Kansas City School of Medicine is an internationally respected clinician, teacher, and researcher specifically in the field of HPV disease prevention. She continues to serve as a consultant to the World Health Organization for HPV vaccination universal recommendations as well as for low and middle resource income countries. She has authored over 100 peer-reviewed articles and book chapters in such journals as the Lancet, New England

Journal of Medicine, Vaccine, and Sexually Transmitted Diseases, *among others. She has been honored as Teacher of the Year at Dartmouth Medical School and New Hampshire Family Physician of the Year in 2006.*

VACCINE SHORTAGES—A PERSPECTIVE
Dean A. Haycock

The sore throat, chills, fever, coughing, and runny nose caused by the latest mutated flu virus used to force me to bed once a year. Finally, I caught on to flu vaccines. I was freed from my annual illness.

Until 2004, I couldn't find anyone to give me a flu shot because there wasn't enough for everyone. For me it was an inconvenience. But for many others—the elderly, the ill—the shortage posed a serious threat. The problem wasn't new. Five of the eight vaccines most commonly given to children were in short supply between 2000 and 2002 and there were more shortages in 2003.

How could something that might mean the difference between life and death for susceptible individuals not be available in one of the most advanced countries in the world? And how could such shortages exist not only for flu vaccines but for more than half a dozen other vaccines for childhood and other diseases?

Such shortages can have a particularly negative impact on disadvantaged kids. American Indian and Alaska Native children, for example, had more than twice the national average chance of not getting a whooping cough vaccination during the 2002–2003 shortage (Groom et al. 2006).

One of the problems is the small number of companies that make vaccines. The Centers for Disease Control and Prevention (CDC) lists just 13 vaccine manufacturers in the United States. And three-quarters of all the vaccines produced in this country—a little under 50—are produced by just three companies: Sanofi Pasteur, Merck & Co., Inc., and GlaxoSmithKline.

This means production or distribution problems, or a decision to stop producing a vaccine because it doesn't make enough money, can result in fluctuating supplies, including shortages.

The CDC monitors supplies and displays vaccine availability on a regularly updated web page called Current Vaccine Shortages & Delays. The site routinely lists minor problems but there is no guarantee that serious shortages won't happen in the future, according to Jeanne Santoli, Chief of Vaccine Supply and Assurance Branch at the CDC.

To limit the consequences of future shortages, the U.S. government buys vaccines from manufacturers and distributes them on a rotating basis to ensure viable, unexpired supplies. This provides a cushion in case vaccine manufacturers are unable to meet the health needs of the public.

Critics of the government claim this is one of the reasons we face vaccine shortages. They claim that the government pays less than it should for the warehoused vaccines. This has the effect of discouraging private manufacturers from producing more and better vaccines. Another problem they see is government regulations that aim to ensure safety but increase production costs.

"To have a viable vaccine industry, we will have to create the incentive for firms to produce them," Devon Herrick, PhD, wrote in a 2004 paper for the National Center for Policy Analysis (NCPA). "The first and foremost incentive," he adds, "has to be the potential for profitability (Herrick 2012). For this to happen the government needs to get out of the business of buying vaccines." The NCPA promotes private alternatives to government regulation and control. More than a quarter of its budget comes from corporations.

But is it intelligent to suggest that companies overwhelmingly committed and devoted to making a profit for themselves should have responsibility for something as important as the production of life-saving vaccines? Can a free economic market really meet the needs of the public if, as Herrick suggests, the most important consideration is that "vaccines should be a moneymaker for drug firms"? Similar concerns have been raised about the pharmaceutical industry in general.

GlaxoSmithKline, Eli Lilly, Pfizer, Abbott Laboratories, and other giant drug companies have been fined billions of dollars for crimes like false advertising, hiding negative scientific results, paying doctors to promote their products, and pushing medications for unapproved uses. The drug companies simply pay the fines and continue to make money.

Critics would like the government to stay out of private industry as much as possible so corporations can make as much money as possible. But greed is not the best incentive for doing good and serving people.

It is clear that too little regulation can threaten the well-being of the country. In 2008, for example, an under-regulated financial market undercut the economy of the entire country so much that the net worth of average U.S. citizens was set back a decade. The negative effects of the Great Recession have lasted for years.

"The notion of the free market is a myth," Nobel Prize–winning economist Joseph Stiglitz said in a 2012 interview with *Newsweek* magazine. "All markets are shaped by laws and regulations, and unfortunately our laws and regulations are shaped in order to create more inequality and less opportunity" (Luscombe 2012). Stiglitz is referring to more inequality and less opportunity for individuals, not for corporations or financial firms.

The problem is not that the government overregulates vaccine production; it is that no single authority has the responsibility for enforcing cooperation between private and public groups involved in vaccine production.

Fortunately, not-for-profit organizations, including the Bill and Melinda Gates Foundation, are now helping to fund research and development of vaccines. To ensure the health of its citizens, however, the government nevertheless should take as much responsibility as necessary for the production of essential vaccines and other medications if private industry fails to do so.

Dr. Grace Lee of the Children's Hospital in Boston concludes: "Our country's current economic crisis lends a special context to the crisis in vaccine financing. It is more important than ever that the government, private insurers, manufacturers, and providers work together to ensure that all children have equitable access to vaccines and that enhancing vaccine delivery is a responsibility shared by all" (Lee et al. 2009).

It's not all about profit.

References

Groom, A. V., et al. "Effect of a National Vaccine Shortage on Vaccine Coverage for American Indian/Alaska Native Children." *American Journal of Public Health* 96, no. 4 (2006): 697–701.

Herrick, Devon. "What's Behind the Flu Vaccine Shortage." http://www.ncpa.org/pub/ba493. Accessed on June 15, 2012.

Lee, G. M., et al. "Vaccine Financing in the United States: An Emerging Crisis." *Archives of Pediatric and Adolescent Medicine* 163, no. 5 (2009):485–487.

Luscombe, B. "10 Questions: Nobel Prize-Winning Economist Joseph Stiglitz on Inventing the 1% and Why They're Bad for the Economy." *Newsweek* 179, no. 23 (2012): 66.

Dean A. Haycock, PhD, is a medical and science writer located in Salem, New York.

SOUNDS OF DEATH: WHOOPING COUGH AND VACCINE REFUSAL
Benjamin Radford

Whooping cough, also known as pertussis, is a highly infectious respiratory disease that by all rights should be doomed by science. Like polio—the crippling disease that plagued children only a few generations ago but has since been eradicated—it is preventable.

It sounds like something from the Middle Ages: whooping cough victims are wracked with prolonged coughing spasms so violent that they sometimes break their ribs. It often (though not always) creates a strange, sickening "whooping" sound as patients struggle to inhale air after such coughing, and is often accompanied by vomiting. If left untreated, the coughing fits can last two or three months, interfering with eating and sleeping. It can also be fatal. Though adults can catch whooping cough, it is most often found in children.

According to the *New York Times*, the spring of 2012 saw a resurgence of pertussis; it "struck Washington State this spring with a severity that health officials say could surpass the toll of any year since the 1940s, before a vaccine went into wide use. . . . The state has declared an epidemic and public health officials say the numbers are staggering: 1,284 cases through early May, the most in at least three decades and 10 times last year's total at this time, 128" (Johnson 2012).

The reasons for the resurgence of this terrible disease are varied. One of them is evolution: the bacteria that causes whooping cough (*Bordetella pertussis* or *Bordetella parapertussis*) have mutated and evolved over time, becoming resistant to traditional antibiotics that once treated it (primarily erythromycin). Overuse of antibiotics has concerned scientists for decades, and antibiotic-resistant strains of diseases clearly show the consequences. The problem is not that the drugs don't work; it's that they work too well and are misused.

But public health officials also see a much bigger problem: drugs that could prevent the disease aren't even being used at all when parents refuse to vaccinate their children. Indeed, as Dr. Steven Novella, a Yale physician, noted on his Science-Based Medicine blog, "there are serious concerns about vaccine refusal as a contributor to the resurgence of whooping cough. Thanks to the anti-vaccine movement there is unsubstantiated fear about the safety of vaccines. In particular there are pockets of vaccine refusal resulting in a loss of herd immunity. Herd immunity results when enough of the population is immune so that an infectious disease cannot spread, so cases become isolated and do not cause an epidemic. Without herd immunity pertussis infections can spread through a population."

Novella also addresses a claim often made by parents who refuse to vaccinate their children—that as long as other kids are vaccinated they don't need to vaccinate their own. "The evidence indicates that unvaccinated children are at higher risk of developing whooping cough than vaccinated children. Existing herd immunity is not sufficient to protect the unvaccinated, even in areas of high vaccine compliance. Further there is early evidence that whooping cough is spreading the most in counties that have a high vaccine refusal rate" (Novella 2012). Parents who vaccinate their children not only make them healthier, they also help protect other people's children.

Anti-Vaccination Fears

Why do some people doubt vaccines? One reason is that their effectiveness cannot be proven on an individual basis. For example, even people who are effectively vaccinated against a disease can still get the disease (no vaccination is completely effective, and for example, you might catch a flu from a different virus strain than the one you were inoculated against); and many unvaccinated people do not get the disease (either because they are already immune or because they were never exposed to it). In other words, one individual's personal experience—however compelling—is not an accurate indicator of the efficacy of a vaccination; instead vaccinations are proven safe and effective in studies of large groups of people. Meanwhile, the institutions best equipped to conduct the necessary large-scale studies (i.e., governments and big drug companies) are also those that the public often distrusts, leading to conspiracy theories.

Fear of vaccination is nothing new; it's been around for centuries. There was vehement resistance to the very first vaccine, created for smallpox in the late 1700s. When the public learned that the vaccine was created by taking pus from the wounds of infected cows and giving it to humans, they were disgusted. Some even believed that the vaccination could actually turn children into cows! In England, vaccination deniers formed an Anti-Vaccination League in 1853, followed by the Anti-Compulsory Vaccination League in 1867. These groups claimed that the smallpox vaccine was dangerous, ineffective, and represented not only a government conspiracy but an infringement on personal rights by the government and medical establishment. Fears over smallpox vaccination have been long since disproven—the vaccination was both safe and effective—but distrust and fear-mongering continue to this day.

Perhaps the most famous current anti-vaccination advocate is Dr. Andrew Wakefield, the lead author of a small 1998 case report suggesting a link between vaccines and the onset of childhood autism. His research was widely cited as scientific proof of vaccine dangers, but he was later found guilty of acting unethically in his research and his paper retracted as "a deliberate fraud."

Vaccine deniers are correct about one thing: there are small but real risks involved in vaccinations, as there are with any drug or medical intervention. They are not hidden but instead well known and information on them easily available from doctors or online. The risks of side effects are far less dangerous than the risks of catching the disease—especially if that disease is preventable.

References

Johnson, Kirk. "Cutbacks Hurt a State's Response to Whooping Cough." *The New York Times,* May 12, 2012, A16. http://www.nytimes.com/2012/05/13/health/policy/ whooping-cough-epidemic-hits-washington-state.html?_ r=2&ref=health. Accessed on July 2, 2012.

Novella, Steven. "Whooping Cough Epidemic." Science-Based Medicine, April 4, 2012. http://www.sciencebased medicine.org/index.php/whooping-cough-epidemic/.

Benjamin Radford is deputy editor of Skeptical Inquirer *science magazine and a Research Fellow with the nonprofit educational organization, The Committee for Skeptical Inquiry. He is author or coauthor of seven books, including* Hoaxes, Myths, and Manias: Why We Need Critical Thinking; Media Mythmakers: How Journalists, Activists, and Advertisers Mislead Us; Tracking the Chupacabra: The Vampire Beast in Fact, Fiction, and Folklore; *and* The Martians Have Landed! A History of Media-Driven Panics and Hoaxes. *Radford is a regular columnist for* LiveScience.com, Discovery News, *and* Skeptical Inquirer *magazine. He has appeared on the Discovery Channel, the History Channel, the National Geographic Channel, the Learning Channel, CBC, CBS, BBC, CNN, and other networks.*

VACCINATION DOUBTS
Louise Kuo Habakus

> "There are unanswered questions about vaccine safety. We need studies on vaccinated populations based on various schedules and doses as well as individual patient susceptibilities that we are continuing to learn about. No one should be threatened by the pursuit of this knowledge. Vaccine policy should be the subject of frank and open debate, with no tolerance for bullying. There are no sides-only people concerned for the well-being of our children."
>
> —Bernadine Healy, MD, former director, National Institutes of Health and former health editor, U.S. News & World Report.

Vaccination evokes strong opinions and emotions. Some are grateful and relieved to get vaccines. Others are angry and resentful about vaccine mandates. Many are caught in the middle—afraid, confused, and looking for answers. Whether you are a parent, student, employee, soldier, or anyone else, you have a stake in this debate. Sooner or later, you will wonder, Should I get a vaccine? Do I have a choice? Who decides?

The late Dr. Bernadine Healy spoke courageously about the need for openness in vaccine safety science and policy. Despite her appeal for "no sides" to this debate, it remains heated and polarized. There are two distinct viewpoints, one "pro-mandate," and the other "pro-choice." The camps usually levy the same insults at one another: irresponsible, dangerous, denialist, corrupt, and antiscience.

The pro-mandate camp strongly supports U.S. vaccination policy. Its key arguments follow:

1. Government officials are best qualified to make vaccination decisions. Only government can ensure that a sufficiently high percentage of people get vaccinated to preserve societal herd immunity.

2. Vaccines are overwhelmingly safe and effective, and the benefits vastly outweigh the risks. Adverse events are vanishingly rare.

3. Science proves the benefit of vaccines beyond a reasonable doubt. No reliable scientific evidence exists that vaccines are responsible for any increase in common childhood health problems, including autism.

4. Vaccine refusers are dangerous and selfish. People who choose not to vaccinate are parasites. They are irrational and threaten others with deadly disease.

5. Only "false prophets" suggest that vaccines may cause disorders like autism. Quack healthcare practitioners concoct unfounded treatments for autism and prey on vulnerable parents desperate for help. People should disdain and shun them.

6. Vaccine exemptions should be abolished. Industry spokesman, Paul Offit, MD, and others suggest that states should

abolish philosophical and religious exemptions. People abuse them and put others at risk. People have a social responsibility to vaccinate.

This article outlines the pro-choice perspective. Here are its key points:

1. Vaccination choice is a human right. Because vaccination poses a risk to life, liberty, and security of a person, only an individual or guardian may decide how, when, and whether to vaccinate.

2. Society as a whole benefits from the cumulative impact of free and informed individual healthcare choices.

3. Vaccine safety science is flawed and incomplete. The Institute of Medicine as well as informed scientists, doctors, and officials have repeatedly acknowledged that fundamental questions about vaccine safety remain unanswered.

4. The U.S. vaccine program is rife with conflicts of interest. Vaccines are big business and all of their promoters—pharma, government, medicine, and science—get their cut. The vaccine program does not put children's safety first.

5. Individuals are entitled to the practitioners and remedies of their choosing, including such biomedical interventions as diet, vitamin and mineral supplementation, chelation, and gastrointestinal treatment.

6. Vaccination exemption rights must expand, not contract. Individuals have the right to free and informed consent for all medical interventions, including vaccination. In practice, not just in theory, individuals must have the right to make their own decisions.

Public health officials assert that vaccines are safe and effective, but the truth is far more complicated. Vaccination is a serious medical intervention for healthy individuals against a disease that might occur. The decision whether to vaccinate has important, potentially life-altering ramifications. While vaccines protect some, they unquestionably harm and cause death to others. Vaccines are legally classified as "unavoidably unsafe." For government to compel a potentially life-threatening product sets vaccination apart from other medical procedures. Public health officials tell us that those who suffer adverse reactions are exceedingly few. The basis for such an optimistic claim is doubtful.

Science on vaccine safety is inadequate. Scientists do not know with certainty the cumulative impact of the childhood vaccination schedule. Vaccines are approved and licensed individually, yet the CDC recommends that doctors give multiple vaccines at once. Furthermore, the CDC recommends vaccines to populations for which there are no safety data, such as flu shots for pregnant women. Research confirms that fewer than 10 percent of doctors report adverse vaccine events. Even so, the government-administered Vaccine Injury Compensation Program has paid $2.5 billion to more than 2,500 families since 1988.

Vaccines are epidemic—they have spread rapidly and extensively to almost all children and many adults in the United States and around the world. In the 1800s and early 1900s, vaccines were a medical intervention of last resort during infectious disease outbreaks. Faced with a smallpox epidemic, the U.S. Supreme Court upheld the constitutionality of a single vaccine mandate for adults in 1905. The penalty for noncompliance was a $5 fine (about $125 today). In the last 50 years, however, governments have imposed multiple preventive vaccines on virtually all children and some adults for the "greater good." Today, the federal government recommends 70 doses of 16 vaccines from birth to age 18. Vaccines and their advertisements are everywhere—from the doctor's office to the Internet to the corner drugstore. All 50 states mandate between 30 and 45 doses of vaccines for children. The penalty for noncompliance is denial of admission to day care and school.

Governments, schools, employers, doctors, and officials concede that Americans have a choice about vaccination, but in practice, they make that choice nearly impossible to exercise. There is pressure to begin vaccinating children from the moment of birth. Formally, all states honor medical exemptions from vaccination as the law requires. Further, 48 states recognize religious exemptions, 20 recognize philosophical exemptions, and some recognize exemptions for documented immunity (blood tests showing sufficient antibodies). Choice is honored in the breach, however. States punish doctors who grant "too many" medical exemptions, schools don't inform parents that exemptions exist, and states impose vaccination on the unwilling through school exclusion and even forced child removal.

Compulsory vaccination for schoolchildren, soldiers, and healthcare workers heightens the pressure to vaccinate all people for whom vaccines are recommended. It also reinforces the stigma for those who do not comply. Government and the medical profession exercise potent financial, legal, and social levers to ensure that people make the "right choice." Should you make the "wrong choice," your child may have far fewer educational options—no public school, often no private school, often no day care, often no access to your doctor, etc. You even risk possible charges of child neglect and the threat of child removal. While in theory the country acknowledges the virtue of vaccination choice, in practice, it indulges the vice of coercive medicine. Renowned human rights scholar Louis Henkin understood: "hypocrisy is the homage that vice pays to virtue." The U.S. vaccine program hypocritically gives lip service to choice while violating the fundamental principle of free and informed consent to medical intervention.

Americans are rightfully concerned. There are no safe vaccines; only difficult choices to weigh and make. Americans want and deserve a more accurate, measured, and responsible national dialogue concerning vaccination. To dismiss as "anti-vaccine" those who advocate for choice, safety, better science, transparency, and restraint does harm to us all. The legitimate battlegrounds in the vaccine debate are between compulsion and choice, transparency and nondisclosure, caution and recklessness, and accountability and impunity.

Our current vaccination schedule is in many ways a grand experiment—we do not know whether widespread, mandatory vaccination will ultimately prove beneficial or harmful. Beyond the science, however, is the question of individual rights. Does any country, and in particular a democracy, have the right to impose vaccination on unwilling individuals, especially in the absence of disease epidemics and adequate safety science? Foremost in the minds of the country's founders was the imperative to protect citizens' inalienable rights. Government today apparently does not trust individuals to serve their own best interests.

The mainstream media portray vaccination concerns as a fringe issue. This is grossly inaccurate. A University of Michigan poll revealed that 89 percent of parents rank vaccine safety as the most important topic in children's health research today (Vaccine and Medication Safety Are Parents' Top Research Priorities 2012). Those deeply concerned about vaccination choice, parental rights, vaccine safety, and undue corporate influence are the majority. Vaccination choice is not a partisan issue, and it is not even just about vaccines. It is about ethics, human rights, science, freedom, dignity, and democracy. It is about the common ideals that Americans hold dear. It is about who we are and what we stand for. And it is literally about the biological integrity of the next generation and those that succeed it.

References

"Vaccine and Medication Safety Are Parents' Top Research Priorities." October 11, 2010, http://www2.med.umich.edu/ prmc/media/newsroom/details.cfm?ID=1760. Accessed on July 3, 2012.

This essay contains excerpts from *Vaccine Epidemic—How Corporate Greed, Biased Science, and Coercive Government Threaten Our Human Rights, Our Health, and Our Children* (Skyhorse 2011), coedited by Louise Kuo Habakus and Mary Holland, with permission by Skyhorse Publishing.

Louise Kuo Habakus is the lead editor of Vaccine Epidemic, *and executive director and cofounder of the Center for Personal Rights, a nonpartisan, nonprofit organization founded to advance the human right to vaccination choice. She was a managing director of Putnam Investments, a corporate vice president for Prudential Financial, and a consultant with Bain & Company. She graduated Phi Beta Kappa from Stanford University, where she also received a graduate degree in international policy studies. In her advocacy work, she lectures and writes frequently, and has appeared in numerous media outlets, including ABC World News Tonight, Fox & Friends, and the* New York Times.

FEDERAL LAW AND MANDATORY VACCINATION
Stephen Lendman

At least three U.S. federal laws should concern all Americans and suggest what may be coming: the Project Bio Shield Act of 2004, the Public Readiness and Emergency Preparedness (PREP) Act, and the Pandemic and All-Hazards Preparedness Act of 2006. Mandatory vaccinations are being hyped for nonexistent threats, like H1N1 (Swine Flu). Vaccines and drugs like Tamiflu endanger human health but are hugely profitable to drug company manufacturers.

The stated purpose of the Project BioShield Act of 2004 is "to provide protections and countermeasures against chemical, radiological, or nuclear agents that may be used in a terrorist attack against the United States by giving the National Institutes of Health contracting flexibility, infrastructure improvements, and expediting the scientific peer review process, and stream-lining the Food and Drug Administration approval process of countermeasures" (Public Law 108-276 2012).

In other words, the FDA may now recklessly approve inad-equately tested, potentially dangerous vaccines and other drugs if ever the Secretaries of Health and Human Services (HHS) or Defense (DOD) declare a national emergency, whether or not one exists and regardless of whether treatments available are safe and effective. Around $6 billion or more will be spent to develop, produce, and stockpile vaccines and other drugs to counteract claimed bioterror agents.

The PREP Act slipped under the radar when George Bush signed it into law as part of the 2006 Defense Appropriations Act. It lets the HHS Secretary declare any disease an epidemic or national emergency requiring mandatory vaccinations. Nothing in the Act lists criteria that warrant a threat. Also po-tential penalties aren't specified for those who balk, but very likely they'd include quarantine and possible fines.

The HHS website also says the Secretary may "issue a decla-ration . . . that provides immunity from tort liability (except for willful misconduct) for claims of loss caused, arising out of, re-lating to, or resulting from administration or use of (vaccine or other pharmaceutical) countermeasures to diseases, threats and conditions determined by the Secretary to constitute a pres-ent, or credible risk of a future public health emergency. . . . " (Public Readiness and Emergency Preparedness Act Questions and Answers 2012).

The industry-run U.S. FDA notoriously rushes inadequately tested drugs to market, putting their efficacy and safety into question, and turning those who use them into lab rats. It in-cludes everyone if a mass vaccination is ordered on the mere claim of a public emergency—no proof required.

The Pandemic and All-Hazards Preparedness Act of 2006 is the other worrisome law. It amended the Public Health Service Act "with respect to public health security and all-hazards pre-paredness and response, and for other purposes" (Public Law

109-417 2012). Even its supporters worry about issues of privacy, liability, and putting profits over public health. Critics express greater concerns about dangerous remedies for exaggerated or nonexistent threats as well as mass hysteria created for political purposes.

At least one other measure is also worrisome—The Model State Emergency Health Powers Act of 2009 (MSEHPA). The act was described by its sponsor, the Center for Law and the Public's Health, a collaborative of Johns Hopkins and Georgetown Universities, as "a primary, international, national, state, and local resource on public health law (and) policy for public health practitioners, judges, academics, policymakers, and others."

MSEHPA is now "track(ing) legal responses to the emerging international response to the 2009 H1N1 (swine flu) outbreak, including declarations of public health emergency at the international, national, state, and local levels. . . . " (News and Updates for May 7, 2009 2012), even though forensic evidence can't confirm any H1N1 deaths. No emergency exists anywhere, and reporting one is all hype to sell dangerous drugs to unsuspecting people globally.

On its website, the American Civil Liberties Union (ACLU) says this about MSEHPA:

It's "written in a way that doesn't adequately protect citizens against the misuse of the tremendous powers that it would grant in an emergency. (It's) replete with civil liberties problems. Its three top flaws are that:

(1) It fails to include basic checks and balances (by) grant(ing) extraordinary emergency powers (that) should never go unchecked. (It) could have serious consequences for individuals' freedom, privacy, and equality."

(2) "It goes well beyond bioterrorism (with) an overbroad definition of 'public health emergency' that may be anything a local or national authority declares for any reason with no conclusive evidence for proof."

(3) "It lacks privacy protections (and) undercut(s) existing protections for sensitive medical information" (Model State Emergency Health Powers Act 2012).

MSEHPA worries other organizations besides the ACLU, both conservative and progressive, including the Free Congress Foundation, American Legislative Exchange Council, Human Rights Campaign, and Health Privacy Project.

Massachusetts May Be a Forerunner of What's to Come

On April 28, 2009, the Massachusetts State Senate unanimously passed a pandemic flu preparation bill that rises to the level of martial law. Among the measures included in the bill were the following:

—"vaccination, treatment, examination, or testing of" all individuals involved in providing health care—as perhaps step one before ordering the same process for all state residents;
—owners or occupiers of all premises "to permit entry into and investigation of the premises";
—closure, evacuation, and decontamination of all suspected facilities; and
—restricting or prohibiting "assemblages of persons" (Bill S.2028 2012).

Other states may be planning similar measures as precursors to mandatory nationwide vaccinations and overall suspension of civil liberty protections.

References

"Bill S.2028. An Act Relative to Pandemic and Disaster Preparation and Response in the Commonwealth." http://www.malegislature.gov/Bills/186/Senate/S02028. Accessed on July 8, 2012.

"Model State Emergency Health Powers Act." American Civil Liberties Union. http://www.aclu.org/technology-and-liberty/model-state-emergency-health-powers-act. Accessed on July 8, 2012.

"News and Updates for May 7, 2009." The Centers for the Law & the Public's Health. http://www.publichealthlaw.net/. Accessed on July 8, 2012.

"Public Law 108-276." http://www.gpo.gov/fdsys/pkg/PLAW-108publ276/html/PLAW-108publ276.htm. Accessed on July 8, 2012.

"Public Law 109-417." http://www.gpo.gov/fdsys/pkg/PLAW-109publ417/html/PLAW-109publ417.htm. Accessed on July 8, 2012.

"Public Readiness and Emergency Preparedness Act Questions and Answers." http://www.phe.gov/Preparedness/legal/pre pact/Pages/prepqa.aspx. Accessed on July 8, 2012.

Stephen Lendman is a research associate at the Centre for Research on Globalization.

HEPATITIS B VACCINE AND MULTIPLE SCLEROSIS
Joan R. Callahan

> A lie travels round the world whilst the truth is putting on its boots.
>
> —Winston Churchill (1932)

Many people sincerely believe that vaccines are dangerous or ineffective or both. This essay focuses on the widespread belief that the hepatitis B vaccine can cause multiple sclerosis (MS) or other chronic diseases. Hepatitis B itself is a serious disease that claims about 1 million human lives every year worldwide, yet it continues to spread, because many people are either unaware of the vaccine or refuse it on the basis of unsubstantiated rumors and fears. The hepatitis B virus (HBV) is about

100 times as infectious as HIV, and both children and adults are at risk, since HBV spreads by ordinary household contact as well as by fluid exchange. Hepatitis B has reached epidemic levels in some parts of the world and has contributed to the increasing rates of pancreatic and liver cancers. The fear of the HBV vaccine has fizzled in the sense that it no longer makes headlines, and the link to MS has been disproven, but vaccination rates remain low nevertheless.

Soon after the hepatitis B vaccine became available in 1982, doctors began to report isolated cases of neurological or other symptoms that developed within weeks or months after vaccination. This health scare went mainstream in the early 1990s, when the vaccine was suspected of causing several diseases. The hepatitis B vaccine was one of several that formerly contained the mercury compound thimerosal, and some doctors questioned the safety of that ingredient. The climax came in 2001, when a French court ordered a vaccine manufacturer to pay damages to two women who developed MS. A higher court overturned that judgment in 2004, and further studies of the vaccine have shown no connection to MS, but media coverage of the case increased public hostility toward vaccines in general. As in the case of the MMR vaccine, many journalists and parents focused on the few studies that faulted the vaccine, while ignoring many others that reached the opposite conclusion.

It is possible that the hepatitis B vaccine may serve as a trigger for neurological problems in people who are already at high risk, but as of 2012 there is no conclusive proof of this effect. Almost any medical treatment has some associated risk, and doctors admit that about 1 in 600,000 persons who receive this vaccine may have an allergic reaction called anaphylaxis. The long-term consequences (if any) are unknown, but no one on record has died from this complication. Given a choice, a temporary, treatable allergic condition seems more acceptable than cancer, cirrhosis, liver failure, or other known consequences of hepatitis B.

When the hepatitis B vaccine became available to the public in 1982, it had already undergone several years of clinical trials. As with any new vaccine or drug, doctors were properly cautious, but the results were encouraging. The first reports of possible neurological problems associated with this vaccine appeared in the medical literature by 1983, and public concern was inevitable. Subsequent reports in the 1990s blamed the vaccine not only for MS, but also for arthritis, skin rashes, and even HIV transmission. None of these reports stood up to scrutiny, but alarming news is hard to retract or forget, and the cumulative weight of inconclusive reports made an impression. Finally, in the late 1990s, the French government yielded to public demand and stopped requiring adolescents to have this vaccine. Anti-vaccination groups in the United States followed suit, demanding an immediate moratorium on mandatory vaccination of children attending public schools.

In 1997, however, analysis of data from 60 million HBV vaccine recipients showed that the incidence of MS was actually slightly *lower* than in the general population. (Of course, this did not prove that the vaccine prevents MS; the difference was probably random.) The vaccination requirement was then reinstated in France. In the United States, the Medical Advisory Board of the National Multiple Sclerosis Society reached the same conclusion: there was no evidence of a statistical or causal link between the hepatitis B vaccine and MS. As of 2012, the American Medical Association recommends this vaccine for everyone under 18, and for adults at high risk. Other influential groups have issued similar statements, but in the minds of true believers, all vaccines are suspect. In a 2010 survey of U.S. parents, nearly 90 percent ranked vaccine safety as the most important topic in children's health research.

Some activists have actually suggested that the hepatitis B vaccine should be reserved for children in specific families or neighborhoods where allegedly high-risk behaviors and unsanitary practices are rampant. Most of the activists themselves, of course, feel that their own families cannot possibly be at risk.

But who should have the task of going door to door, interviewing people, and inspecting their homes to make this determination? The whole point of requiring everyone to be vaccinated, irrespective of socioeconomic status or lifestyle choice, is to avoid the connotation of blame and simply stop the disease. Anyone can get sick.

Consequences

Although the hepatitis B vaccine has been available for nearly 30 years, many people avoid it because of these unproven health scares. By some estimates, about one-third of the global population—more than 2 billion people—are hepatitis B carriers who can transmit the disease to others by fluid exchange or household contact. In 2008, an Australian baby made world headlines when his parents concealed his whereabouts to shield him from mandatory hepatitis B vaccination. The mother already had the disease, and the child's future health was in immediate danger, yet public opinion favored the parents' right to refuse medical treatment.

There is no way to tell how many people have died needlessly from liver disease, or infected their own children, as a result of what now appears to be irresponsible scare-mongering. The day after this book goes to press, someone may conclusively prove that the vaccine is dangerous. For the moment, however, we have no such proof, only an epidemic to fight.

What Went Wrong?

The 2001 French court case discussed earlier seemed to legitimize the hepatitis B vaccine health scare, when in fact judges are not doctors, and the evidence was extremely weak even before the judgment was reversed on appeal. Another factor that helps keep this scare alive is the catastrophic nature of MS, which (like autism) affects young people and is incurable at present.

The main problem, however, seems to be the usual gang of ambulance chasers and tabloid journalists who identify salable health scares and construct data to keep them going. Studies have shown that even healthcare workers in some countries now avoid hepatitis B vaccination because of perceived risk.

In 2004, for example, one vocal group that opposes hepatitis B vaccination claimed that the vaccine is more dangerous than the disease, citing "Merck's package insert showing the frequency of vaccine damage at a rate of 10.4%." This statement would be alarming, if true—but if the vaccine predictably "damaged" 10 percent of recipients, it would not be on the market. In fact, the Merck package insert stated:

> Injection site reactions and systemic complaints were reported following 0.2 percent and 10.4 percent of the injections, respectively. The most frequently reported systemic adverse reactions (>1% injections), in decreasing order of frequency, were irritability, fever (>101°F oral equivalent), diarrhea, fatigue/weakness, diminished appetite, and rhinitis.

These are minor side effects that last for a few hours or days, not for the rest of the person's life, and they are not necessarily related to the vaccine. In clinical trials, a comparable percentage of subjects who take a placebo report similar symptoms.

But if so many consumers reject the hepatitis B vaccine, what will happen if researchers someday develop an equally safe and effective vaccine to prevent HIV? The rejoicing will be premature, and decades of research effort will be in vain, if unfounded health scares block public acceptance of that vaccine too.

Further Readings

"Continue to Vaccinate Against Hepatitis B." *Prescrire International* 18 (2009): 131.

DeStefano, F., et al. "Hepatitis B Vaccine and Risk of Multiple Sclerosis." *Expert Review of Vaccines* 1 (2002): 461–466.

Duclos, P. "Adverse Events after Hepatitis B Vaccination." *Canadian Medical Association Journal* 147 (1992): 1023–1026.

François, G., et al. "Vaccine Safety Controversies and the Future of Vaccination Programs." *Pediatric Infectious Disease Journal* 24 (2005): 953–961.

Fraunfelder, F. W., et al. "Hepatitis B Vaccine and Uveitis: An Emerging Hypothesis Suggested by Review of 32 Case Reports." *Cutaneous and Ocular Toxicology* 29, no. 1 (November 30, 2009): 26–29.

Gout, O. "Vaccinations and Multiple Sclerosis." *Neurological Sciences,* 22 (2001): 151–154.

Herroelen, L., et al. "Central-Nervous-System Demyelination after Immunisation with Recombinant Hepatitis B Vaccine." *Lancet* 338 (1991): 1174–1175.

Kalb, C., and D. Foote. "Necessary Shots?" *Newsweek,* September 13, 1999.

Löbermann, M., et al. "Vaccination and Multiple Sclerosis." *Nervenarzt* 81, no. 2 (October 17, 2009): 181–193. [In German]

MacIntyre, C. R., and J. Leask. "Immunization Myths and Realities: Responding to Arguments Against Immunization." *Journal of Paediatrics and Child Health* 39 (2003): 487–491.

Mikaeloff, Y., et al. "Hepatitis B Vaccination and the Risk of Childhood-Onset Multiple Sclerosis." *Archives of Pediatric and Adolescent Medicine* 161 (2007): 1176–1182.

Mikaeloff, Y., et al. "Hepatitis B Vaccine and the Risk of CNS Inflammatory Demyelination in Childhood." *Neurology* 72 (2009): 873–880.

Nadler, J. P. "Multiple Sclerosis and Hepatitis B Vaccination." *Clinical Infectious Diseases* 17 (1993): 928–929.

Offit, P. A. "Thimerosal and Vaccines—A Cautionary Tale." *New England Journal of Medicine* 357 (2007): 1278–1279.

Pless, R. P. "Recent Differing Expert Opinions Regarding the Safety Profile of Hepatitis B Vaccines: Is There Really a Controversy?" *Expert Opinion on Drug Safety* 2 (2003): 451–455.

Ramagopalan, S. V., et al. "Association of Infectious Mononucleosis with Multiple Sclerosis: A Population-Based Study." *Neuroepidemiology* 32 (2009): 257–262.

Rougé-Maillart, C. I., et al. "Recognition by French Courts of Compensation for Post-Vaccination Multiple Sclerosis: The Consequences with Regard to Expert Practice." *Medicine, Science and Law* 47 (2007): 185–190.

Tardieu, M., and Y. Mikaeloff. "Multiple Sclerosis in Children: Environmental Risk Factors." *Bulletin de l'Académie Nationale de Médecine* 192 (2008): 507–509. [In French]

Terney, D., et al. "Multiple Sclerosis after Hepatitis B Vaccination in a 16-Year-Old Patient." *Chinese Medical Journal* 119 (2006): 77–79.

Topuridze, M., et al. "Barriers to Hepatitis B Coverage among Healthcare Workers in the Republic of Georgia: An International Perspective." *Infection Control and Hospital Epidemiology* 31 (2010): 158–164.

Joan R. Callahan is the award-winning author of numerous biological journal papers, environmental reports, and science books. She received her PhD from the University of Arizona and has worked as a consultant and researcher for over 30 years, most recently as an epidemiologist for the Naval Health Research Center and as a contractor for the National Institute of Standards and Technology. Her latest books include Biological Hazards *(Oryx Press, 2002) and* Emerging Biological Threats *(Greenwood Press, 2009).*

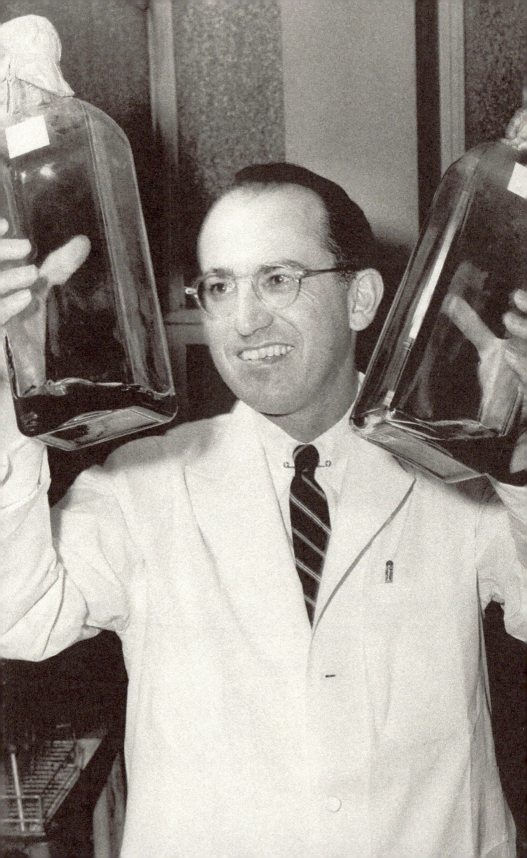

This chapter contains brief sketches of individuals and organizations who are important in understanding the history of vaccination laws, policies, and procedures in the United States and around the world. The number of such individuals and organizations is legion, and only some especially significant organizations and individuals, or those typical of other organizations and individuals, are included.

Baruch S. Blumberg (1925–2011)

Blumberg was awarded a share of the 1976 Nobel Prize in Physiology or Medicine for his discovery of the virus that causes hepatitis B. That discovery made possible the development of a vaccine against the disease, an achievement for which Blumberg himself was largely responsible.

Blumberg made this discovery, sometimes called one of the most important medical discoveries of the 20th century, quite by accident. At the time, he was engaged in an effort to discover why some ethnic groups appear to be more susceptible to some infectious diseases than are other ethnic groups. His attempts to resolve this puzzle involved taking blood samples from individuals from a great variety of ethnic groups throughout the world. One of his findings in this research

Dr. Jonas Salk brandishes two bottles containing a culture used to grow a successful vaccine for polio. (AP/Wide World Photos)

had to do with a somewhat different question, the nature of a disease known at the time as *serum hepatitis*, or *hepatitis B*. Scientists had known for some time that two forms of hepatitis exist, one transmitted by the ingestion of contaminated foods, so-called *infectious hepatitis*, or *hepatitis A*, and serum hepatitis, or hepatitis B. Little was known about the cause of either disease.

In 1967, Blumberg discovered that individuals infected with hepatitis B in various parts of the world had antibodies in their blood for an antigen first discovered in the blood of Australian aborigines (and, therefore, called *Australian antigen* at the time). He eventually showed that this antigen consisted of a characteristic fragment of the outer shell of a virus, now known to be the virus that causes hepatitis B. With this information, Blumberg and his colleagues (in particular, American microbiologist Irving Millman) were able to design and produce a vaccine against the hepatitis B virus, which was licensed for use in the United States by the U.S. FDA in 1969. More sophisticated vaccines have since been developed and approved by the FDA. Blumberg's discovery of the hepatitis B virus and his development of the corresponding vaccine are thought to have saved untold thousands of lives annually.

Baruch Samuel Blumberg was born in Brooklyn, New York, on July 28, 1925. He was the second of three children of Ida and Meyer Blumberg and the grandson of immigrants to the United States from Europe. He attended a yeshiva (Hebrew school) in Flatbush for his primary education and the Far Rockaway High School. He served in the U.S. Navy during World War II, which provided him with an opportunity to gain his college education under military sponsorship at Union College, Schenectady, New York. Blumberg graduated from Union in 1946 with his BS in physics. He then continued his studies in mathematics at Columbia University, but, at the suggestion of his father, switched to a medical program at the College of Physicians and Surgeons of Columbia in

1947. He received his MD from Columbia in 1951, and then remained at the Columbia Presbyterian Medical Center to complete his internship and residency. In 1955, Blumberg entered a doctoral program in biochemistry at Balliol College at Oxford University, England, from which he received his PhD in 1957.

Blumberg's first professional assignment was at the National Institutes of Health (NIH) in Bethesda, Maryland, where he became involved in the formation and development of a new division on Geographic Medicine and Genetics. The mission of this division was to investigate the ways in which a person's or a population's genetic makeup might affect their health and illness patterns, in general, and their susceptibility to infectious diseases, in particular. It was this background that eventually led Blumberg into the research that led to his discovery of the hepatitis B virus and vaccine.

In 1964, Blumberg was appointed associate director for clinical research at the Fox Chase Cancer Center in Philadelphia, a post he held until 1986. He also served at Fox Chase as distinguished scientist and senior advisor to the president. Beginning in 1964, Blumberg also had a long relationship with the University of Pennsylvania, where he was Associate Professor of Medicine, Human Genetics, and Anthropology (1964–1970), Professor of Medicine (1970–1977), Professor of Human Genetics (1974–1977), Professor of Anthropology (1975–1977), and University Professor of Medicine and Anthropology (1977–2011). He continued his connection with Balliol College, where he served as Master from 1989 to 1994. In 1999, Blumberg's career took a somewhat different direction when he accepted the post of founding director of the Astrobiology Institute of the National Aeronautics and Space Administration (NASA) at the Ames Research Center in Moffett Field, California. He was also senior advisor to the NASA administrator in Washington, DC, from 2000 to 2001. After leaving the Astrobiology Institute, Blumberg continued his affiliation with NASA by taking a post as Distinguished

Scientist at the NASA Lunar Science Institute at Ames Research Center.

Because of Blumberg's special expertise in the field of medical anthropology, he was in demand at universities and research centers around the world. He had been visiting professor or researcher at the University of Kentucky, Indiana University, Stanford University, University of Washington, University of Otago (New Zealand), Trinity College of Oxford University, University of Bangalore, University of Singapore, and the Stazione Zoologica Anton Dohrn of Naples. In addition to the Nobel Prize, he had been awarded the Passano Award, the Karl Landsteiner Memorial Award, the Richard & Hinda Rosenthal Foundation Award, the Molly & Sidney Zubrow Award, the Sammy Davis Junior National Liver Institute Award, the Showa Emperor (Japan) Memorial Award, and the Gold Medal Award of the Canadian Liver Foundation and Canadian Association for the Study of the Liver.

Blumberg died of a heart attack on April 5, 2011, shortly after giving the keynote speech at the International Lunar Research Park Exploratory Workshop being held at the Ames Research Center.

Dale and Betty Bumpers Vaccine Research Center

NIAID Office of Communications and Government
Relations
6610 Rockledge Dr., MSC 6612
Bethesda, MD 20892–6612
Phone: (301) 402–1663
URL: http://www.niaid.nih.gov/about/organization/vrc/Pages/default.aspx
E-mail: niaidnews@niaid.nih.gov

The Dale and Betty Bumpers Vaccine Research Center is generally known simply as the Vaccine Research Center (VRC). It was established within the National Institute of Allergy and Infectious Diseases of the U.S. National Institutes of Health in

2001, largely as a consequence of the efforts and influence of the then-Senator Dale Bumpers of Arkansas, and his wife Betty. Both Bumpers had long been interested in the importance of vaccination in protecting the health of children and adults and had long lobbied for increased federal participation in the support of research efforts for the development and distribution of new vaccines. Senator Bumpers was also a long-time advocate of funding for research on HIV/AIDS and methods for protecting against the disease. Betty Bumpers was also one of the cofounders of the vaccination support group Every Child by Two (see entry on the next page).

Since its founding, the mission of the VRC has evolved somewhat so that today it is focused primarily on the development and distribution of a vaccine against the human immunodeficiency virus (HIV) and the disease it causes, acquired immune deficiency syndrome (AIDS). The center is working to discover the underlying mechanisms by which immunity to the HIV virus might be established, to identify specific candidates that might be available for an HIV vaccine, and to develop animal and human testing protocols for those candidate vaccines. The center makes use of researchers and facilities on the NIH campus in Bethesda, Maryland, as well as supporting and coordinating research efforts at academic institutions, industrial facilities, and clinical settings both throughout the United States and around the world.

Center research also focuses on the design and development of vaccines for viruses that might be related to or similar to the HIV virus. It is working, for example, in conjunction with the NIH Laboratory of Virology and Laboratory of Infectious Diseases on a vaccine against Ebola and Marburg viral infections, as well as on the ongoing development of seasonal vaccines against influenza. A detailed description of the center's long-term strategic plan for the development of vaccines is available online at http://www.niaid.nih.gov/about/organization/vrc/Documents/vrcsp.pdf. Scientific reports on developments at the center's research laboratories are published in a variety of professional journals, to which links are available on its website at http://www.niaid.nih.gov/about/organization/vrc/publications/Pages/default.aspx.

Current director of the VRC is Dr. Gary J. Nabel, who earned his BS, MD, and PhD degrees from Harvard University. Prior to his selection as director of the VRC, Nabel was Henry Sewall professor of internal medicine, professor of biochemistry, and Howard Hughes Medical Institute investigator at the University of Michigan in Ann Arbor, and director of the Center for Gene Therapy and codirector of the Center for Molecular Medicine at the University of Michigan.

Every Child By Two
1233 20th St. N.W., Suite 403
Washington, DC 20036–2304
Phone: (202) 783–7034
Fax: (202) 783–7042
URL: http://www.ecbt.org/index.cfm
E-mail: http://www.ecbt.org/aboutecbt/contactus.cfm

Every Child By Two (ECBT) is an organization founded in 1991 by Rosalyn Carter and Betty Bumpers, former first ladies, respectively, of the states of Georgia and Arkansas. The organization was created largely in response to a measles epidemic that had killed 120 individuals that year, the majority of them children. Most, if not all, of those deaths probably could have been prevented if children and adults had been vaccinated against the disease to which they eventually succumbed. The primary goal of the organization is to work toward informing all Americans of the necessity of childhood vaccinations and to promote the circumstances under which that objective can be achieved. Carter and Bumpers have individually received numerous awards for their work on behalf of immunization, including honors such as election to the National Women's Hall of Fame, the Hepatitis Foundation International Humanitarian Award, and an Honorary Fellowship with the American Academy of

Pediatrics, for Bumpers, and a Humanitarian Award from the Save the Refugees Fund, the Nathan S. Kline Medal of Merit from the International Committee Against Mental Illness, and an Award of Merit for Support of the Equal Rights Amendment from the National Organization for Women, for Carter.

One major objective of ECBT is to promote laws that require mandatory immunization of children, a goal that has been largely accomplished as all states now require certain types of immunizations as a condition of school attendance. The organization also works with a number of immunization groups to promote such policies and to ensure that healthcare providers receive the funding needed to carry out such requirements. The organization also works with the Centers for Disease Control and Prevention (CDC) to conduct educational programs for healthcare providers and to develop electronic immunization registry programs.

The ECBT provides a wealth of information for parents and healthcare providers on all aspects of immunization programs. The section for parents, for example, provides basic information on the nature of vaccines, appropriate schedules for the vaccination of children, ways of dealing with financial aspects of immunizations, and vaccine safety. The section intended for healthcare providers provides information on immunization schedules, currently available vaccines and their safety, vaccination registries, and self-assessment strategies for immunization programs.

An important aspect of the ECBT's work is the development of immunization registries and the distribution of information about such registries. An immunization registry is a confidential, computerized record of vaccination histories that parents and healthcare providers can use to keep track of the vaccination histories of children. Immunization registries are also called immunization information systems (IIS). These systems were created by the CDC and are now available in every state. In addition to storing basic information about immunization histories, registries can be used to identify areas with low immunization rates, provide reminders to parents of necessary immunization dates, provide data and statistics for research projects, and integrate immunization services with other public health functions, such as vision screening and lead screening.

The resources and contacts section of ECBT's website provides useful information for parents and healthcare providers on a number of topics of value to both groups, including vaccine information statements from the CDC, a booklet on immunization registries, state and local government resources, information about the federal Special Supplemental Nutrition Program for Women, Infants, and Children (WIC) and its screening protocol, special information about and resources related to influenza immunization, information about vaccine developers and research, and the so-called Purple Book, a handbook for clinicians responsible for immunization programs.

ECBT also sponsors, cosponsors, and provides information on a number of conferences and courses on immunization held in the United States and around the world each year, such as (in 2012) a course on clinical vaccinology, the First International Immunization Conference (a webinar meeting), a course on epidemiology and vaccinology offered by the CDC, and the 2ndGlobal Congress for Consensus in Pediatrics and Child Health.

One of the most useful services offered by ECBT for both the general public and healthcare providers is its "Daily Clips" section, which provides brief summaries of important news articles on immunization, with links to the articles themselves. Examples of the type of information provided were recent articles on the lack of relationship between vaccines and autism, the effects of withholding chickenpox vaccinations on children's risk for the disease, recent data on the incidence of measles infections, the association between the H1N1 virus and bacterial infections, and the safety of swine flu vaccines.

In 2004, ECBT coauthored with the Trust for America's Health an important report on the status of immunization in the United States, *Closing the Gap*. That report described the importance of childhood immunization, reviewed immunization rates in the United States at the time of the report, reviewed some factors involved that contributed to the "immunization gap," and recommended improvements in U.S. policies toward immunization that would contribute to "closing the gap" between desired and actual immunization rates.

Ian Frazer (1953–)

Frazer invented a vaccine against the human papillomavirus (HPV), which is the causative agent in the vast majority of cervical cancer, the third most common type of cancer among women worldwide. The virus has also been implicated in a number of other types of cancers of the genital system, including vaginal, vulvar, uterine, and ovarian cancer, as well as anal cancer in men. HPV is also the most common sexually transmitted infection (STI), responsible for genital warts and other types of oral and genital infections. The invention of a vaccine to prevent the transmission of HPV holds the promise for saving millions of lives annually worldwide from cervical and other types of cancer.

Ian Hector Frazer was born in Glasgow, Scotland, on January 6, 1953. At the age of three, he moved with his family to Edinburgh, where his father took a position in biochemistry at Edinburgh University, while his mother continued her career as a medical researcher. With that type of background, it is hardly surprising that young Ian soon became interested in science. In a 2006 interview with Australian television channel ABC1, Frazer noted that he was "really fascinated by how things worked, what made them happen, why they didn't always happen, and that became a driving force in what I actually did at school." He attended George Watson's College, a private primary and secondary school in Edinburgh before enrolling at the University of Edinburgh. Torn between a career in physics and medicine, he finally chose the latter because he thought it provided more research opportunities. He eventually earned his bachelor of science degree in pathology in 1974 and his bachelor of medicine and bachelor of surgery in 1977, both from Edinburgh. He completed his residencies at Edinburgh Eastern General Hospital, the Edinburgh Royal Infirmary, and the Roodlands General Hospital in Haddington, Scotland.

In 1981, Frazer emigrated to Australia to take a position as senior research officer at the Walter and Eliza Hall Institute in Melbourne. He left the Hall Institute in 1985 to become director of the Division of Clinical Immunology at the Princess Alexandra Hospital in Brisbane, a post he held until 1999. Between 1989 and 1993, Frazer also served simultaneously as associate professor in the Department of Medicine at the University of Queensland. In 1994, he was promoted to full professor at the University of Queensland. In 1991, Frazer also accepted an appointment as director of the Center for Immunology and Cancer Research (now the Diamantina Institute) at the University of Queensland, a post he continues to hold. In 1994, he added the title of professor in the Department of Medicine at the university.

Frazer's interest in an HPV vaccine dates to the late 1980s when he first discussed the problems of developing such a vaccine with Chinese virologist Jian Zhou. The basic problem the two researchers faced was a classic challenge for inventors of a vaccine: to develop a product that will convince the human immune system of the presence of a harmful substance (the HPV virus) without actually using material sufficiently virulent to induce the disease itself. The problem was eventually resolved by Jian's wife, Xiao-Yi Sun, who used the methods of recombinant DNA to produce a synthetic particle that closely resembled the shell of the HPV virus. The synthetic particle was sufficiently similar to the virus itself that it produced an immune response when injected into a human as did the HPV virus itself. After more than five years of testing, the synthetic vaccine was approved for human use in the United States by the FDA in 2006. It is now available in two proprietary formulations known as Gardasil® and Cervaris®.

(Although sometimes given lesser attention, Jian's contribution to the development of the vaccine was substantial. In fact, he is often referred to as an "equal partner" in the project. Jian's life was tragically cut short in 1999 when, at the age of 42, he died as a result of complications arising out of a routine medical procedure in Australia.

In the years following licensing of the HPV vaccine, Frazer has received a number of awards and honors including the Howard Florey Medal for Medical Research, Prime Minister's Prize for Science, Balzan Prize for Preventive Medicine, Australian Medical Association Gold Medal, William B. Cooley Award, CSIRO Eureka Prize for Leadership in Science, Centenary Medal for services to cancer research, Ramaciotti Medal, American Academy of Dermatology Lila Gruber Award for Dermatology, Novartis Prize for Clinical Immunology, Golden Plate Award of the International Achievement Summit, International Life Award for Scientific Research, Merck Sharp & Dohme Howard Florey Medal, Clunies Ross Award of the Academy of Technological Sciences and Engineering, Distinguished Fellowship Award of the Royal College of Pathologists, and John Curtin Medal. In 2006, he was named Australian of the Year and Queenslander of the Year, and in 2012, he was named a National Living Treasure by the National Trust of Australia.

Maurice Hilleman (1919–2005)

Hilleman was an American bacteriologist who developed more than three dozen different vaccines, more than any other researcher in history. Robert Gallo, one of the discoverers of the virus responsible for AIDS, has called Hilleman "the most successful vaccinologist in history." Another colleague has called him "the Pope of vaccines." Among the most widely used of Hilleman's vaccines are those for use against measles, mumps, hepatitis A, hepatitis B, meningitis, pneumonia, *Haemophilus influenzae* bacteria, and rubella. They are credited with having saved countless number of lives worldwide each year, with the measles vaccine alone being responsible for having saved more than a million lives since its introduction in 1968.

Maurice Ralph Hilleman was born on a farm near Miles City, Montana, on August 30, 1919. He was the eighth child born to Gustav and Anna Hilleman. His twin sister died at birth, and his mother died two days later. Hilleman later told one of his biographers that this early experience always made him feel that "he had escaped an appointment with death." He was raised by his uncle, Robert Hilleman, a chicken farmer who lived near his family's home. He later said that his exposure to chickens, whose eggs are widely used in vaccine research, was a factor in his later success in vaccinology.

After graduating from high school, Hilleman felt that he had little chance of attending college, as the Great Depression was then at one of its lowest levels. He was, however, able to earn a scholarship to Montana State College (now Montana State University), from where he earned his bachelor's degree in 1941. He then continued his studies at the University of Chicago, which granted him his PhD in microbiology and virology in 1944. In 1944, Hilleman was hired by the E. R. Squibb & Sons company, where he worked as a research associate in the virology laboratory. His most important accomplishment during his three years at Squibb was the development of a vaccine against Japanese B encephalitis, a debilitating disease that occurred among American servicemen and women during World War II.

In 1947, Hilleman joined the faculty at the Army Medical Services Graduate School (AMSGS) at the Walter Reed Army Medical Center as chief of the virus department. A year later, he was promoted to chief of the Respiratory and Virus Research and Diagnosis Section at AMSGS, a post he held until

1956. During his stint at Walter Reed, he identified the genetic changes in the flu virus that presaged a massive pandemic of Hong Kong flu in 1957. He then developed a vaccine to combat the new strain of flu virus and made possible the production of more than 40 million doses of the vaccine, thus preventing the uncontrolled spread of the disease.

On New Year's Day of 1958, Hilleman assumed a new position at Merck & Company, as director of the newly created department of virus and cell biology research. He remained at Merck for the rest of his professional career. Even after retiring officially at the age of 65 in 1984, he continued to work at the company as a consultant and advisor. During his long tenure at Merck, Hilleman was instrumental in the development of about three dozen vaccines, perhaps the most famous (although not necessarily the most important) was a vaccine for mumps. In 1963, his daughter Jeryl Lynn came down with a case of the mumps. Hilleman took the family illness as an opportunity to learn more about and develop a vaccine against the disease. He used material taken from his daughter's throat to culture the mumps virus and, from that specimen, was able to develop a vaccine against the disease. The so-called Jeryl Lynn strain of the mumps vaccine is still used today, with more than 150 million doses having been produced since the 1960s, preventing an estimated 1 million cases of the disease worldwide annually.

Throughout his career, Hilleman was involved in a wide variety of academic, public service, and professional organizations and associations. For example, he was a member of the Russian-United States Collaboration on Biological Weapons Control of the National Academy of Science, the AIDS Vaccine Design and Evaluation Group of the National Institute of Allergy and Infectious Diseases, the Overseas Medical Research Laboratories Committee of the U.S. Department of Defense, the Study Group on Cerebrospinal Meningitis Control, and the Working Group on Immunology and Epidemiology of the Special Virus Cancer Program. He also received a large number of honors and awards during his lifetime, including the Prince Mahidol Award from the King of Thailand for the advancement of public health, the Mary Woodard Lasker Award for Public Service, the Sabin Gold Medal and Lifetime Achievement Awards, and a special lifetime achievement award from the World Health Organization (WHO). He was also given honorary doctorates by Montana State College, the University of Maryland, the University of Leuven, and Washington and Jefferson College. The Merck Company named its virus production facility in Durham, North Carolina, in honor of Hilleman in 2008, and the Merck Foundation, in collaboration with the University of Pennsylvania School of Medicine and the Children's Hospital of Philadelphia (CHOP), established the Maurice R. Hilleman Chair of Vaccinology in 2005. In 2007, American pediatrician and author Paul Offit published a biography of Hilleman, *Vaccinated: One Man's Quest to Defeat the World's Deadliest Diseases*. Hilleman died in Philadelphia on April 11, 2005, as a result of cancer. At the time of his death, he was adjunct professor of pediatrics at the University of Pennsylvania School of Medicine in Philadelphia.

Immunization Action Coalition
1573 Selby Ave., Suite 234
St. Paul, MN 55104
Phone: (651) 647–9009
URL: http://www.immunize.org/
E-mail: admin@immunize.org

The Immunization Action Coalition (IAC) claims to be one of the first broad-based Internet resources on the subject of immunization and currently the largest resource of its kind in the world, serving an average of 12,000 visitors per day. It was created in 1994 in order to increase vaccination rates by providing accurate, up-to-date information on vaccines and the diseases they are designed to prevent. The organization's website is probably the largest and most complete source of information on every aspect of immunization on the web today. The coalition's resources are subdivided into three distinct fields, one for health professionals (www.immunize.org), one for the general public and health professionals (www.vaccineinformation.org), and one, an online database of local, state, regional, national, and international immunization organizations (www.izcoalitions.org).

The IAC website organizes its resources into six major categories: Handouts for Patients and Staff, Clinic Resources, Vaccine Information Statements, Diseases and Vaccines, Talking about Vaccines, and Topics. Some of the topics covered in the first of these categories are "Administering Vaccines," "Documenting Vaccinations," "Medical Management," "Patient Schedules," "Questions & Answers," "Recommendations," "Screening Questionnaires," "Standing Orders," "Storage and Handling," "Supplies Checklist," "Talking with Parents," "Translations," and "Vaccine Index." The Clinic Resources section covers topics such as "Administering Vaccines," "Coding and Billing," "Documenting Vaccination," "Scheduling Vaccines," "Screening for Contraindications," "Storage and Handling," and "Vaccine Recommendations."

The Vaccine Information Statements provide detailed explanation of all available immunizations in English or Spanish or, for a number of immunizations, in any one of 40 other languages, including Arabic, Armenian, Bosnian, Farsi, French Hmong, Ilokano, Indonesian, Japanese, Laotian, Marshallese, Nepali, Polish, Punjabi, Samoan, Tagalog, Thai, Turkish, Urdu, and Yiddish. The section on Diseases and Vaccines provides information on the two dozen infectious diseases for which vaccines are available.

One of the most interesting sections of the IAC website is the one on Talking about Vaccines, in which a number of articles deal with topics of general interest, such as ways in which medical professionals can talk with parents about their concerns over vaccination, the importance of vaccinations, issues of vaccine safety, the role of adjuvants and other ingredients in vaccines, mitochondrial disorders, the role of vaccination vis-a-vis alternative medicine, religious concerns, autism, the issue of multiple injections, the use of thimerosal in vaccines, and responses to proposed alternative schedules of vaccination.

The final section of the IAC website provides information on a number of other somewhat disparate issues, such as vaccination issues for children adopted from foreign countries, vaccination policies and practices for healthcare personnel and for the elderly, issues of mandatory vaccination and exemptions in state laws, special vaccination of issues for men who have sex with other men, questions and issues of needle safety, vaccinations and pregnancy, travel vaccination requirements, and vaccination issues related to tattooing and body piercing.

A particularly useful service of the coalition is a searchable database of local, regional, and state immunization coalitions. A search for all such coalitions in the state of California, for example, produces 13 results, ranging from the state California Immunization Coalition to the regional Central Valley Immunization Coalition to the local San Diego Immunization Coalition to the special interest coalitions for Los Angeles children and the Los Angeles County Asian & Pacific Islander Hepatitis B Task Force.

Edward Jenner (1749–1823)

Jenner is generally regarded as the father of vaccination, the person who first recognized that exposure to the relatively mild disease of cowpox could provide a person with protection from the far more serious disease of smallpox. He was by no means the first person to have recognized this fact, but he was the first person to test his hypothesis in a controlled, scientific manner, which he followed up by challenging children treated with a cowpox vaccine with the smallpox virus itself. This combination of factors is largely responsible for the general acknowledgment of his role as the creator of the first vaccine against one of the world's most terrible infectious diseases.

Edward Anthony Jenner was born in Berkeley, Gloucestershire, England, on May 17, 1749. He was the eighth of nine children born to Stephen Jenner, the vicar of Berkeley, and his wife Sarah. He attended primary school at Wotton-under-Edge and Cirencester and, during his early years, was inoculated against smallpox by variolation. At the age of 14, he was apprenticed to one Daniel Ludlow, a surgeon who worked in Chipping Sodbury, South Gloucestershire. At the conclusion of that apprenticeship in 1770, he began his formal medical studies at St. George's Hospital in London, where he studied under the renowned surgeon Dr. John Hunter. When Jenner completed his studies in London in 1772, he returned to Berkeley, where he established a practice in medicine and surgery. Although he later practiced in London and Cheltenham, he remained largely a Berkeley resident for the rest of his life.

As did almost any physician of the time, Jenner offered his patients protection against smallpox by the process of variolation, in which material taken from the smallpox sore of an infected person is transferred to an incision in an uninfected person's body. Although the procedure was generally successful in providing immunity against the disease, it carried a substantial risk of actually producing the disease in the uninfected individual. In thinking about a possible alternative for this age-old procedure, Jenner reflected on the well-known fact that milkmaids appeared to develop a natural immunity against smallpox because they were frequently infected by the much less dangerous cowpox, a close relative of smallpox. Jenner asked himself what would happen if he intentionally infected a child with cowpox material. The opportunity to test this hypothesis presented itself on May 14, 1796, when Jenner's gardener and his wife agreed to allow their eight-year-old son, James Phipps, to undergo inoculation with cowpox material. A short time after the experiment, Jenner then injected young James with smallpox material itself. When the boy did not contract the disease, Jenner was convinced that his hypothesis was correct.

He then proceeded to inoculate anyone else in his region who wanted and agreed to the new procedure, which he named *vaccination* (after the Latin word *vaca* for "cow").

Reasonably enough, the British medical profession was skeptical about Jenner's discovery. The general public was also suspicious of the practice, and Jenner was made the butt of many jokes and criticisms in newspapers and magazines and in speeches made by medical authorities, government officials, religious leaders, and members of the general public. Vaccination slowly became accepted, however, and in 1840 the British government banned its only major competitive procedure, variolation. From that point on, vaccination with cowpox material became essentially the only procedure for providing immunity to smallpox in most parts of the world. The British government also took concrete notice of Jenner's work by awarding him two honoraria, an award of £10,000 in 1802 for his research on vaccination, and a second award in the amount of £20,000 in 1807 for his studies in the field of microbiology. These monetary awards allowed him to live comfortably at a time when his regular practice was regularly interrupted by the demands of studying and educating the general public and medical profession about his discovery.

National leaders from every part of the world recognized Jenner's achievements. For example, in 1804, Emperor Napoleon ordered that a special gold medal be struck to recognize his discovery, and the Empress of Russia presented him with a ring to express her appreciation for his work. He even received a certificate of appreciation and a string of wampum beads from a council of North American Indian Chiefs of the Five Nations in 1807.

In 1803, Jenner returned to London to accept an appointment as president of the newly created Royal Jennerian Institution, an organization established to promote and make available vaccination against smallpox throughout the nation. During this time, he also joined and became active in the Medical and Chirurgical Society, later to become the Royal Society of Medicine. The society now offers the Edward Jenner medal, in Jenner's honor, to distinguished work in epidemiological research. Adding to his honors, Jenner was appointed Physician Extraordinary to King George IV in 1821, and was chosen to be mayor and justice of the peace in Berkeley. In 1806, he was also elected a foreign member of the Royal Swedish Academy of Sciences.

Jenner suffered a stroke on January 25, 1823 that left him partially paralyzed. He never fully recovered from that event and suffered a second stroke a day later, from which he died at his home in Berkeley.

Interestingly enough, Jenner had long retained a special interest in natural history to which he returned from time to time throughout his life. For example, he was elected a fellow of the Royal Society in 1788, a decade before his vaccination discoveries, largely as the result of a paper he had presented to the society on the life and habits of the nested cuckoo. Then, late in life, he returned to his interest in birds by offering a paper on "Observations on the Migration of Birds" that was published in the *Philosophical Transactions of the Royal Society of London* a few months after his death, in November 1823.

Albert Z. Kapikian (1930–)

Kapikian has been called "the father of human gastroenteritis virus research" because of the more than five decades he has devoted to gastroenterological diseases caused by a variety of viruses. His work has led to the identification of new pathogenic viruses and to the invention of vaccines against diseases of the gut caused by those viruses. One of his major contributions has been the demonstration of the power of electron microscopy in studying viruses and their role in disease. One of his early breakthroughs was the discovery and identification of the Norwalk virus, a pathogen that causes a highly contagious disease that can be transmitted by person-to-person contact, the ingestion of contaminated food, or by contact with a contaminated surface. The disease is characterized by stomach pain, nausea, and vomiting that can quickly become debilitating. Kapikian first reported the properties of the virus, now known as the norovirus, in 1972. A year later, Kapikian and his colleagues, Stephen Feinstone and Robert Purcell, used electron microscopy technology again to discover the virus responsible for hepatitis A.

Arguably, Kapikian's greatest accomplishment was his development of a vaccine against the rotavirus, a pathogen that is responsible for diarrhea among young children. The devastating effects of the disease are thought to be responsible for nearly half a million deaths of children under the age of five each year throughout the world. Kapikian's research team worked for more than 25 years on the development of a vaccine to protect against the disease. It was finally approved for use and licensed by the FDA in 2008.

Albert Zaven Kapikian was born on May 9, 1930, in New York City, to Armenian immigrants. He attended Queens College, which granted him his BS degree in 1952, and Cornell University, from which he received his MD in 1956. He then completed his internship at Meadowbrook Hospital in Hempstead, New York. In 1957, Kapikian took a position at the National Institute of Allergy and Infectious Diseases (NIAID), where he has remained throughout his professional career. In 1967, he was appointed head of the epidemiology section of the Laboratory of Infectious Diseases, a post he continues to hold well past the normal age of retirement for most individuals. In addition to his work at NIAID, Kapikian has served as guest worker in virology at the Royal Postgraduate Medical School of the University of London (1970) and as resident professor in Child Health and Development at the School of Medicine and Health Services of George Washington University (1977 to the present).

Kapikian's work in vaccinology has earned him a number of honors and awards, including the 2011 Maurice Hilleman/ Merck Award, 2005 Sabin Gold Medal, 2001 Cornell University Alumni Award of Distinction, 1993 Pan American

Society Diagnostic Virology Award, 1998 Children's Vaccine Initiative (CVI) Pasteur Award for Recent Contributions to Vaccine Development (with Roger I. Glass and Ruth Bishop), 1987 Behring Diagnostics Award of the American Society for Microbiology, and 1974 Stitt Award of the U.S. Association of Military Surgeons. Kapikian has twice received the Public Health Service Meritorious Service Award.

Pearl Kendrick (1890–1980) and Grace Eldering (1901–1988)

The names of Pearl Kendrick and Grace Eldering will forever be connected in the history of immunization. The two researchers, employees of the Michigan Department of Health, developed a vaccine for whooping cough (pertussis) at a time when the disease killed as many as 6,000 boys and girls in the United States each year. As their biographer, Carolyn G. Shapiro-Shapin, has written, the two women "developed standardized diagnostic tools; modified and improved extant vaccines; conducted the first successful, large-scale, controlled clinical trial of pertussis vaccine; and participated in international efforts to standardize and disseminate the vaccine."

Pearl Luella Kendrick was born on August 24, 1890, in Wheaton, Illinois, to Milton H. and Ella (Shaver) Kendrick. Milton Kendrick was a Methodist minister, whose changing church assignments caused the family to move a number of times during Pearl's childhood. She is said to have suffered from a case of whooping cough at the age of three, at about the time her family moved to New York State. She attended high school in Sherburne, New York, from which she graduated in 1908. She then attended Greenville (Illinois) College for a year before returning to New York State and enrolling at Syracuse University. She was awarded her BS in zoology from Syracuse in 1914. She is said to have chosen zoology as her major at least partly because she "wanted to get this business of evolution settled in her head," deciding, that is, whether her religious and creationist or Darwinian explanation of nature was correct.

After graduation, Kendrick taught a variety of subjects in a number of schools in New York before accepting a job as principal at St. Johnsville, New York. In 1919, she left the education profession to take up an assignment as a laboratory assistant with the New York State Department of Health. She held that position for only about a year before resigning and accepting a similar appointment with the Michigan Department of Health at its new regional laboratory in Grand Rapids. She is said to have been offered the position at least partly because women were willing to work the same jobs as men in scientific research (and elsewhere), but at lower wages. She maintained her professional association with the Grand Rapids laboratory for the rest of her professional career. While continuing her research, she took graduate courses through the University of Michigan, eventually completing her doctorate in microbiology at the Johns Hopkins University during a sabbatical year in 1932.

Efforts to develop a vaccine against pertussis began soon after the discovery of the causative agent in 1906 by Belgian immunologist Jules Bordet (for whom the agent is named) and Belgian bacteriologist Octave Gengou. None of the vaccines became very popular, however, because no evidence was available as to their efficacy. Kendrick and Eldering broke through that barrier, not only by developing a new type of vaccine, but also by designing controlled trials with experimental and control groups to demonstrate the vaccine's efficacy. In 1939, Kendrick and Eldering published a series of papers that positively confirmed the success of their new vaccine, resulting in the rapid adoption of the vaccine by public health authorities throughout the United States and around the world.

In fact, Kendrick and Eldering remained important advocates, advisors, and consultants for pertussis immunization programs around the world in the remaining years of their lives. Kendrick served, for example, as consultant on pertussis issues in Mexico in 1940 and 1942, and as a consultant on behalf of WHO in a number of countries between 1949 and 1965. After her retirement from the Grand Rapids laboratory in 1961, she also served as consultant on pertussis in the Soviet Union in 1962. From 1951 to 1960, Kendrick also served as lecturer in the Department of Epidemiology at the University of Michigan School of Public Health in Ann Arbor. She died of bone cancer in Grand Rapids on October 8, 1980.

Grace Eldering was born on September 5, 1900, in Myers, a small town in eastern Montana. Like her colleague and companion, Kendrick, Eldering developed a case of pertussis early in life, at the age of five, about which, she later said, she never forgot the "endless, painful coughing." She grew up in the small town of Rancher, Montana, on the Yellowstone River, and attended the University of Montana, where she received her bachelor's degree with majors in chemistry and biology in 1927. Although she had hopes of becoming a doctor, she did not possess the financial resources to pursue that career; so she settled, instead, for a career in medical research. In 1928, she moved to Michigan and volunteered in the Michigan Department of Health's Bureau of Laboratories in Lansing. Six months later she was put on the payroll at the laboratories, and four years later she was transferred to the Grand Rapids laboratory of the Department of Health. There she met Kendrick, and the two began their long collaboration on the pertussis vaccine. Much of the work carried out by the two women was conducted after regular laboratory hours, when they had completed their normal work assignments.

As was the case with Kendrick, Eldering continued her graduate studies in extension courses through the University of Michigan, finally earning her doctor of science degree from Johns Hopkins in 1941. She was appointed director of the Grand Rapids laboratory upon her partner's retirement in 1951. Kendrick and Eldering shared both their public and private lives together for more than 50 years. Eldering died in Grand Rapids on August 31, 1988. Both Eldering and Kendrick were inducted into the Michigan Women's Hall of Fame in 1983.

Shibasaburo Kitasato (1852–1931)

An obituary of Kitasato written on his death in 1931 called him "one of the last, if not the very last, of that small coterie of research workers who laid so well the foundations of bacteriology and its daughter science, immunology." He was involved in the discovery and development of a number of vaccines for use against plague, diphtheria, tetanus, and anthrax.

Shibasaburo Kitasato (in Japanese, Kitasato Shibasaburō) was born in the village of Okuni, Higo Province (now Oguni Town in Kumamoto Prefecture), on the island of Kyushu, Japan, on January 29, 1852. (Some sources give his birth year as 1853.) His father was Korenobu Kitasato, mayor of Okuni. After completing his secondary education, Kitasato entered the medical program at Igakusho Hospital (now Kumamoto University Medical School), where his primary mentor was Dutch physician C. G. van Mansvelt. Van Mansvelt is said to have had a very strong influence on Kitasato, providing him with private instruction not only in medicine, but also in a variety of topics related to the Western world, about which Kitasato was largely uninformed. When van Mansvelt left Igakusho, he suggested to Kitasato that he (Kitasato) transfer to the Tokyo Medical School (now the University of Tokyo School of Medicine) for the remainder of his medical training, which Kitasato did. He received his MD from Tokyo in 1883.

Kitasato's first job was with the recently established Public Health Bureau in Tokyo. (Note: Authorities differ as to some details—especially dates and names—of this stage of Kitasato's life.) His superior at the bureau, Masanori Ogata, had just returned from a visit to Germany, where he had learned about the latest developments in theory and practice in the field of bacteriology, information which he shared with Kitasato. In 1885, Ogata recommended that and then arranged for Kitasato to travel to Berlin to work in the laboratory of Robert Koch, generally regarded as one of the founders of the science of microbiology. Kitasato spent six years at Koch's laboratory, a time during which he made some important breakthroughs in the field of vaccinology. His first important breakthrough came in 1889 when he announced that he had found a way to culture the bacterium, *Clostridium chauvoei*, which causes the blackleg disease in cattle. Shortly thereafter, also in 1889, he announced an even more important discovery, a procedure for culturing the bacterium, *Clostridium tetani*, which causes tetanus. Most bacteriologists had despaired of finding a way of culturing the pure bacterium because it always occurred only in association with other bacteria. Kitasato found that, if he heated the bacterial mixture to very high temperatures, all species would die off except *C. tetani*, thus producing a pure culture of the bacterium. This step was essential to the eventual production of a vaccine against the organism.

In 1890, Kitasato published a series of papers with German physiologist Emil von Behring on a method for vaccinating children against diphtheria and tetanus. The method depended on von Behring and Kitasato's discovery that the bacteria that cause these two diseases produce soluble toxins that can be found in serum taken from an infected animal. If that serum is injected into an uninfected animal, it will cause the disease itself or, in smaller amounts, it will stimulate the animal's immune system to start producing antitoxins, thus providing immunity against the disease. A key element in this research was Kitasato's series of experiments determining the precise amount of toxin-laden serum needed to produce an immune reaction without killing an animal. Many observers point to this series of papers as the birth of the science of immunology.

In 1891, Kitasato returned to Japan and founded his own institute for bacteriological research. The government at first provided financial support for the institute and eventually took control of it, naming it the Japanese Institute for Infectious Diseases. Over the years, Kitasato and the institute gained international fame for the number of famous researchers who worked and studied there. Kitasato maintained his relationship with the institute until 1914, when it was transferred from the Public Health Bureau to the Ministry of Education. In protest against this bureaucratic change, Kitasato and his staff resigned from the institute and created their own private research facility in Tokyo, the Kitasato Institute of Infectious Diseases (later, Kitasato University).

Kitasato added another major accomplishment to his record in 1894 when he traveled to Hong Kong to search for the organism causing an outbreak of the bubonic plague there. Within weeks of his arrival, he had discovered the causative bacterium, only a short time before a colleague, Alexandre Yersin, made the same discovery. Because scholars at the time thought Kitasato's description of the organism was not sufficiently precise, recognition for the discovery and naming of the organism, *Yersina pestis*, were awarded to Yersin. Many modern scholars believe, however, that Kitasato deserves at least equal credit for this important accomplishment.

In 1917, Kitasato was appointed the first dean of the new medical school at Keio University, a school he helped found. In the same year, he made his first foray into the field of politics, being appointed by the Emperor to the House of Peers. In 1924, he was given an even higher honor when he was named danshaku (baron) by the Emperor. A year later, he also received the highest honor available to a Japanese scientist, the Harben Gold Medal of the Royal Institute of Public Health. Kitasato also served as the first president of the Japanese Medical Society when it was founded in 1923. He died at home in Nakanojo, Gumma Prefecture, Japan, on June 13, 1931.

Douglas R. Lowy and John T. Schiller

Lowy and Schiller were joint recipients of the 2011 Sabin Gold Medal for their research into vaccines that can be used for the prevention of cancer. The two researchers have worked together at the U.S. National Institutes of Health National Cancer Center, where they have produced more than 100 joint research papers on various aspects of vaccinology. They are best known today for their development of a vaccine against the HPV, the pathogen responsible for the vast majority of cervical cancer cases, as well as cancers of the vulva, vagina, anus, and penis. In 2006, the FDA issued a license for the use of that vaccine, sold under the name of Gardasil® in the United States.

Lowy and Schiller's invention of the HPV vaccine involved two major breakthroughs. In the first of these breakthroughs, they found that a critical protein in a bovine form of the papillomavirus was able to self-assemble into a structure that was not in itself infectious, but that was capable of producing an immune response in an animal. They then found that the comparable protein in the HPV did not undergo a similar self-assembly, but that they could modify the gene that codes for the HPV to bring about a similar result. The virus-like particle produced in this way proved to be both safe (it did not cause the disease) and efficacious (it did provoke the desired immune response), making it the ideal candidate for the HPV vaccine.

Douglas R. Lowy was born in New York City on May 25, 1942. Both his parents were physicians, but he had no intention of following in their paths when he enrolled at Amherst College, in Amherst, Massachusetts. Instead, he majored in art, history, and French, earning his bachelor of arts degree in 1964. When he enrolled for graduate studies at New York University (NYU), however, he began to change his mind, largely because of a growing interest in microbiology. When he received his MD in 1968, he was still uncertain as to whether he wanted to practice medicine or pursue a career in medical research. As a result, he decided to "hedge his bets," as he told an interviewer for *Bethesda* magazine in 2012, and completed programs in internal medicine at Stanford University and dermatology at Yale University. He also kept his toe in research by opening his own research laboratory in the Laboratory of Viral Diseases at the National Institute of Allergy and Infectious Diseases (NIAID) between 1970 and 1973. He finally made up his mind in 1975 when he accepted an appointment at the

NIH as a researcher in the National Cancer Institute (NCI). He was later made chief of the Laboratory of Cellular Oncology, and chief of the Basic Research Laboratory. He currently holds the position of deputy director of the Center for Cancer Research at NCI. In addition to the Sabin Gold Medal, Lowy has been awarded the Wallace P. Rowe Award for Excellence in Virology Research of the NIAID and the Dorothy P. Landon-AACR (American Association for Cancer Research) Prize for Translational Cancer Research, the Novartis Prize for Clinical Immunology, the American Medical Association's Nathan Davis Award for Outstanding Government Service, and the Service to America–Federal Employee of the Year Award of the nonpartisan Partnership for Public Service (all along with Schiller).

John T. Schiller was born in Madison, Wisconsin, the son of a tractor salesman with a childhood quite different from that of New York–born Lowy. He was fascinated with science from an early age and earned his bachelor of science degree in molecular biology from the University of Wisconsin at Madison in 1975. He continued his graduate studies at the University of Washington at Seattle, from which he received his master's degree and PhD in microbiology in 1982. In looking for a postdoctoral program in tumor virology, Schiller kept hearing mention of Lowy's laboratory, and decided to apply for a position there. He was accepted and began his program in the Laboratory of Cellular Oncology in 1983. He has remained with the NCI ever since, becoming a senior staff fellow in 1986 and senior investigator in 1992. In 1998, he was appointed chief of the Neoplastic Disease Section of the NCI, a post he continues to hold.

As of 2012, more than 90 million doses of Gardasil had been distributed worldwide. As Dr. Peter Hotez, president of the Sabin Vaccine Institute said upon awarding Lowy and Shiller the Gold Medal, "[m]illions of lives will be positively affected by Lowy and Schiller's dedication in developing the world's first vaccines against cervical cancer."

Jacques Miller (1931–)

Miller has been described as the father of modern immunology, largely because of his discoveries about the details as to how the mammalian immune system works. The first of those discoveries came in 1961 when he elucidated the role of the thymus in the immune process, an organ for which scientists had previously found little function in the human body. The second important discovery occurred in 1967 when Miller found that mammals have two distinct types of white blood cells, now known as T-cells and B-cells. These designations arise out of the origin of the two types of cells, the *t*hymus (for T-cells) and *b*one marrow (for B-cells). Understanding the role played by T-cells and B-cells is an essential step forward in the design and development of potential vaccines used in immunization programs.

Miller was born as Jacques Francis Albert Pierre Meunier in Nice, France, on April 2, 1931. His family left Nice while Jacques was still a young boy to move to Shanghai, where his father took a job as manager of a Franco-Chinese bank. When he became old enough, Jacques was sent to Switzerland for his schooling. He remained there only a short time, however, because of the increasing threat posed by the spread of World War II to all parts of Europe. Miller later explained that the war was an important factor in his choosing medicine as a career. "There was a war going on and I felt I didn't want to kill people," he told an interviewer from the journal *The Lancet*. "I thought if I did medicine I could patch them up." He later refined his medical goals and decided to focus on research rather than clinical work. Part of the motivation for that decision was the loss of a sister to tuberculosis in 1940. He told *The Lancet* reviewer that going through that experience made him realize that he might be able to do more good in the world as a medical researcher than as a practicing physician. And thus was his career path determined.

In 1941, as the war began to spread to Asia, the Meunier family moved again, this time to Australia, where they changed their name to *Miller*. There Jacques attended St. Aloysius' College in Sydney (a secondary school), after which he continued his studies at the University of Sydney in medicine. He was awarded his bachelor of science (medical) degree in 1954 and his bachelor of medicine and bachelor of surgery in 1956 from Sydney. Partway through his bachelor's studies at Sydney, Miller also took a year off to earn a bachelor of science degree in bacteriology at the university. Upon completing his medical studies in 1956, Miller fulfilled his residency requirements at the Royal Prince Albert Hospital in Sydney. At that point, he decided to follow up on his earlier commitment to becoming involved in medical research. In 1958, he was awarded a Gaggin Research Fellowship that allowed him to continue his studies at the Chester Beatty Research Institute of the University of London. He was awarded his PhD in experimental pathology in 1960 for research on leukemia in mice in which he found that mice without a thymus were unable to generate an immune response against disease. It was this research that provided science with the first definitive evidence of the role of the thymus in the mammalian body.

In 1963, Miller came to the United States, where he spent a year working at the NIH. He then returned to London where he completed the requirements for his DSc degree in experimental pathology and immunology. During his stay in London, he also served as associate professor of experimental pathology at the University of London.

In 1966, Miller returned to Australia to take charge as Head of Experimental Pathology at the Walter and Eliza Hall Institute of Medical Research (WEHI) in Melbourne. He remained in that post until his retirement in 1997, at which time he was named Emeritus Professor at WEHI and the University of Melbourne. Officially retired, Miller has continued to work three to four days a week in his research laboratory. In addition to his assignment at Melbourne, Miller has served as visiting scholar and visiting professor at a number of other institutions around the world, including the Basel Institute for Immunology in

Switzerland, the Centre d'Immunologie INSERM-CNRS de Marseille-Luminy in France, and the Deutsches Krebsforschungszentrum in Germany.

During his long and productive career, Miller has received a host of honors and awards, including the Gairdner Foundation International Award, Scientific Medal of the Zoological Society of London, Paul Ehrlich and Ludwig Darmstaedter Prize, Rabbi Shai Shacknai Memorial Prize, International St Vincent Prize of the World Health Organization, Sandoz Prize for Immunology, Peter Medawar Prize of the Transplantation Society, Croonian Prize of the Royal Society, J. Alwyn Taylor International Prize for Medicine, Copley Medal of the Royal Society of London, and Prime Minister's Prize for Science. He was elected a fellow of the Royal Society of London in 1970 and a foreign associate member of the United States National Academy of Science in 1982. In 2003, he was appointed a Companion of the Order of Australia.

National Vaccine Information Center
407 Church St., Suite H
Vienna, VA 22180
Phone: (703) 938–0342
URL: http://www.nvic.org/
E-mail: contactNVIC@gmail.com

The National Vaccine Information Center (NVIC) was founded in 1982 by a group of parents whose children had been injured or died as a result of having received legal and recommended immunizations. The organization is chartered as a 501(c)3 charitable organization that receives all of its funding from donations by individuals and philanthropic foundations. NVIC claims not to advocate either for or against the use of vaccines, but to provide information on immunization to the general public. Its mission is to promote the availability of "all preventive health care options, including vaccines, and the right of consumers to make educated, voluntary health care choices." Its goal is to prevent injuries and deaths from immunizations and to defend the "informed consent effort in medicine." (Critics of the organization have a somewhat different view of its goals, with journalist Michael Specter having called it "the most powerful anti-vaccine organization in America.")

NVIC claims to have achieved a number of goals in its more-than-two-decades career, perhaps most important of which was passage of the National Childhood Vaccine Injury Act of 1986. That act recognizes that injury and death may sometimes be caused by vaccination, and that parents and survivors of such incidents deserve to be compensated for their emotional and financial losses. The special "vaccine court" established by the act now regularly awards billions of dollars to such individuals under provisions of the 1986 act. The organization also takes credit for improvement of vaccines, including the purified pertussis DtaP. vaccine approved for use by the FDA in 1996 and the inactivated polio virus vaccine approved for use by the FDA in 1999.

The organization has also sponsored and cosponsored a number of national and international conferences dealing with immunization issues, including the first International Scientific Workshop on Neurological Complications of Pertussis and Pertussis Vaccination in 1989, as well as the first, second, third, and fourth International Public Conference on Vaccination, in 1997, 2000, 2002, and 2009, respectively. The sense of these conferences is reflected in the title of the fourth conference, "Show Us the Science & Give Us the Choice." Its most recent major conference was Medical Science and Public Trust, dealing with the policy, ethics, and legal issues related to immunization in the 20th and 21st centuries, held in February 2011.

NVIC has also traditionally had an aggressive educational program aimed at parents, legislators, and medical professionals. One of its primary educational mechanisms is an online newsletter, the *NVIC Vaccine E-newsletter*, which is freely available to anyone interested in the topic. Its website also includes the NVIC Advocacy Portal through which interested individuals can become involved in efforts to ensure that all parents are permitted informed consent on immunization issues. A third resource operated by the organization is the Vaccine Reaction Registry, an online site at which parents can report adverse events that they believe are attributable to immunization. Finally, NIVC also maintains the Cry for Vaccine Freedom Wall, a website on which parents can share related individual stories about adverse immunization events that occurred in their lives.

The NVIC website contains a great deal of valuable information on immunization-related topics, such as Ask 8, eight essential questions to ask before having one's child vaccinated; Diseases and Vaccines, a comprehensive explanation of infectious diseases against which vaccines are available, along with a description and discussion of such vaccines; Vaccine Ingredient Calculator, a device by which parents can determine precisely the composition of vaccines to which their children may be exposed; and a Searchable Reaction Database, on which a person can track down specific adverse events that may be associated with an immunization event. An online video presentation, "Ask Nurse Vicky," also covers essential background information about immunization and possible adverse events with which the procedure may be associated.

The Law and Policy portal on the NVIC website is also an excellent resource for detailed information on federal and state laws dealing with immunization, along with links to a number of reports and policy statements on vaccination produced over the years by the U.S. Institute of Medicine. Information about possible current legislative actions on various aspects of immunization is also available through this portal.

President of the NVIC and perhaps its best known representative is Barbara Loe Fisher, one of the founders of the organization. In addition to a very busy speaking and writing schedule, Fisher is the author or coauthor of three books on immunization risks, *DPT: A Shot in the Dark* (1985), *The Consumer's*

Guide to Childhood Vaccines (1997), and *Vaccines, Autism & Chronic Inflammation: The New Epidemic* (2008). She maintains a blog on the NVIC website, "Vaccine Awakening," that regularly deals with current vaccination issues.

Ruth S. Nussenzweig (1928–)

Nussenzweig has spent most of her professional career in the search for a vaccine against malaria, one of the most destructive infectious diseases in the world. WHO estimates that about 650,000 people die annually worldwide from the disease, with many times that number living with the disease. Malaria is caused by a parasite (called a *sporozoite*) that is transmitted from one person to another person by the bite of the *Anopheles* mosquito. When an infected mosquito bites a person, it injects sporozoites into that person's bloodstream, through which they travel to the liver. In the liver, sporozoites release bodies known as merozoites, which return to the blood stream and attack red blood cells. They cause those cells to burst apart, releasing additional merozoites to the blood, where they attack other red blood cells. This bodily change causes high fevers, chills, and flu-like symptoms that may develop into anemia, leading to coma and death.

When Nussenzweig was still a young researcher, she became interested in finding a vaccine for malaria, but was somewhat discouraged by warnings of her colleagues that such a vaccine was "impossible." One problem was that exposure to malaria at one point in a person's life did not lead to an immunity to the disease; a person can contract malaria three, four, or more times. Nussenzweig has told an interviewer that she was also handicapped in her efforts because she knew of only one paper dealing with a malaria vaccine written early in the 20th century. She persevered in her attempts, however, and eventually found that she could reduce the virulence of sporozoites by exposing them to X-rays. When these sporozoites were injected into an animal (first mice, then monkeys, and finally humans), they provided immunity against malaria. The principle she developed became the basis of about half of the more than five dozen malaria vaccines currently undergoing laboratory and field testing.

Ruth Sonntag Nussenzweig was born in Vienna, Austria, on June 20, 1928. Both of her parents were physicians. At the age of 11, the Nussenzweig family fled Austria for Brazil in order to escape Nazi persecution of Jews. They settled in São Paulo, where Ruth attended primary and secondary school before enrolling at the University of São Paulo to study medicine. She received her MD from the University of São Paulo in 1953, and then continued her studies there in parasitology. She was awarded PhD in that field in 1968.

Shortly after her arrival in São Paulo, Ruth met Victor Nussenzweig, who later also attended the University of São Paulo School of Medicine. The two of them became close friends and were eventually married in 1953. They have remained co-workers in the field of malaria, as well as husband and wife for nearly 60 years. Their three children are also all medical doctors. After completing their studies in São Paulo, the Nussenzweigs decided to complete their postgraduate work in France, he at the Institut Pasteur in Paris, and she at the College de France. After two years in France, they returned to Brazil, but found their efforts to continue their research programs in São Paulo "frustrating," as Ruth mentioned in a speech presented in 2008. They decided to go abroad once more to find a more congenial research setting, which is what they found in the United States.

In 1965, Ruth accepted an appointment at the NYU Medical Center (now the Langone Medical Center), where she has remained ever since. She was named Professor of Preventative Medicine in 1972 and has also served as head of the Division of Parasitology and professor and chair of the Department of Medical and Molecular Parasitology. She is currently C.V. Starr Professor of Medical Parasitology and Pathology. In addition to her work at NYU, Dr. Nussenzweig has served on the Scientific and Technical Advisory Committee of WHO and worked with the Pew Foundation. She is also the author and coauthor of more than 200 peer-reviewed papers, many with her husband and/or one or more of her children.

Both Ruth and her husband have received a number of honors in recognition of their work in parasitology and vaccinology. In 2008, she was awarded the Gold Medal of the Sabin Vaccine Institute, one of the highest honors available to researchers in the field. In the same year, the Department of Pathology at the NYU School of Medicine held a special symposium in honor of the accomplishments of Ruth and Victor Nussenzweig in honor of their 80th birthdays.

Paul A. Offit (1951–)

Offit is a pediatrician who specializes in infectious diseases. He is currently Maurice R. Hilleman Professor of Vaccinology and Professor of Pediatrics at the University of Pennsylvania and Chief of the Division of Infectious Diseases and Director of the Vaccine Education Center at CHOP. He has been for many years the primary spokesperson in defense of widespread, and usually mandatory, vaccination for both children and adults. In a nominating letter on behalf of membership in the American Pediatric Society, a colleague wrote that Offit "has led the academic and practicing pediatric communities, and in fact the entire medical establishment, in speaking out against the inaccurate and dangerous messages of the anti-vaccine movement. No other individual," the writer went on, "has done as much to bring reason and evidence-based thinking to the public discussion of vaccine safety, in spite of death threats to himself and his family."

Paul A. Offit was born in Baltimore, Maryland, on March 27, 1951. At the age of five, Offit spent three weeks in a polio ward, recovering from foot surgery. He later said that that experience "caused me to see children as very vulnerable and helpless." It was a major influence in his later decision to pursue a career in medicine. After graduating from high school, he enrolled at Tufts University, in Medford, Massachusetts, from which he received his BS in 1973. He then continued his studies at the University of Maryland Medical School, which awarded him MD in 1977. Offit completed his internship and residency in pediatrics at CHOP between 1977 and 1980, followed by a fellowship in infectious diseases at CHOP from 1980 to 1982. After completing his training, Offit accepted an appointment as instructor in pediatrics at the University of Pennsylvania School of Medicine in 1982, where he has remained ever since. He was promoted to chief assistant professor in pediatric in 1984, associate professor in 1992, and full professor in 2000. Simultaneously with his research and teaching in Pennsylvania, Offit has served as research associate and clinical assistant professor at Stanford University and as research investigator, assistant professor, and adjunct associate professor at the Wistar Institute of Anatomy and Biology, a research and educational institution in Philadelphia.

Offit's primary research accomplishment was the development of a vaccine against the rotavirus that causes gastroenteritis, a condition responsible for the death of hundreds of thousands of children worldwide each year. He has said that his interest in that project began when a six-year-old child under his care died of the disease in 1979 while he was still a pediatric resident in Philadelphia. He and his colleagues worked for more than 25 years in developing the vaccine, whose trade name is Rota Teq. Rota Teq was licensed for use with children by the FDA in 2006.

Offit is a very popular speaker on the topic of vaccines. Over the past three years, he has averaged more than 20 major speeches on the topic throughout the United States. He is also a very productive writer with more than 80 scholarly papers and more than 60 articles in popular magazines and newspapers on vaccines and vaccination. In addition, he is the author or coauthor of 11 books, including *Vaccines: What Every Parent Should Know*; *The Vaccine Handbook: A Practical Guide for the Clinician*; *The Cutter Incident: How America's First Polio Vaccine Led to a Growing Vaccine Crisis*; *Vaccinated: One Man's Quest to*

Defeat the World's Deadliest Diseases; *Autism's False Prophets: Bad Science, Risky Medicine, and the Search for a Cure*; *Vaccines and Your Child: Separating Fact from Fiction*; and *Deadly Choices: How the Anti-Vaccine Movement Threatens Us All.*

Among Offit's many awards and honors are the J. Edmund Bradley Prize for Excellence in Pediatrics of the University of Maryland Medical School, Lederle Young Investigator Award in Vaccine Development, Research Achievement Award of CHOP, Gold Medal Award from CHOP, Jonas Salk Bronze Medal from the Association for Professionals in Infection Control and Epidemiology, Stanley A. Plotkin Award for Outstanding Achievement in Vaccines of the Pediatric Infectious Diseases Society, Dr. Charles Mérieux Award for Achievement in Vaccinology and Immunology from the National Foundation for Infectious Diseases, Humanitarian of the Year Award of the National Meningitis Association, William Osler Patient Oriented Research Award of the University of Pennsylvania School of Medicine, President's Certificate for Outstanding Service of the American Academy of Pediatrics, and Ralph D. Feigin Award for Excellence. Offit has also been named Canon Ely Distinguished Professor at Boston Children's Hospital, Stevens Distinguished Visiting Professor at LeBonheur Children's Hospital and the University of Tennessee Medical Center, Lori Haker Visiting Professor at the Medical College of Wisconsin, and Ashley Weech Visiting Professor at Children's Hospital of Cincinnati. He is also a member of a number of international, national, and regional associations, such as American Society for Microbiology, American Society for the Advancement of Science, American Society for Virology, Union of Concerned Scientists, Society for Experimental Biology and Medicine, The American Association of Immunologists, Pediatric Infectious Disease Society, The Society for Pediatric Research, American Gastroenterological Association, International Society for Vaccines, and Association for the Prudent Use of Antibiotics.

Louis Pasteur (1822–1895)

Pasteur was one of the giants of the 19th century. He made important contributions in the fields of chemistry, microbiology, and medicine, including the development of a number of vaccines for humans and other animals. In 1880, he invented the first laboratory-produced vaccine in an act of serendipity, the unplanned and unexpected discovery of a scientific phenomenon. The event occurred when one of Pasteur's laboratory associates failed to carry out his instructions for inoculating chickens being used in an experiment during the summer vacation period. When Pasteur came back from vacation, he made the unexpected discovery that chickens that had been inoculated with an outdated sample of potentially fatal cholera bacteria did not die from the procedure but, instead, were protected from later exposure to the disease. Pasteur reasoned that the explanation for this phenomenon might be that the chickens had been exposed to a weakened version of the cholera bacteria (in the outdated sample), which caused their immune systems to begin producing antibodies to the cholera bacteria. In such a case, researchers should be able to make a vaccine consisting of weakened (attenuated) germs that would challenge an animal's immune system to produce antibodies against a disease without actually contracting the disease itself. After discovering a method for attenuating cholera bacteria to just the right level of virulence, Pasteur announced just such a vaccine that solved a problem that had plagued chicken farmers since time immemorial.

A year after his discovery of a chicken cholera vaccine, Pasteur shifted his attention to a second disease of long concern to farmers, anthrax, a disease that affected cows, sheep, goats, and other domestic animals. Pasteur applied the same principle to this research that he did in his work on chicken cholera, producing a sample of anthrax pathogens that were weak enough not to produce the disease in animals, but were virulent enough to stimulate production of antibodies in vaccinated animals. In a series of tests conducted in May 1882, he confounded his critics who thought Pasteur was a charlatan with his new approach to disease prevention by vaccinating one group of sheep with his vaccine, and leaving a second group of sheep unprotected. As he had expected, Pasteur was able to show that the vaccinated sheep had become resistant to anthrax, while the unvaccinated group had not.

Perhaps Pasteur's greatest accomplishment was his application of pathogen attenuation to a vaccine designed for humans against the disease of rabies. Although he had been working on such a vaccine for a considerable period of time, he had not yet tested the vaccine on humans when, on July 6, 1885, nine-year-old Joseph Meister was brought to him after having been mauled by a rabid dog. Given that Meister was almost certainly going to die from the attack, Pasteur decided to test his new rabies vaccine on the boy. The experiment was a success, and Joseph did not contract rabies.

Louis Pasteur was born on December 27, 1822, in Dole, France, a town in eastern France near the Swiss border. He was the third child of Jean-Joseph Pasteur, a tanner, and his wife, Jeanne-Etienne Roqui Pasteur. When Louis was still a young child, the Pasteur family moved first to Marnoz, and then to Arbois, where he attended the Collège d'Arbois primary school and then the Besançon Royal High School. After completing his secondary education, Pasteur matriculated at the Ecole Normale Supérieure in Paris, one of the nation's most prestigious institutes of higher education. He was awarded his PhD in chemistry and physics for his studies in crystallography and the chemistry of arsenius acid in 1847.

Pasteur's first professional appointment was as professor of chemistry at Strasbourg University in 1849. Five years later, he was appointed professor of chemistry and dean of the newly created Faculty of Science at Lille Science University. He held that post for only three years before accepting the position of Scientific Director at the Ecole Normale Supérieure in Paris. Pasteur stayed at his new position for a decade, resigning only in 1867 as the result of student unrest at the school which resulted in closing of the school and resignation of all staff and professors, including Pasteur. While still serving at the Ecole Normale Supérieure, Pasteur had also accepted a teaching appointment at the famous school of fine arts, the Ecole des Beaux-Arts in Paris, where he taught geology, physics, and chemistry to students majoring in painting, sculpture, architecture, and other fine arts. He also resigned this post in 1867.

After leaving his posts at the Ecole Normale Supérieure and the Ecole des Beaux-Arts in 1867, Pasteur was appointed to the chair in organic chemistry at the Sorbonne, where he remained until 1872. At that point, bothered by health problems and overwhelmed with research, speaking, and writing obligations, he applied for early retirement from the Sorbonne.

No short biographical sketch can begin to capture the enormity of Pasteur's contribution to a variety of fields of scientific research. His research on fermentation transformed the business of beer- and wine-making and the world's understanding of a number of dairying process. His studies of silkworm diseases saved the silk industry from disaster and collapse. The list of honors and awards he received would cover many pages of this book. They include a special prize on his studies of racemic acids from the Société de Pharmacie de Paris; Rumford Medal of the Royal Society of London; Montyon Prize for Experimental Physiology, Zecker Prize in Chemistry, Alhymbert Prize, and Jean Reynaud Prize, all of the Académie des Sciences; Gold Medal of the Comite Central Agricole de Sologne (for research on diseases associated with wine); Grand Prize Medal of the Exposition Universelle (Paris) (for wine preservation technology); Honorary MD from the University of Bonn; Commander of the Imperial Order of the Rose, Brazil; Copley Medal of the Royal Society of London (for his research on fermentation and silkworm diseases); Grand Cross of the Legion of Honor; and Grand Cordon of the Order of Isabella the Catholic, Spain. He was elected chevalier, commander, and grand officer of the Imperial Order of the Legion of Honor; member of the Académie des Sciences (mineralogy section); fellow of the Royal Society; member of the Académie de Médecine; member of the Académie Française; and member of the Académie des Sciences and, later, perpetual secretary of the academy.

Pasteur died at his home at Marnes-la-Coquette, Hauts-de-Seine, France, on September 28, 1895, following a series of strokes. He is perhaps best remembered today by way of the Institut Pasteur in Paris, founded in 1887 for the purpose of conducting research on the treatment and prevention of infectious diseases.

Stanley A. Plotkin (1932–)

Plotkin is a highly regarded research vaccinologist, who has worked on vaccines for cytomegalovirus, polio, rabies, and rotavirus. In the 1960s, he developed a rubella vaccine that replaced earlier versions of the vaccine and has since become the vaccine of choice against the disease throughout the world. Plotkin is also editor of *Vaccines*, the standard textbook in the field, now in its fifth edition (Saunders/Elsevier). He is also the author or coauthor of more than 600 peer-reviewed papers on the subject of vaccinology.

Stanley Alan Plotkin was born in New York City on May 12, 1932. He attended NYU, from which he received his BA, and the State University of New York Medical School in Brooklyn, from which he received his MD in 1956. He completed his internship at the Cleveland (Ohio) Metropolitan General Hospital and his residency in pediatrics at CHOP and the Hospital for Sick Children in London, England. He then spent three years at the Epidemic Intelligence Service of the CDC (now the Centers for Disease Control and Prevention) in Atlanta, Georgia.

In 1959, Plotkin accepted an appointment as instructor at the University of Pennsylvania School of Medicine. He remained at Pennsylvania until 1991, advancing through the ranks as assistant and associate professor and, finally, Professor of Pediatrics and Microbiology. In 1960, he also joined the staff at the Wistar Institute of Anatomy and Biology as an associate member. He also remained at Wistar until 1991, at which time he held the post of Professor of Virology. During this period, Plotkin was also Director of Infectious Diseases and Senior Physician at CHOP.

In 1991, Plotkin left his academic and clinical assignments to join the staff of the French vaccine manufacturer, Pasteur Mérieux Serums & Vaccins, later to become Pasteur Mérieux Connaught, and now, Sanofi Pasteur. The company is said to be the world's largest company devoted solely to the manufacture of vaccines. Plotkin worked for seven years with the company as Medical and Scientific Director. He then left Sanofi Pasteur to open his own consulting firm, Vaxconsult, L.L.C., which provides advice to vaccine manufacturers, biotechnology companies, and nonprofit research organizations. He currently holds the titles of Emeritus Professor at the University of Pennsylvania and Adjunct Professor at the Johns Hopkins University.

Plotkin's most notable research accomplishment was his development of a vaccine against rubella in the 1960s. At the time, a number of researchers were working on a vaccine that used an attenuated virus, produced by passing the virus through a number of generations in some nonhuman cell, such as those from duck embryos, rabbit kidneys, and dog kidneys. Plotkin and his colleagues decided to use human fibroblast cells as their attenuating medium. They passed the virus through 25 generations in these cells and found that the virus had become sufficiently attenuated so that it could not cause the disease itself, but it was able to stimulate the human immune system to start making antibodies against the virus. The procedure was not widely accepted at first, partly because of the way in which the vaccine was produced. But it soon became widely popular, and is now the primary forms of the vaccine used against rubella around the world.

Plotkin has served in a number of professional capacities, including chairman of the Infectious Diseases Committee and the AIDS Task Force of the American Academy of Pediatrics, liaison member of the Advisory Committee on Immunization Practices, and chair of the Microbiology and Infectious Diseases Research Committee of the NIH. He has been awarded a number of honors, including the Bruce Medal in Preventive Medicine of the American College of Physicians, the Distinguished Physician Award of the Pediatric Infectious Diseases Society, the Clinical Virology Award of the Pan American Society for Clinical Virology, the Richard Day Master Teacher in Pediatrics Award of the Alumni Association of New York Downstate Medical College, the Marshall Award of the European Society for Pediatric Infectious Diseases, the French Legion of Honor Medal, the Distinguished Alumnus Award and the Gold Medal of CHOP, the Sabin Gold Medal, the Fleming (Bristol) Award of the Infectious Diseases Society of America, the medal of the Fondation Mérieux, the Finland Award of the National Foundation for Infectious Diseases, and the Hilleman Award of the American Society for Microbiology. He has also been awarded honorary doctoral degrees from the University of Rouen (France) and the Complutense University of Madrid (Spain).

Gaston Ramon (1886–1963)

Ramon made a number of important contributions to the field of immunology in the first half of the 20th century. Foremost among these was his development of safe vaccines for both diphtheria and tetanus, two of the most devastating infectious diseases of the time. He also developed a method for determining the potency of a vaccine and produced one of the first effective conjugate vaccines.

One of the most serious problems associated with the use of existing vaccines in the early 20th century was their potential for producing the very diseases against which they were designed to protect. As long as an active virus or bacterium was used in a vaccine, the possibility always existed that a person's immune system might not be able to hold off the pathogen, and he or she would develop the disease caused by the agent. Researchers explored a number of methods of reducing this risk. Ramon's solution was to inactivate the toxin responsible for diphtheria (and later tetanus) by heating it and treating it with a solution of formaldehyde in water called formalin. The use of formalin appeared risky at the time (as it still does) because formaldehyde is toxic, and its use in vaccines would appear only to increase the risk of vaccination. By adjusting the concentration of formalin used, however, Ramon was able to produce a vaccine that was able to activate a person's immune system, without causing damage to that person's body. This approach to the production of vaccines is still in use today.

Gaston Ramon was born in the town of Bellchaume, in the department of Yonne, in the Burgundy region of France, on September 30, 1886. Young Gaston is said to have been very bright and curious about the natural world, presaging his later career in scientific research. He attended high school in the nearby city of Sens, where his father was a baker, before attending the veterinary school at Alfort, in the Val de Marne, from 1906 to 1910. Upon Ramon's graduation from Alfort, one of his instructors, Henri Vallée, introduced Ramon to Emile Roux, then director of the prestigious Institut Pasteur in Paris. Roux assigned Ramon to the task of vaccinating horses stockaded at the institute for the production of anti-diphtheria, anti-tetanus, and anti-gangrene vaccines. One of the discoveries made by Ramon in this work was that vaccines often did not "travel well." That is, by the time they were transported from the place they were produced to the places where they were actually used (such as a battlefield), they had undergone degradation and were no longer suitable for use. Ramon found that the addition of very small amounts of formalin acted as a preservative for vaccines (as it was for many other products then and now), increasing the amount of time during which they were still safe and effective.

After World War I, Ramon was able to obtain a small laboratory in an annex to the Institut Pasteur, where he continued his research on vaccines. Over the next three decades, he made four major discoveries in the field of immunization. The first, and perhaps most important, was his discovery that the use of formalin, along with mild heating, not only preserved a vaccine, but also reduced the risk of adverse events as a result of their application. His second discovery was that toxins and toxoids (Ramon called them *anatoxine diphtérique*, or "anatoxins") could be titrated against each other in such a way as to determine with great accuracy the potency of the toxoid and, therefore, the vaccine in which it was being used.

Ramon's third contribution to immunology was his theory of adjuvancy (which he called *adjuvantes et stimulantes de l'immunité*, or "adjuvants and stimulants of immunity"). This theory was based on Ramon's observation that the addition of certain substances, such as tapioca, alum, or calcium chloride, to a vaccine appeared to increase the potency of that vaccine. Ramon's discovery remains an essential component of vaccinology in today's world. Finally, working with Christian Zoeller, Ramon developed the first combination vaccine (which they called an "associated vaccine") consisting of more than one antigen. The advantage of such a vaccine, in wide use today, is that it provides immunity to more than one infectious disease at a time. The MMR (mumps-measles-rubella) multivalent vaccine in use worldwide today is an example of such a vaccine.

Ramon maintained his association with the Institut Pasteur in one capacity or another throughout most of his professional career. He was named director of the institute's annex at Garches in 1926, a post he held until 1944. In 1934, Ramon was also named assistant director of the Institut Pasteur in Paris, a post he also kept until 1940. In that year, he was named director of the Institut Pasteur, and a year later, honorary director of the institute. He served at Institut Pasteur until his retirement in 1948. In 1947, Ramon was given the honorary title of director of research at the Institut National D'Hygiene (French Health

Institute), and a year later he was named director of the Office International des Epizooties (International Epizootic Office) in Paris. Ramon retired from active research and administration in 1958. He died in Paris on June 8, 1963.

Ramon was elected to the French Academy of Medicine in 1934 and the French Academy of Sciences in 1943. He was awarded the Clotilde Liard award by the former association in 1924 and the Bréant and Général Muteau awards by the latter society in 1925 and 1937, respectively. In 1958 he received the Gold Medal of the French National Centre for Scientific Research (CNRS), the highest scientific research award given in France.

Benjamin A. Rubin (1917–2010)

Rubin is best known as the inventor of the so-called pronged vaccinating needle used primarily for inoculation against small-pox. He applied for a patent for this invention in 1965, during a period when world public health authorities were initiating a massive effort to eradicate smallpox from the planet. Only a year after Rubin received his patent, in fact, WHO put into motion an international program for providing smallpox vac-cinations throughout the world in an effort to finally eradicate the disease. That goal was ultimately achieved in 1977, when the last case of smallpox was diagnosed in Somalia. WHO then waited two more years before finally declaring that the disease had been successfully eradicated from earth.

In his patent application, Rubin explained the problems in-volved in traditional methods of vaccinating against smallpox. Those methods involved placing a small drop of vaccine on the skin and then poking small holes in the skin with a sharp needle. After about 20 jabs, excessive vaccine was wiped off the skin. The procedure was, in the first place, uneconomical because some vaccine was always wasted in the last step of the procedure. It was also inexact, since it was difficult always to control the depth of the jabs, making it uncertain as to how much of the vaccine actually penetrated the skin.

Rubin's solution to this problem was to start with a conventional sewing needle, and then to grind down the eye of the needle until the tip of the eye was broken off. The result of this process was a fork-shaped needle of precise size that could be used to pick up an exact amount of vaccine. The needle was then used to penetrate the skin and deliver exactly the correct amount of vaccine with the loss of essentially no product during the inoculation. One of the great advantages of Rubin's invention was that it was simple to use, making it convenient to carry out smallpox vaccinations in virtually any setting, just the product needed to make the WHO eradication program a reality. The U.S. Patent Office issued Rubin patent #3,194,237 on July 13, 1965, for this invention.

Benjamin Arnold Rubin was born in New York City on September 27, 1917. He attended public schools in New York City before matriculating at the City College of New York (CCNY), from which he earned his bachelor of science degree in biology and chemistry in 1937. He then continued his studies at Virginia Polytechnic Institute, from which he received his master of science degree in 1938, and at Yale University, which granted him his PhD in microbiology in 1947. The delay between his MS and PhD was caused by the onset of World War II, during which Rubin served as a microbiologist for the U.S. Army from 1940 to 1944. After the war, he worked for one year at the Schenley Research Institute and from 1945 to 1947 at the Yale Office of Scientific Research and Development.

Upon completing his PhD program, Rubin took a position as associate microbiologist at the Brookhaven National Laboratory, where he remained until 1952. He then became chief microbiologist at the Syntex South America Corporation in Mexico (1952–1954) and assistant professor of public health at the Baylor University College of Medicine (1954–1960). In 1960 he joined the Wyeth Laboratories of American Home Products as manager of the Biological Product Development Department, where he worked for the next 24 years. In 1984, he left Wyeth to return to the academic world as professor of microbiology at the Philadelphia College of Osteopathic Medicine. He retired from that post in 1996. During his time at Wyeth, Rubin also served as a consultant in the Space Biology Program at General Electric from 1967 to 1975.

Rubin received the John Scott Award and Medal in 1981, an award given to individuals who have made "useful inventions" in their careers. In 1993, he was awarded the Procter Medal of the Pharmaceutical Trade Association, an award given for individuals who have "contributed to the alleviation of human suffering." Rubin was also named to the Inventors Hall of Fame in 1992. He died in Philadelphia on March 8, 2010, at the age of 92.

Albert Sabin (1906–1993)

Sabin was lead researcher on a team that produced the second polio vaccine approved for use in the United States by the FDA. The vaccine differed from an earlier polio vaccine developed by Jonas Salk in the early 1950s in that it contained attenuated polioviruses, while the Sabin vaccine was made of dead viruses. The vaccine was attenuated by passing it through nonhuman cells, during which process the virus mutates into a nonlethal form. Thus, while it is still capable of producing an immune response in humans, it is no longer capable of producing the disease itself. Today the Sabin vaccine is often the vaccine of choice for immunization against polio in many countries of the world, although the Salk vaccine is still the vaccine of choice in the United States. The Sabin vaccine is also different from the Salk vaccine in that it is given orally, while the Salk vaccine is administered by inoculation.

Albert Bruce Sabin was born in Bialystok, Poland, on August 26, 1906, to Jacob and Tillie Saperstein. The family immigrated to the United States in 1921 because of the persecution of Jews then very common in Eastern Europe (as well as other parts of the continent). Upon their arrival in the United States, the family changed their last name to "Sabin," and settled in

Paterson, New Jersey. Sabin's father worked there in the textile industry, while his mother remained at home as a homemaker. Sabin graduated from Paterson High School in 1923, continuing his education at NYU, from which he received his MD in 1931. As was the case with Salk, Sabin was actually more interested in medical research than in becoming a practicing physician. After completely his internship and residency at Bellevue Hospital, in New York City, he began his research career first at the Lister Institute for Preventative Medicine, in London, and later at the Rockefeller Institute for Medical Research, in New York City (now Rockefeller University). In 1939, Sabin accepted an appointment as associate professor of pediatrics at the University of Cincinnati College of Medicine, with a joint appointment at the Children's Hospital Research Foundation in Cincinnati. He was to spend the rest of his professional career in Cincinnati, serving later as Professor of Research Pediatrics and Distinguished Service Professor at the university.

Sabin's career was interrupted in 1943 by World War II, when he joined the U.S. Army Medical Corps as a member of the Epidemiological Board's Virus Committee. This assignment took him to a number of locations around the world where he studied the transmission of a number of infectious diseases. This work led to his development of vaccines for dengue fever, Japanese B encephalitis, and sandfly fever. Sabin was discharged from the military service in September 1945, after which he returned to his research on a polio vaccine in Cincinnati. A decade later, the vaccine was ready for tests on humans, the first of whom were Sabin himself and some of his colleagues. The more extended test on large numbers of humans was not possible in the United States in the late 1950s because of possible conflicts with the Salk vaccine, which had just been approved for use. Instead, Sabin and his colleague arranged for the needed test of his vaccine in Russia and Eastern Europe, where it was eventually given to more than 100 million individuals. The success of that large-scale test eventually led to the vaccine's approval by the FDA in 1962. Since that date, both the Salk and Sabin vaccines have been used in various parts of the world, leading to a point at which polio may soon be entirely eradicated from the planet.

Sabin finally retired officially from his Cincinnati posts at the age of 80 in 1986. By that time, he was suffering from almost constant pain caused by calcification of the spine. The condition was eventually resolved successfully by surgery in 1992. Even after his official retirement, however, Sabin continued to work in a variety of other capacities, including the post of Senior Medical Science Advisor at the Fogarty International Center at the NIH in Washington, DC. His spinal problems finally forced Sabin to retire completely in 1988. He died in Washington on March 3, 1993, at the age of 86, of heart failure.

In addition to his work in Cincinnati, Sabin served as president of the Weizmann Institute of Science in Rehovot, Israel, from 1970 to 1972, as consultant to the U.S. National Cancer Institute in 1974, and as Distinguished Research Professor of Biomedicine at the Medical University of South Carolina from 1974 to 1982. He was awarded 46 honorary doctoral degrees from institutions in the United States and around the world, including NYU, Temple University, Ohio State University, Albert Einstein College of Medicine, George Washington University, Federal University of Rio de Janeiro (Brazil), Hebrew University of Jerusalem (Israel), University of Newcastle-upon-Tyne (England), National University of Plata (Argentina), and University of Messina (Italy). He also received many honors and awards during his lifetime, including the James D. Bruce Memorial Award of the American College of Physicians; the Robert Koch Medal of the Robert Koch Foundation; the NYU Gold Medal; the Orden del Merito de Duarte, Sanchez y Melia, Gran Cruz of the Dominican Republic; the Crosse Rossa Italiana, Medaglia d'Oro of Rome, Italy; the Guilherme Fernando Halfed Medal, Juiz de Fora, Brazil; and the Presidential Medal of Freedom (the highest civilian award presented by the President of the United States). The Albert B. Sabin Education Center at Cincinnati Children's Hospital and the Sabin Vaccine Institute in Washington, DC, are both named in Sabin's honor.

Jonas Salk (1914–1995)

Salk was an American medical researcher who specialized in the field of virology. He is best known today for his discovery and development of the first vaccine against poliomyelitis, better known simply as polio. Salk first became interested in the development of vaccines while still a medical student at NYU. As part of his studies, he was invited to investigate the possibility of developing a vaccine against influenza, an ongoing public health problem in the United States and the rest of the world. Salk envisioned a vaccine consisting of the virus that causes influenza that had been treated to prevent the disease itself, but that retained enough of its original characteristic features to fool the human immune system into producing an immune response against the inactivated virus. After receiving his degree from NYU, Salk continued his research on a flu vaccine at the University of Michigan School of Medicine and the University of Pittsburgh Medical School through the late 1940s and early 1950s. On April 12, 1955, his longtime mentor, Thomas Francis, Jr., announced at a press conference at the University of Michigan that Salk's long search for a polio vaccine had been proved successful.

Jonas Edward Salk was born in New York City on October 28, 1914, to Daniel and Dora Press Salk, the oldest of three sons. The Salks were Russian-Jewish immigrants who had only high school educations themselves, but insisted that their three sons would always have every educational opportunity available to them. Jonas attended Townsend Harris High School in Flushing, New York, a school for exceptional students associated with Queens College. He graduated from Harris at the age of 16 in 1930, and then enrolled at CCNY. There he intended to major in the law, but was convinced by his mother to transfer to pre-medicine instead. Upon completing his studies at CCNY, Salk continued his studies at the NYU College of Medicine, where his primary advisor was Francis. It was under Francis' urging that Salk first began his studies of viruses, a career choice with which he was to remain for the rest of his professional life.

After receiving his MD from NYU in 1939, Salk was chosen as one of only 12 medical graduates to do his internship at the Mount Sinai Hospital in New York City. He completed that stage of his training in 1942 and then accepted an appointment at the University of Michigan School of Medicine. Much of his initial work on the development of a polio vaccine was completed at Michigan. In 1947, Salk left Michigan to take a position as associate professor of bacteriology at the University of Pittsburgh, where he eventually completed his research on and testing of the polio vaccine leading to the 1955 announcement back in Ann Arbor.

Salk's invention of a polio vaccine brought enormous relief to people around the world since it provided the first opportunity ever for avoiding a terribly disabling and often fatal disease. However, that news was not always good. Producing the vaccine in commercial quantities was a daunting industrial task, and the first year during which the vaccine was available was accompanied by reports of a number of deaths and disabling disease events associated with it. Experts also debated the relative merits and disadvantages of Salk's approach and that of Albert Sabin, who shortly after Salk's success, had produced an alternative type of vaccine that used an altered form of the live virus. Today, both vaccines are in use throughout the world and have been responsible for eradicating the disease in many nations. In 1994, for example, WHO declared that polio had been eradicated from the Western Hemisphere. Comparable success was experienced in other locations. In China the number of polio cases dropped from 5,065 in 1990 to five in 1994, after a massive immunization campaign in 1992 and 1993. No cases of polio were found in China until

2011, when travelers from regions that were not polio free entered the country.

Salk continued to serve at Pittsburgh for more than two decades, where he was named research professor of bacteriology in 1949, professor of preventative medicine in 1954, and Commonwealth professor of experimental medicine in 1957. In 1963, Salk left Pittsburgh to found his own research institution, the Salk Institute for Biological Studies in La Jolla, California. A major thrust of his work there was research on autoimmune responses in the human body, reactions in which the body's immune system attacks its own body as if it were a "foreign invader." One of his last projects was an effort to develop a vaccine against HIV/AIDS disease. For the purpose of conducting research in this area, he founded the Immune Response Corporation with venture capitalist Kevin Kimberlin. This effort was not successful, however, and the corporation disbanded in 2007. Salk died in La Jolla on June 23, 1995, of heart failure.

During his lifetime, Salk received many honors, some of them the highest recognition that can be given to a science. They included the Lasker Award in 1956, the Jawaharlal Nehru Award and the Congressional Gold Medal in 1975, the Gold Plate Award of the Academy of Achievement in 1976, and the Presidential Medal of Freedom in 1977. He was elected to the Polio Hall of Fame in 1958 and the California Hall of Fame in 2007. In one sense, his greatest recognition has come in the naming of public schools in his honor in Mesa, Arizona; Sacramento, California; Bolingbrook, Illinois; Merrillville, Indiana; Old Bridge, New Jersey; Levittown, New York; Tulsa, Oklahoma; and Spokane, Washington.

In addition to nearly 170 scientific papers, Salk was the author of four books, *Man Unfolding* (1972), *Survival of the Wisest* (1973), *World Population and Human Values: A New Reality* (1981), and *Anatomy of Reality: Merging of Intuition and Reason* (1983).

Viera Scheibner (1935–)

Scheibner is a micropaleontologist who has expressed strong feelings about the risks and ineffectiveness of vaccines. (Micropaleontology is the study of very small fossils, usually less than about one millimeter in diameter. Such fossils are valuable clues to the structure and composition of the early Earth.) She is highly respected and frequently quoted by anti-vaccinationists around the world. Her academic qualifications to speak on the subject and her fair-mindedness, however, have been a matter of considerable criticism by members of the medical profession. In one review of her work in the Australian journal *The Skeptic*, for example, the author concluded that "the gaps in her research in this area [vaccination] call into question her objectivity and cast doubts on her ability to speak as an expert witness." In 1997, the Australian Skeptics society awarded her the "Bent Spoon Award," presented annually to the Australian "perpetrator of the most preposterous piece of pseudoscientific piffle." Among vaccination deniers, however, Scheibner is very influential, much sought after as a spokesperson against required immunization. In defending her presence on the popular online encyclopedia, Wikipedia, for example, one supporter chastised the "allopathic editors" with their "links to AMA shill quackwatch and other sites attacking her," who tried to have the site deleted.

Viera Scheibner (originally, Scheibnerová) was born on March 27, 1935, in Bratislava, Czechoslovakia (now Slovak Republic). Her parents were both employed by the Law Courts in Bratislava. She matriculated at the Jan Masaryk University in Brno in 1953 with plans to major in medicine. A year later, however, she transferred to the School of Natural Sciences at Jan Amos Comenius University in Bratislava, from which she earned her bachelor's degree in 1958. She then continued her doctoral studies at Comenius, earning her PhD in micropaleontology in 1964. Scheibner's first teaching assignment was as Lecturer in the Department of Geology and Paleontology at Comenius University from 1958 to 1961. She was later promoted to Senior Lecturer (1962–1967) and Docent (equivalent to Senior Associate Professor; 1967–1968) at Comenius.

In 1968, Scheibner, her husband, and her two children emigrated to Australia, where she took a position as micropaleontologist at the Geological Survey of New South Wales (now called the Department of Mineral Resources). In 1971 she was promoted to Research Scientist (1971–1973), then to Senior Research Scientist (1973–1976), and then to Principal Research Scientist (1976–1987). She retired from her post at New South Wales in 1987. During her professional career, Scheinber authored 47 peer-reviewed papers and two monographs on topics in micropaleontology. From 1972 to 1976, she participated in the Deep Sea Drilling Project (DSDP) sponsored by the Scripps Institute of Oceanography.

Scheibner became interested in vaccination issues partially as a result of the work of her second husband, Leif Karlsson, a Swedish biomedical electronics engineer whom she married in 1985. While working with Karlsson on a new device for the monitoring of infant breathing patterns, she noticed a pattern of abnormal breathing among children who had recently been vaccinated. She began to wonder about the possible connection between the diphtheria-pertussis-tetanus (DPT) vaccine the children had received and the apparently abnormal breathing pattern. She presented her findings at the Second Immunisation Conference of the Public Health Association of Australia in Canberra in May 1991. She then turned her attention to a possible connection between vaccination and sudden infant death syndrome (SIDS) and came to the conclusion that "vaccination is the single biggest cause of SIDS" in an article in a 2004 issue of the *Journal of the Australasian College of Nutritional and Environmental Medicine*. (Critics point out that the period during which Scheibner was making this claim, vaccination rates in Australia increased from 53% to 92%, while SIDS deaths fell by 81% over the same period of time.)

In addition to her papers on micropaleontology, Scheibner has written two books on vaccination issues, *Vaccination: 100 Years of Orthodox Research Shows That Vaccines Represent a Medical Assault on the Immune System* (Santa Fe, NM: New Atlantean Press, 1993) and *Behavioural Problems in Childhood: The Link to Vaccination* (Turramurra, NSW: Taycare Printing, 2000). (Both books are self-published originally.) She has also written a number of articles on vaccination and health problems purported to be related to the practice, most of which have been published in chiropractor, homeopathic, and other alternative medical journals. She is also widely sought after as a speaker and consultant by groups of anti-vaccinationists. Scheibner has also written more than three dozen letters to the online version of the *British Medical Journal* on topics ranging from the unreliability of scientific papers as evidence and vaccination as the cause of shaken baby syndrome to the problem of measles outbreak among those vaccinated for the disease and the possible source of otherwise unexplained fractures. She has also written for other journals on topic such as adverse effects of adjutants in vaccines, little known facts about poliomyelitis vaccinations, and problems with the Gardasil vaccine. She has written in her own autobiography that she has "gathered a solid, extensive and irrefutable block of scientific evidence documenting vaccines as ineffective to prevent diseases, and which time and again issued warnings about a variety of real dangers, including brain haemorrhages and other brain damage, and retinal haemorrhages and other ophthalmological injuries and including death." (For a detailed response to this claim, see Stephen Basser, "Anti-immunisation scare: The Inconvenient Facts," at http://www.skeptics.com.au/wordpress/wp-content/uploads/theskeptic/1997/1.pdf.)

Vaccine Education Center
The Children's Hospital of Philadelphia
34th Street and Civic Center Boulevard
Philadelphia, PA 19104

Phone: (215) 590–1000
URL: http://www.chop.edu/service/vaccine-education-center/
home.html
E-mail: http://www.chop.edu/service/vaccine-education-center/
contactus.html

The Vaccine Education Center was established at CHOP in 2000 for the purpose of providing accurate and up-to-date information about infectious diseases and the vaccines that are available for preventing them. Children's Hospital is the oldest pediatric hospital in the United States, with a long commitment to all types of services for children of all ages and backgrounds. It continues to have one of the largest pediatric research and educational programs in the country. Current director of the Vaccine Education Center is Dr. Paul A. Offit, Chief of Infectious Diseases at CHOP. Offit is a well-known writer, speaker, and advocate for vaccination programs. The center is funded by Children's Hospital, with no financial support by any vaccine-producing corporation.

The primary contribution of the Vaccine Education Center is its rich website, which contains a great deal of information on infectious diseases and vaccines for parents, children, healthcare providers, and the general public. One page of the website, for example, lists each of the vaccines currently available, with a description of its function. Another page reviews the vaccine schedule that is recommended for young children. Other pages provide information on vaccine safety frequently asked questions, vaccines recommended for adults, information for travelers to foreign countries, and special information for educators. An important section of the website offers Q&A sheets on a number of topics, such as "The Facts about Childhood Vaccines," "Aluminum in Vaccines," "Vaccines and Autism," "Too Many Vaccines? What You Should Know," and fact sheets on most infectious diseases, including influenza, meningococcus, rotavirus, shingles, and HPV. Special booklets are also available on *Vaccines and Your Baby*, *Vaccines and Teens*, and *Vaccines and Adults*.

The center's website also provides a reference page with links to other organizations and lists of print and electronic resources on vaccine-related topics. The In the News page also provides up-to-date reviews of vaccine-related topics of current interest, such as the relationships (or lack of it) between vaccinations and autism, the effects of vaccines on brain chemistry, current adult vaccination rates, and troubling trends in the incidence of measles outbreaks. The center has recently established a new program, Parents PACK—Possessing, Accessing, and Communicating Knowledge about vaccines—designed to provide parents with accurate information about vaccinations and to make available a single resource center with which they can interact to obtain answers to specific questions and concerns. Parents PACK has a free monthly newsletter that carries current news on vaccine-related issues.

Vaccination Risk Awareness Network, Inc.
P.O. Box 169
Winlaw, BC
Canada V0G 2J0
Phone: (250) 355–2525
URL: http://vran.org/
E-mail: info@vran.org

The Vaccination Risk Awareness Network, Inc. (VRAN) was formed in 1982 as the Committee Against Compulsory Vaccination (CACV) in Ontario, Canada. The group was founded in opposition to the newly adopted School Pupils Act, which required that all students in the province be vaccinated before being allowed to attend school. The original act had no provision for exemptions, so parents who objected to having their children vaccinated for religious, health, philosophical, or other reasons had no recourse to the provisions of the act. Members of CACV met with sympathetic members of the Parliament to develop language for the bill that would include such exemptions, and an amendment was adopted containing those provisions in December 1984. The organization eventually decided to continue its operations on a broader front, and reorganized as VRAN, in 1992.

The fundamental philosophy that underlies the work of the VRAN is that potentially serious adverse effects are an inherent part of vaccination, and that parents and other adults should be fully aware of the nature of those adverse effects. With that information, individuals should then have the right to make decisions as to whether they or their children should have vaccinations and, if so, under what circumstances and according to what schedule. (A very useful outline of VRAN's philosophical underpinnings and program of action can be found in its Policy Statement on Vaccination, on its website at http://vran. org/about/policy-statement-on-vaccination/.) In addition, anyone who has experienced an adverse event as the result of being vaccinated needs to be compensated for such an event, and one of VRAN's objectives is to educate parents and other adults as to the procedures available for reporting and being compensated for adverse vaccination events.

In addition to its role in educating the general public about possible problems associated with vaccination, VRAN claims that it acts as a watchdog organization that identifies actions by government and health officials that violate the right of individuals to be exempted themselves, or to have their children exempted from vaccination laws and regulations. The organization provides a mechanism on its website by which individuals who have experienced such problems can report violations to VRAN (see http://vran.org/report-a-reaction/).

VRAN's website provides information about vaccination in six general areas: About Vaccines, Health Risks, Autism, Exemptions, Personal Stories, and Alternatives. The About Vaccines section contains a great deal of detailed information about all aspects of vaccines, including information on specific diseases and vaccines available for each disease, the recommended Canadian vaccination schedule, pet vaccines, and vaccine ingredients and production. The Health Risks section reviews information available about a number of conditions thought to be associated with vaccines, including cancer, Gulf War Syndrome, obesity and diabetes, and SIDS. The Autism section discusses some of the controversy associated with the putative association between vaccines and behavioral disorders, but tends to focus on research that appears to support the association. The Exemptions section provides an interesting and useful review of Canadian law dealing with vaccination and outlines procedure for exemptions where vaccination regulations are in place. The Alternatives section provides links to a number of print and electronic articles that deal with a wide-ranging number of topics, some only peripherally related to vaccination.

While VRAN does not publish print material of its own, it does have a link to a number of books, pamphlets, and other materials on the topic of compulsory vaccination on the Resources page of its website. The organization does produce a newsletter that contains articles on vaccination, disease trends, news from around the world, vaccine reactions, injury testimonials, and alternative health information. The newsletter is available to members only.

Emil von Behring (1854–1917)

Von Behring was awarded the Nobel Prize for Physiology or Medicine in 1901, the first such prize given in that category. His award read "for his work on serum therapy, especially its application against diphtheria, by which he has opened a new road in the domain of medical science and thereby placed in the hands of the physician a victorious weapon against illness and deaths." Von Behring's work depended on the discoveries of a number of other researchers and was completed with the assistance of other colleagues, including especially Japanese immunologist Shibasaburo Kitasato.

That work began with the realization that some pathogenic bacteria release a substance that is responsible for the disease they produce in a soluble form that remains in the bloodstream of an infected animal. For example, blood taken from an animal with diphtheria can be filtered so that all diphtheria bacteria are removed from the fluid. The soluble substance produced by the bacteria, however, remains in the bloodstream. When that filtrate is injected into an uninfected animal, that animal also contracts the disease. Von Behring called the disease-provoking substance a *toxin*.

Von Behring also realized that injecting a toxin into an uninfected animal causes that animal's immune system to begin producing antibodies against the toxin, thus providing immunity for the animal against that disease. Von Behring called those antibodies *antitoxins*. Moreover, inoculating an animal that already has a given disease, such as diphtheria, with diphtheria toxin, may prevent the disease from becoming any worse and may actually cure the infection. Von Behring called the process of treating an infected animal by this method *serum therapy*.

Von Behring's work on the diphtheria toxin caused him to consider the possibility of producing a vaccine that could be used to prevent the disease in humans. One of the options that occurred to him was a vaccine consisting of a mixture of diphtheria toxin and antitoxin, combined in a ratio that would initiate the immune response in a person without actually causing the disease. After many years of research, involving to a considerable extent the testing of mixtures containing differing proportions of toxin and antitoxin, he produced just such a vaccine in 1913.

Emil Adolf von Behring was born in Hansdorf, Prussia (now Ławice, Poland), on March 15, 1854. He was the eldest son of 13 children of a schoolmaster who, for obvious reasons, was not able to send his son to a university. Emil instead matriculated at the Akademie für das militärärztliche Bildungswesen (Army Medical College of Berlin) following his graduation from secondary school. He received his medical degree in 1878 and passed the state medical exam two years later. Over the next decade, he served in a number of local army posts, carrying out research in addition to his clinical duties. In 1888, the high command ordered von Behring to return to Berlin, where he was to join the laboratory of the eminent bacteriologist Robert Koch. This move was motivated by the army's concern about the risks that infectious diseases posed to troops in the field and its desire to find ways to protect its men against those diseases. Over the next six years, von Behring worked with Koch, Paul Ehrlich, Friedrich Löffler, Alexandre Yersin, Emile Roux, and a number of other researchers on problems of identifying the causative agents of disease and methods for bringing them under control. It was during this period that von Behring and Kitasato completed their historic studies on diphtheria (primarily von Behring) and tetanus (primarily Kitasato).

In 1894, von Behring was appointed Professor of Hygiene at Halle University, where he remained for just one year. He then moved on to the comparable chair at the University of Marburg, where he remained for the rest of his professional career. One of the least pleasant features of the story of von Behring's work on the diphtheria vaccine was his success in largely excluding Ehrlich, his coworker on the project, from receiving any of the substantial financial rewards and popular recognition (including the Nobel Prize) for an accomplishment that probably should have been shared more equally between them.

Von Behring's health began to deteriorate after 1900, and he restricted himself largely to the study of tuberculosis and the search for a vaccine against that disease. In 1904, he founded his own company, Behringwerke, for the manufacture of vaccines and sera. The company was a great success and made von Behring a rich man in his late years. The company continues to operate today, now as Dade Behring Holdings Inc., the world's largest corporation devoted solely to the manufacture and distribution of clinical diagnostics. Von Behring died at his estate in Marburg on March 31, 1917.

Andrew Wakefield (1957–)

Wakefield is a gastroenterologist who reported on an association between the use of the MMR vaccine in a paper published in *The Lancet* medical journal in 1998. Wakefield and his 12 coauthors concluded from their studies of 12 autistic children that they had found a new medical disorder that was associated with "gastrointestinal disease and developmental regression in a group of previously normal children, which was generally associated in time with possible environmental triggers." The most prominent of those "environmental triggers," according to Wakefield and his team, was exposure to the MMR vaccine. A number of research teams attempted to replicate those findings in later studies, generally without success.

In 2004, a reporter for the London *Sunday Times* newspaper, Brian Deer, wrote an article in which he raised questions about possible conflicts of interest in Wakefield's research, an article that led to a much more detailed review of the research by the British General Medical Council (GMC). After an exhaustive study of the Wakefield research, the GMC presented a list of conclusions about Wakefield's work in January 2010 that included a list of four counts of dishonesty, 12 counts of abuse of developmentally challenged children, and three dozen charges of professional misconduct. The GMC struck Wakefield's name from the British medical register, and he is now prohibited from practicing medicine in the United Kingdom. At the same time, *The Lancet* withdrew Wakefield's original paper, and 11 of his 12 coauthors retracted their approval of the research underlying the paper.

Andrew Jeremy Wakefield was born in 1957 to a family with a long history in medicine. His mother was a general practitioner and his father, a neurologist. He attended King Edward's School in Bath and then matriculated at St. Mary's Hospital Medical School (now the Imperial College School of Medicine). He received his MD in 1981 and was made a fellow of the Royal College of Surgeons in 1985. A year later, Wakefield received a Wellcome Trust Traveling Fellowship that allowed him to take a position at the University of Toronto, where he engaged in research on tissue rejection in organ transplantations. At the conclusion of his fellowship, Wakefield returned to England, where he joined the staff of the Royal Free Hospital in London. His special area of interest there was on liver transplantation procedures. It was during this period, in about 1996, during which Wakefield and his team began the controversial research on the relationship among exposure to the MMR vaccine, gastrointestinal disorders, and autism that led to their 1998 paper.

For parents of autistic children, and for those concerned about the possibility of their children's becoming autistic, Wakefield's research was a Godsend. It provided an answer to the vexing question which had puzzled researchers for years: What is it that causes autism? Wakefield's answer to that question was somewhat more nuanced than sometimes appeared in the popular press. "For the vast majority of children," he said, "the MMR vaccine is fine. But," he went on, "I believe there are sufficient anxieties for a case to be made to administer the three vaccinations separately. I do not think that the long-term safety trials of MMR are sufficient for giving the three vaccines together." That statement was sufficient to seal Wakefield's place in the history of medical discoveries for many parents.

In the midst of the controversy surrounding his work, Wakefield left the United Kingdom in 2001 and moved to the United States, where he is also not licensed to practice. Instead, he took a research position at the International Child Development Resource Center, in Melbourne, Florida, an organization that seeks to find and treat the causes of childhood developmental disorders. In 2004, a group of parents and professionals sympathetic to Wakefield's research established a new facility for him in Austin, Texas, known as Thoughtful House (now The Johnson Center for Child Health and Development). Wakefield served there until 2010 when he resigned, apparently in response to the actions taken against him by the GMC.

Wakefield has never admitted to any false doing in his research and has called Deer "a hit man who was brought in to take [me] down." He has written and spoken extensively about his research on vaccines and autism and about the campaign to deny him of his career and his life. He has recounted his side of this story in a popular book, *Callous Disregard: Autism and Vaccines: The Truth Behind a Tragedy* (Skyhorse Publishing, 2010). In 2012, Wakefield filed suit against Brian Deer for "false and defamatory accusations" against him contained in Deer's articles on the MMR-autism controversy. Although largely dismissed by the medical profession and a large portion of the general public, Wakefield remains immensely popular among a group of individuals for whom the idea of a vaccine-MMR connection is eminently reasonable and likely. Even at the end of 2012, a number of blogs were available on the Internet at which Wakefield's supporters could express their belief in and hopes for his theories about the causes of autism.

Lady Mary Wortley Montagu (1689–1762)

Lady Montagu was an aristocrat, socialite, writer, and early spokesperson for feminist issues. She is perhaps best known today for her advocacy of vaccination as protection against smallpox. Although her suggestions were largely derided and ignored by the general public and most public health experts in Great Britain, she was able to convince members of the royal family of the necessity, safety, and effectiveness as a protection against smallpox and, thus, eventually established the practice with the royal imprimatur in Great Britain.

Lady Montagu was born as Mary Pierrepont in London on May 15, 1689. She was the eldest daughter of Evelyn Pierrepont, the fifth Earl of Kingston-upon-Hull, and Lady Mary Fielding, daughter of William, Earl of Denbigh. She was reputed to have been a bright child who mastered Latin by the age of eight. After her mother's death in childbirth for her fourth child, Mary was raised first by her paternal grandmother, and later by her father. One historian has observed that her father always "enjoyed the company of women" and, after his four daughters were grown, "married women younger than any of them." In any case, Mary assumed the responsibilities of "head of the household" at a very young age, hardly before she was even a young woman herself.

When she came of age, Mary's father promised her hand in marriage to an older man, Clotworthy Skeffington, who was, according to one writer, "boorish," but apparently quite wealthy. In violation of her father's wishes and promises to that man, Mary eloped instead with one Edward Wortley Montagu, a lawyer and later lifelong Member of Parliament. Mary and Wortley Montagu had corresponded for seven years before they decided to marry. The couple eventually had one son, also named Edward Wortley Montagu, in 1713.

In December 1715, Lady Wortley Montagu contracted smallpox. Although she survived the disease, she (like many individuals who contracted smallpox) was badly scarred, leaving her without eyelashes and a deeply pitted skin. (Her younger brother had also died of the disease earlier.) This event was a devastating occurrence for a young woman of 26 years who had become locally famous for her charm and good looks.

In early 1716, King George I appointed Wortley Montagu his ambassador to the Ottoman Empire. The Wortley Montagus left for their new position in August of that year, stopping for a period of time along the way in both Venice and Adrianople (now Edirne, Turkey) for short visits. The Wortley Montagus remained in Constantinople for only two years, having been recalled to London in October 1718. However, those two years were probably the most famous and productive years in Mary Wortley Montagu's life. During that time, she wrote a series of letters to relatives and friends in England later to become known as the Letters from Turkey. In the letters, she provided one of the most comprehensive and incisive descriptions of Islamic life then available to the Western world. While in Constantinople, the Wortley Montagus also had a second child, a daughter also named Mary Wortley Montagu, in 1718.

From a medical and health perspective, the most important aspect of Mary Wortley Montagu's letters was her description of smallpox vaccination, a procedure largely unknown and unused in England at the time. She described how old women with special knowledge of the procedure traveled from house to house every September offering to carry out a procedure they called *engrafting*. That procedure involved the placement of small amounts of smallpox material into a half dozen open veins. She noted that individuals who had the treatment often developed small numbers of barely visible scars, but that no one she knew of had ever died of the procedure. She was so convinced of the value of the procedure (and so struck by her own experience and that of her brother) that she had her own son vaccinated against the disease.

After the Wortley Montagus returned to England in 1718, she pursued her interest in vaccination. In 1721, a smallpox epidemic struck England, and Mary insisted on having her then three-year-old daughter vaccinated against the disease. She also encouraged the then-princess of Wales (and later Queen Caroline) to conduct a series of tests of the vaccination process. In the first test, a group of seven prisoners awaiting execution were vaccinated against and then exposed to smallpox, with all surviving (and then being granted their freedom). In a second test, six orphan children were also vaccinated and challenged with the disease, with all subjects again surviving. Based on the results of these tests, the princess convinced King George I to have two of his grandchildren (the princess' children) to be vaccinated against smallpox. They received the procedure and survived.

The Wortley Montagus lived, apparently happily, for another 20 years in England. In 1739, Mary decided, for reasons that are not clear, to leave England on her own and take up residence in Italy. She never saw her husband again, although they corresponded regularly and apparently remained on good terms. In spite of the damage that smallpox had done to her famous beauty, Mary apparently remained attractive to many men and is reputed to have engaged in a number of amorous affairs. One of the most famous of those affairs was that involving Francesco Algarottim, Count Algarotti, with whom she exchanged a number of rather vivid love letters during her time in Italy. Mary finally returned to England in 1761, largely at the urging of her daughter. By that time, however, she had developed breast cancer and survived only a short while. She died in London on August 21, 1762 at the age of 73.

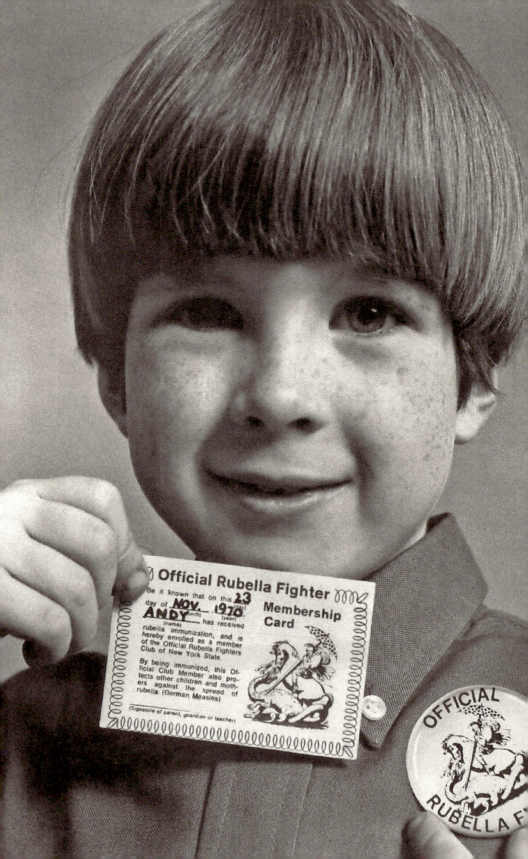

Official Rubella Fighter
Be it known that on this **23**
day of **NOV.** **1970**
(month) (year)
ANDY has received
(name)
rubella immunization, and is
hereby enrolled as a member
of the Official Rubella Fighters
Club of New York State.

By being immunized, this Official Club Member also protects other children and mothers against the spread of
rubella (German Measles).

(Signature of parent, guardian or teacher)

Membership Card

OFFICIAL
RUBELLA F

This chapter provides some relevant data and documents concerning the history of immunization practices throughout the world. The Data section provides basic information on current and historical trends on immunization practices in the United States and other parts of the world. The Documents section which follows is arranged in chronological order and includes excerpts from important committee and commission reports; from bills, acts, and laws; and from important legal cases.

Data

Table 5.1: National and State Vaccination Coverage among Children Aged 19–35 Months—United States, 2010

The Centers for Disease Control and Prevention (CDC) conducts annual surveys to determine the extent to which American children are being vaccinated against certain common diseases. Table 5.1 shows these data for a number of diseases for 2010, the most recent year for which data are currently available.

Table 5.2: Recommended Immunization Schedule

Recommended immunization schedules are announced and updated by both international and national organizations on a regular basis. The schedule most recently announced in the United States (December 23, 2011) is shown in Table 5.2.

A boy displays his "Official Rubella Fighter Membership Card" and button after being immunized for rubella during the "rubella umbrella" campaign of the late 1960s, a predecessor to later government-sponsored measles eradication campaigns. (Centers for Disease Control)

Table 5.1   National and State Vaccination Coverage among Children Aged 19–35 Months—United States, 2010

State	MMR (≥1 dose; %)	PCV (≥4 doses; %)	Hep B (birth; %)	Hep A (≥2 doses; %)	Rotavirus (%)	Hib (%)
United States	91.5	83.3	64.1	49.7	59.2	72.7
Alabama	95.4	86.1	70.7	50.5	63.4	72.4
Alaska	88.4	75.7	71.2	44.7	47.1	66.1
Arizona	87.7	79.9	80.4	51.0	60.7	71.1
Arkansas	90.5	79.5	82.4	34.2	48.5	74.5
California	91.4	83.5	53.0	53.4	58.9	71.0
Colorado	89.3	81.6	57.6	42.0	55.0	68.3
Connecticut	97.8	91.1	60.0	48.5	61.8	79.4
Delaware	94.0	87.9	69.3	62.0	82.1	71.9
District of Columbia	94.7	88.0	63.5	55.8	52.7	78.8
Florida	94.1	88.1	52.3	49.6	59.7	80.5
Georgia	91.5	86.3	74.9	64.4	59.0	74.7
Hawaii	93.2	83.0	71.5	44.9	52.1	76.0
Idaho	87.2	79.7	65.2	44.2	50.4	66.3
Illinois	90.5	87.1	66.1	45.2	60.3	75.1
Indiana	92.3	80.2	77.9	46.9	54.3	71.6
Iowa	93.8	87.6	52.3	55.8	66.1	77.8
Kansas	90.0	85.3	80.1	49.7	58.9	78.6
Kentucky	89.5	77.7	83.3	45.6	57.5	68.9
Louisiana	89.7	84.3	61.6	51.4	57.9	70.9
Maine	90.9	81.6	72.0	27.2	42.1	72.7

Maryland	90.5	75.6	69.0	46.0	53.4	65.9
Massachusetts	92.3	90.4	67.3	51.1	70.9	78.1
Michigan	91.1	88.1	80.3	45.0	54.3	81.3
Minnesota	92.7	88.7	46.8	49.3	67.5	75.7
Mississippi	93.8	84.3	69.1	40.7	56.9	77.9
Missouri	90.4	76.2	64.8	44.4	59.3	67.9
Montana	85.1	72.6	67.8	35.5	54.9	64.9
Nebraska	94.2	90.4	66.7	60.3	73.2	79.9
Nevada	87.0	70.8	66.6	54.8	49.4	61.3
New Hampshire	95.8	93.2	62.8	59.7	73.1	81.0
New Jersey	86.1	82.4	37.2	40.8	53.9	62.6
New Mexico	88.8	78.2	60.0	51.1	53.9	68.3
New York	89.3	72.8	50.5	37.7	48.5	64.1
North Carolina	94.5	87.5	75.0	48.1	69.6	77.1
North Dakota	92.6	89.4	79.5	61.1	73.4	79.8
Ohio	93.6	81.8	73.5	46.2	57.2	76.2
Oklahoma	91.0	74.5	66.4	56.6	44.4	62.9
Oregon	92.8	87.7	61.7	55.6	52.8	73.4
Pennsylvania	92.3	87.2	71.5	54.8	66.1	77.1
Rhode Island	95.8	82.3	69.7	54.2	76.7	74.1
South Carolina	91.7	88.1	67.4	47.4	62.9	76.9
South Dakota	92.1	76.4	62.4	33.1	46.8	67.0

(Continued)

Table 5.1 *(Continued)*

State	MMR (≥1 dose; %)	PCV (≥4 doses; %)	Hep B (birth; %)	Hep A (≥2 doses; %)	Rotavirus (%)	Hib (%)
Tennessee	93.9	84.3	55.3	59.9	65.9	77.8
Texas	91.8	83.0	69.6	54.9	61.9	70.9
Utah	85.5	78.7	79.8	49.6	65.6	69.5
Vermont	92.7	84.2	21.4	38.0	51.8	69.7
Virginia	92.3	84.9	58.3	50.0	66.9	72.8
Washington	89.8	82.9	77.3	44.9	50.9	71.2
West Virginia	92.0	74.3	66.7	54.0	51.0	64.1
Wisconsin	93.2	88.4	61.4	52.1	64.7	82.7
Wyoming	92.5	79.6	58.4	33.5	53.5	64.7

Key:
MMR = measles, mumps, rubella
PCV = pneumococcal conjugate vaccine
Hep B = hepatitis B
Hep A = hepatitis A
Hib = Influenza

Source: Centers for Disease Control and Prevention. "National and State Vaccination Coverage among Children Aged 19–35 Months–United States, 2010." *Morbidity and Mortality Weekly Report* 60, no.34 (September 2, 2011): 1157–1163. http://www.cdc.gov/mmwr/preview/mmwrhtml/mm6034a2.htm?s_cid=mm6034a2_w.

Table 5.2 Recommended Immunization Schedule[1]

Vaccine	Age											
	Months									Years		
	Birth	1	2	4	6	9	12	15	18	19–23	2–3	4–6
Hepatitis B	Hep B	Hep B					Hep B					
Rotavirus			RV	RV	RV							
Diphtheria, tetanus, pertussis			DTaP	DTaP	DTaP			DTaP				DTaP
Haemophilus influenzae type b4			Hib	Hib	Hib		Hib					
Pneumococcal			PCV	PCV	PCV		PCV					
Inactivate poliovirus			IPV	IPV			IPV					IPV
Influenza								Influenza (yearly)				
Measles, mumps, rubella							MMR					MMR
Varicella							Varicella					Varicella
Hepatitis A							Hep A (Dose 1)				Hep A series	

[1]Recommendations age birth–6 years. For recommendations, age 7–18, see source chart cited below.

Key:
Hep B = Hepatitis B vaccine
RV = Rotavirus vaccine
DTaP = Diphtheria and tetanus toxoids and acellular pertussis (DTaP) vaccine
Hib = *Haemophilus influenzae* type b conjugate vaccine
PCV = Pneumococcal vaccines
IPV = Inactivated poliovirus vaccine
MMR = Measles, mumps, and rubella vaccine
Hep A = Hepatitis A vaccine

Note: Detailed recommendations contain a number of special provisions and recommendations. See source chart below for full details of recommended schedule.

Source: Centers for Disease Control and Prevention. "Recommended Immunization Schedules for Persons Aged Through 18 Years, United States, 2012." http://www.cdc.gov/vaccines/recs/schedules/downloads/child/0-18yrs-11x17-fold-pr.pdf

Table 5.3: Approved Vaccines and Their Effectiveness

A number of vaccines have been approved for use in the United States over the past half century or more, all with rather dramatic effects on the diseases for which they were designed. Table 5.3 summarizes some basic information about these vaccines.

Table 5.4: Coverage of Two Major Vaccination Schedules Worldwide, 1980–2010

The fraction of children who have received the vaccines generally recommended by public health authorities varies world-

Table 5.3 Approved Vaccines and Their Effectiveness

Disease	Date Vaccine Approved	Estimated Annual Deaths, 20th Century	Estimated Annual Deaths, 2010	Percent Reduction in Deaths
Tetanus	1943	580	26	96
Polio	1955/1963	16,316	0	100
Measles	1963	530,217	63	>99
Mumps	1967	162,344	2,612	98
Rubella	1969	47,745	5	>99
		152	0	100
Hepatitis B	1981	66,232	9,419	86
Haemophilus influenzae type b conjugate	1987	20,000	240	99
Hepatitis A	1995	117,333	8,493	93
Varicella	1995	4,085,120	408,572	90
Diphtheria (DTP)	1970	21,053	0	100
Pertussis (DTP)	1970	200,752	27,538	86
Tetanus (DTP)	1970	580	26	96
Smallpox	1931	29,005	0	100
Rotavirus	2006	62,500[1]	28,125[1]	55

[1]Hospitalizations

Source: Hinman, Alan R., Walter A. Orenstein, and Anne Schuchat. "Vaccine-Preventable Diseases, Immunizations, and MMWR—961–2011." *Morbidity and Mortality Weekly* 60, no. 4 (October 7, 2011): 49–57.

wide, depending on a variety of factors. The World Health Organization regularly conducts surveys to determine this information for all regions of the world. Table 5.4 summarizes these data for two major vaccine schedules, one in which children have received three doses of the DPT vaccine, and another in which they have received some form of a measles-antigen-containing vaccine.

Table 5.4 Coverage of Two Major Vaccination Schedules Worldwide, 1980–2010

DTP3 Coverage

UNICF Region	1980	1981	1982	1983	1984	1985	1986	1987	1988	1989
Central and Eastern Europe and CIS	76	84	81	79	79	81	75	80	78	74
East Asia and Pacific	6	8	8	46	57	65	68	68	83	87
Eastern and Southern Africa	9	17	18	31	37	40	44	51	52	55
Industrialized Countries	62	72	74	76	82	80	88	89	89	90
Latin America and the Caribbean	37	42	47	49	56	56	56	59	62	64
Middle East and North Africa	24	25	31	33	40	57	63	65	76	81
South Asia	5	6	11	13	16	19	21	29	38	49
West and Central Africa	1	5	6	7	13	20	25	31	36	42

UNICF Region	1990	1991	1992	1993	1994	1995	1996	1997	1998	1999
Central and Eastern Europe and CIS	75	79	80	75	85	82	85	88	90	91
East Asia and Pacific	89	87	85	8i3	82	79	81	82	82	82
Eastern and Southern Africa	62	57	56	61	66	67	68	66	65	65
Industrialized Countries	89	89	88	87	91	91	94	91	92	89
Latin America and the Caribbean	68	78	77	78	80	83	82	83	86	89
Middle East and North Africa	84	78	80	81	79	81	83	82	83	85
South Asia	67	57	55	59	64	68	64	62	65	64
West and Central Africa	49	37	40	36	41	38	34	32	38	40

(Continued)

Table 5.4 (Continued)

UNICF Region	2000	2001	2002	2003	2004	2005	2006	2007	2008	2009	2010
Central and Eastern Europe and CIS	93	93	91	87	92	94	94	98	95	95	95
East Asia and Pacific	83	83	82	84	85	85	89	90	92	94	94
Eastern and Southern Africa	66	69	70	70	73	74	75	77	78	77	80
Industrialized Countries	91	90	91	92	92	93	93	93	92	93	93
Latin America and the Caribbean	91	90	91	92	92	93	93	93	92	93	93
Middle East and North Africa	87	87	85	86	86	88	88	88	90	90	91
South Asia	64	63	62	64	67	71	71	74	75	76	76
West and Central Africa	44	41	43	46	51	55	58	62	65	72	72

MCV Coverage

UNICF Region	1980	1981	1982	1983	1984	1985	1986	1987	1988	1989
Central and Eastern Europe and CIS	73	82	85	89	89	89	78	80	84	83
East Asia and Pacific	1	1	1	53	60	67	56	67	82	85
Eastern and Southern Africa	8	17	20	34	38	42	48	51	53	58
Industrialized Countries	52	59	61	66	70	72	75	74	81	84
Latin America and the Caribbean	42	49	48	48	52	60	61	60	66	70
Middle East and North Africa	20	23	30	29	33	55	58	61	73	78
South Asia	0	0	1	3	5	6	14	25	33	44
West and Central Africa	4	8	9	9	15	24	32	37	43	50

(Continued)

Table 5.4 (Continued)

UNICF Region	1990	1991	1992	1993	1994	1995	1996	1997	1998	1999
Central and Eastern Europe and CIS	85	83	81	82	81	82	85	89	90	91
East Asia and Pacific	89	85	82	79	75	78	83	82	82	83
Eastern and Southern Africa	61	58	57	60	66	64	67	66	67	64
Industrialized Countries	83	82	81	82	86	88	90	90	89	90
Latin America and the Caribbean	76	80	83	82	82	85	84	89	90	92
Middle East and North Africa	79	78	79	80	80	81	84	83	85	85
South Asia	56	47	53	59	66	69	64	57	54	56
West and Central Africa	50	47	41	41	44	44	41	40	41	40

Region											
Central and Eastern Europe and CIS	93	94	92	91	92	95	96	96	96	96	96
East Asia and Pacific	83	83	83	84	85	85	9	91	93	94	95
Eastern and Southern Africa	64	67	68	68	71	69	73	76	76	77	79
Industrialized Countries	91	91	91	92	92	93	93	93	93	93	93
Latin America and the Caribbean	93	94	93	95	94	93	95	94	95	94	93
Middle East and North Africa	86	85	85	85	86	86	86	87	87	89	90
South Asia	57	58	58	60	64	68	73	76	77	77	77
West and Central Africa	46	44	44	49	52	56	59	59	62	68	71

Key: DPT3 Coverage = Immunization for third in trivalent DPT vaccine

MCV Coverage = Measles-containing vaccine

CIS = Commonwealth of Independent States (somewhat comparable to former Soviet Union)

Source: UNICEF. "Immunization Summary: A Statistical Reference Containing Data Through 2010." Geneva: World Health Organization, 2012. http://www.childinfo.org/files/immunization_summary_en.pdf. Used by permission of the World Health Organization and the United Nations Children's Fund (UNICEF).

Documents

Letter from Lady Mary Wortley Montagu about Variolation in Turkey (1717)

In 1717, Lady Wortley Montagu accompanied her husband, the newly named British ambassador to the court of the Ottoman Empire, to Turkey. There she observed the traditional process of variolation practiced by groups of older Turkish women. She wrote to her sister about the practice, expressing her approval of it and her intent to "spread the word" about variolation if and when she returned to Great Britain.

A propos of distempers, I am going to tell you a thing that I am sure will make you wish yourself here. The small-pox, so fatal, and so general amongst us, is here entirely harmless by the invention of ingrafting, which is the term they give it. There is a set of old women who make it their business to perform the operation every autumn, in the month of September, when the great heat is abated. People send to one another to know if any of their family has a mind to have the small-pox; they make parties for this purpose, and when they are met (commonly fifteen or sixteen together), the old woman comes with a nut-shell full of the matter of the best sort of small-pox, and asks what veins you please to have opened. She immediately rips open that you offer to her with a large needle (which gives you no more pain than a common scratch), and puts into the vein as much venom as can lie upon the head of her needle, and after binds up the little wound with a hollow bit of shell; and in this manner opens four or five veins. The Grecians have commonly the superstition of opening one in the midde [*sic*] of the forehead, in each arm, and on the breast, to mark the sign of the cross; but this has a very ill effect, all these wounds leaving little scars, and is not done by those that are not superstitious, who choose to have them in the legs, or that part of the arm that is concealed. The children or young patients play together all the rest of the day, and are in perfect health to the eighth. Then the fever begins to seize them, and they keep their beds two days, very seldom three. They have very rarely above twenty or thirty in their faces, which never mark; and in eight days' time they are as well as before their illness. Where they are wounded, there remain running sores during the distemper, which I don't doubt is a great relief to it. Every year thousands undergo this operation; and the French embassador [*sic*] says pleasantly, that they take the small-pox here by way of diversion, as they take the waters in other countries. There is no example of any one that has died in it; and you may believe I am very well satisfied of the safety of this experiment, since I intend to try it on my dear little son.

I am patriot enough to take pains to bring this useful invention into fashion in England; and I should not fail to write to some of our doctors very particularly about it, if I knew any one of them that I thought had virtue enough to destroy such a considerable branch of their revenue for the good of mankind. But that distemper is too beneficial to them not to expose to all their resentment the hardy wight [*sic*] that should undertake to put an end to it. Perhaps, if I live to return, I may, however, have courage to war with them. Upon this occasion admire the heroism in the heart of Your Friend, &c.

Source: Melville, Lewis. "Lady Mary Wortley Montague: Her Life and Letters (1689–1762)." http://www.gutenberg. org/files/10590/10590.txt. Accessed on May 12, 2012.

Boylston's Inoculation Efforts in Colonial Boston (1726)

One of the earliest and strongest proponents of inoculation against smallpox in the early Colonies was Dr. Zabdiel Boylston, who conducted an extended series of experiments and inoculations in the 1720s. During this period, he carried out 244 inoculations, and two of his colleagues performed an additional 36 inoculations, with only six deaths among their subjects. (In the following passage, Boylston explains the circumstances of those six fatalities.) In 1726, Boylston wrote an account of his work, which described in

*some detail the inoculations he carried out in Boston and nearby
towns and the results produced.*

I began the practice indeed from a short Consideration
thereof; for my Children, whose Lives were very dear to me,
were daily in danger of taking the Infection, by my visiting the
Sick in the natural Way; and although there arose such a Cloud
of Opposers at the Beginning, yet finding my Account in the
Success, and early Circumstances of my Patients (with the En-
couragement of the good Ministers) I resolved to carry it on for
the saving of Lives, not regarding any, or all of the Menaces,
and Opposition that were made against it.

I have not, in this Practice, left any room for any one to cavil,
and say, that my Experiments have not been fair, and full Proofs,
that inoculating the Small-Pox is a perfect Means of moderat-
ing that Distemper, to the greatest Demonstration. This, the
warmest Opposers of that Practice, who have seen any fair Trials
made, are convinc'd of; and the only Difficulty of convincing all
Mankind, is how to make them Eye-witnesses to a Number sick
of the Small-Pox in both ways of Infection; and this would do it
at once, and very much to their Satisfaction in, and Approbation
of this Method. And here it should be considered how rashly our
Patients, even whole Families together, rushed into this, without
any Physical Preparation, or other needful Provision, especially
in such cold Season as November and December, being convinced of the Success of this Method. . . . I have not used this
Practice only to the healthful and strong, but to the weak and
diseased, the aged and the young: Not only to the rich, but have
carried it into the houses of the poor, and laid down whole Families; an tho' thro' my own Hurry in Business, and their living
out of Town, I have been forced to leave them to the Manage-
ments of inexperienced Nurses, yet they all did very well.

And as to the six who died under Inoculation, I would ob-
serve that Mrs. Dixwell, we have great Reason to believe, was
infected before. Mr. White, thro' splenetic Delusions, died
rather from Abstinence than the Small-Pox. Mrs. Scarborough

and the Indian Girl died of accidents by taking cold. Mrs. Wells and Searle were Persons worn out with Age and Diseases, and very likely these two were infected before. Neither can it be said that there was one found sound and healthful Person amongst them. . . .

When the World has had Experience of the good Effects of this Method, it will no longer remain a Doubt; but it will be made use of, and acknowledged to be the most certain procurative Means to produce the better Sort; & the only preventive Remedy against the worst and confluent Sort.

And it is, and shall be acknowledged, to the Praise and Glory of God! that whereas a most wild, cruel, fierce, and violent Distemper, and which has destroy'd Millions of Lives, is now (by that happy Discovery of its Transplantation) become tractable, safe, and gentle.

Source: Boylston, Zabdiel. *Small-Pox Inoculated in New England.* London: S. Chandler, 1726, 12, 58. http://pds.lib. harvard.edu/pds/view/8290362?n=1&imagesize=1200&jp 2Res=.25&printThumbnails=no.

An Act to Secure General Vaccination (1855)

In 1855, the Commonwealth of Massachusetts adopted the first law requiring that all children be vaccinated before enrolling in school. The text of that law is reprinted below, in its original and uncorrected form.

Chap. 0414 An Act to secure General Vaccination.

Be it enacted by the Senate and House of Representatives, in General Court assembled, and by the authority of the same, as follows:

Sect. 1. Parents and guardians of youth, shall cause the children under their care to be vaccinated before they attain the age of two years.

Sect. 2. The school committee of the several towns and cities, shall not allow any child to be admitted to, or connected with the public schools, who has not been duly vaccinated.

Sect. 3. The selectmen x)f [*sic*] the several towns, and the mayor and aldermen of every city, shall enforce the vaccination of all the inhabitants of said towns and cities; and every parent or guardian of youth who shall not cause his or her child or ward to be vaccinated, (the said child or ward being more than two years of age,) shall be liable to a fine of five dollars for each and every year's neglect, to be recovered on complaint of the selectmen of the town, or of the mayor and aldermen of the city, for the benefit and use of said town or city.

Sect. 4. The selectmen of the several towns, and the mayor and aldermen of every city, shall enforce re-vaccination whenever they shall judge the public health requires the same: provided, that none shall be required to be re-vaccinated who shall prove, to the satisfaction of said selectmen, or mayor and aldermen, that they have been successfully vaccinated, or re-vaccinated, within five years next preceding; and any neglect of such requirement of the selectmen, or of the mayor and aldermen, shall render the person or persons guilty of such neglect, liable to a fine as above, to be recovered as aforesaid, for the use of said town or city.

Sect. 5. It shall be the duty of all incorporated manufacturing companies, of all the superintendents of almshouses, State reform schools, lunatic hospitals, and of all other places where the poor or sick are received, and of masters, of houses of correction, jailers, or keepers of prisons, the warden of the State Prison, and of the superintendents or officers Of all other institutions supported wholly or in part by the State, to cause all the inmates of the above-named institutions to be properly vaccinated. And all persons hereafter received into such institutions shall be vaccinated immediately on their entrance, unless such persons can show sufficient evidence of previous vaccination within the term of five years.

Sect. 6. The towns and cities shall be at the expense of furnishing the means of vaccination to such of their own citizens as may be unable to meet the same. All public institutions and incorporated manufacturing companies, named in section five, shall provide the means of vaccination at the expense of said institutions and corporations.

Sect. 7. This act shall take effect on and after its passage. [Approved by the Governor, May 19, 1855.]

> **Source:** The State Library of Massachusetts. "1855 Chap. 0414. An Act to Secure General Vaccination." http://archives.lib. state.ma.us/bitstream/handle/2452/97237/1855acts0414. txt?sequence=1

Jacobson v. Massachusetts, 197 U.S. 11 (1905)

In February 1902, an outbreak of smallpox in the city of Cambridge, Massachusetts, prompted the city council to adopt a regulation requiring all citizens of the city to be vaccinated against the disease. One such citizen, Henning Jacobson, refused to be vaccinated, claiming that the city's regulation violated his Constitutional rights, particularly those guaranteed by the Preamble to the Constitution. When Jacobson was arrested, he brought suit against the Commonwealth, a case that he lost in trial court, the court of appeals, and the Massachusetts Supreme Court. He then appealed his conviction to the U.S. Supreme Court, which ruled in 1905 that the state was justified and constitutionally permitted to require universal vaccination against infectious diseases. The decision was the first occasion on which the U.S. Supreme Court invoked the rights of a state to adopt public health laws. [Omitted citations are indicated by brackets, {}.]
[The Court begins its opinion by pointing out that the Preamble to the Constitution is not the source of any substantive powers granted by the Constitution itself, so that Jacobson's appeal to the Preamble is in and of itself moot. It then goes on to consider any respect in which the Constitution may limit the rights of a state to require immunization of its citizens against disease. It poses the question:]

Is the [Massachusetts state] statute [requiring vaccination] . . . inconsistent with the liberty which the Constitution

of the United States secures to every person against depriva-
tion by the State?

[The Court first affirms that:]

According to settled principles, the police power of a State
must be held to embrace, at least, such reasonable regulations
established directly by legislative enactment as will protect
the public health and the public safety. {} It is equally true
that the State may invest local bodies called into existence
for purposes of local administration with authority in some
appropriate way to safeguard the public health and the public
safety. The mode or manner in which those results are to be
accomplished is within the discretion of the State, subject,
of course, so far as Federal power is concerned, only to the
condition that no rule prescribed by a State, nor any regulation adopted by a local governmental agency acting under
the sanction of state legislation, shall contravene the Constitution of the United States or infringe any right granted or
secured by that instrument.

[The issue facing the Court, then, is:]

We come, then, to inquire whether any right given or secured by the Constitution is invaded by the statute as inter-
preted by the state court.
*[The Court recognized that some state health laws mainly infringe
on a person's personal liberties, but declared that such a situation
may be necessary in dire health conditions. It concluded that:]*

If the mode adopted by the Commonwealth of Massachusetts for the protection of its local communities against smallpox proved to be distressing, inconvenient or objectionable to
some—if nothing more could be reasonably affirmed of the
statute in question—the answer is that it was the duty of the
constituted authorities primarily to keep in view the welfare,
comfort and safety of the many, and not permit the interests

of the many to be subordinated to the wishes or convenience of the few. There is, of course, a sphere within which the individual may assert the supremacy of his own will and rightfully dispute the authority of any human government, especially of any free government existing under a written constitution, to interfere with the exercise of that will. But it is equally true that, in every well ordered society charged with the duty of conserving the safety of its members the rights of the individual in respect of his liberty may at times, under the pressure of great dangers, be subjected to such restraint, to be enforced by reasonable regulations, as the safety of the general public may demand.

[The Court concludes with a warning as to the limitations of its ruling.]

Until otherwise informed by the highest court of Massachusetts, we are not inclined to hold that the statute establishes the absolute rule that an adult must be vaccinated if it be apparent or can be shown with reasonable certainty that he is not at the time a fit subject of [*sic*] vaccination or that vaccination, by reason of his then condition, would seriously impair his health or probably cause his death. No such case is here presented. It is the case of an adult who, for aught that appears, was himself in perfect health and a fit subject of vaccination, and yet, while remaining in the community, refused to obey the statute and the regulation adopted in execution of its provisions for the protection of the public health and the public safety, confessedly endangered by the presence of a dangerous disease

We now decide only that the statute covers the present case, and that nothing clearly appears that would justify this court in holding it to be unconstitutional and inoperative in its application to the plaintiff in error. .

[Jacobson was ordered to pay the $5 fine assessed when he first refused to be vaccinated.]

Source: *"Jacobson v. Massachusetts—*197 U.S. 11 (1905)." http://supreme.justia.com/cases/federal/us/197/11/case. html. Accessed on March 19, 2012.

Poliomyelitis Vaccination Assistance Act, P.l. 377 Chapter 863 (1955)

Almost as soon as the first polio vaccine became available in 1955, the U.S. Congress passed a law providing financial assistance to states to encourage the widespread vaccination of individuals against the disease. The act is significant because it is the first time that the U.S. Congress becomes involved in the immunization of U.S. citizens. The relative sections of the law are as follows:

SEC. 2. There is hereby authorized to be appropriated, to remain available until February 15, 1956, such sums as may be necessary for making payments to States which have submitted, and had approved by the Surgeon General, applications for grants under this Act.

SEC. 3. (a) From the sums appropriated pursuant to section 2, the Surgeon General shall allot to each State which has an application approved pursuant to section 4:

(1) an amount equal to 33% [*sic*] per centum of the number of unvaccinated eligible persons in such State multiplied by the product of (A) the cost of the poliomyelitis vaccine per eligible person, and (B) the State's allotment percentage; and

(2) an additional amount equal to 20 per centum of allotments available to the State under paragraph (1) of this subsection, such additional amount to be available for expenditure only in accordance with the provisions of section 6 (b) of this Act.

[Section (b) then provides more details as to how funds will be distributed.]

State Applications for Funds

[Remaining sections of the act prescribe the way funds allotted to states are to be used for vaccination programs. Among these provisions, as an example, is the following:]
(b) [State applications must provide]

that in poliomyelitis vaccination programs conducted by public agencies in the State no means test or other discrimination based on financial ability of individuals will be imposed to limit the eligibility of persons to receive vaccination against poliomyelitis. . . .

Source: Public Law 377–August 12, 1955, 704–705.

Vaccination Assistance Act of 1962 (42 USC Sec. 247b)

The Poliomyelitis Vaccination Assistance Act and the newly introduced Sabin vaccine proved to be so effective in preventing polio that the U.S. Congress decided in 1962 to pass a more comprehensive act authorizing the use of federal funds to initiate and support immunization programs against a number of infectious diseases. The main provisions of the act were as follows:

Sec. 247b. Project grants for preventive health services
(a) Grant authority
The Secretary may make grants to States, and in consultation with State health authorities, to political subdivisions of States and to other public entities to assist them in meeting the costs of establishing and maintaining preventive health service programs.

[Among the specific provisions of the act are the following:]

(i)   Technical assistance
The Secretary may provide technical assistance to States, State health authorities, and other public entities in connection with the operation of their preventive health service programs . . .

(A)   research into the prevention and control of diseases that may be prevented through vaccination;

(B)   demonstration projects for the prevention and control of such diseases;

(C)   public information and education programs for the prevention and control of such diseases; and

(D)   education, training, and clinical skills improvement activities in the prevention and control of such diseases for health professionals (including allied health personnel). . . .

(A)   providing immunization reminders or recalls for target populations of clients, patients, and consumers;

(B)   educating targeted populations and health care providers concerning immunizations in combination with one or more other interventions;

(C)   reducing out-of-pocket costs for families for vaccines and their administration;

(D)   carrying out immunization-promoting strategies for participants or clients of public programs, including assessments of immunization status, referrals to health care providers, education, provision of on-site immunizations, or incentives for immunization;

(E)   providing for home visits that promote immunization through education, assessments of need, referrals, provision of immunizations, or other services;

(F)   providing reminders or recalls for immunization providers;

(G)   conducting assessments of, and providing feedback to, immunization providers;

(H)   any combination of one or more interventions described in this paragraph; or

(I)   immunization information systems to allow all States to have electronic databases for immunization records. .

Source: 42 USC Sec. 247b. http://uscode.house.gov/down
load/pls/42C6A.txt.

National Childhood Vaccine Injury Act of 1986 (Public Law 99–660)

In 1986, the U.S. Congress passed the National Childhood Vaccine Injury Act, which had three major objectives: ensuring an adequate supply of safe and effective vaccines, providing a mechanism for stabilizing the price of vaccines, and creating a program for compensating individuals who developed medical problems as a consequence of being vaccinated. The program was designed as a no-fault alternative to the traditional tort system in which individuals who claimed to have been injured as a result of being vaccinated have to sue a vaccine manufacturer for compensation. The law is very long and complicated, but contains the following essential elements. Citations and footnotes are omitted in this selection. [Omissions of text are indicated by ellipses (. . .).]

Part 2—National Vaccine Injury Compensation Program Subpart a—Program Requirements

§300aa–10. Establishment of Program
(a) Program established
There is established the National Vaccine Injury Compensation Program to be administered by the Secretary [of Health and Human Services] under which compensation may be paid for a vaccine-related injury or death.
(b) Attorney's obligation
It shall be the ethical obligation of any attorney who is consulted by an individual with respect to a vaccine-related injury or death to advise such individual that compensation may be available under the program for such injury or death.
(c) Publicity
The Secretary shall undertake reasonable efforts to inform the public of the availability of the Program . . .

300aa–11. Petitions for compensation
(a) General rule

(1) A proceeding for compensation under the Program for a vaccine-related injury or death shall be initiated by service upon the Secretary and the filing of a petition containing the matter prescribed by subsection (c) of this section with the United States Court of Federal Claims. The clerk of the United States Court of Federal Claims shall immediately forward the filed petition to the chief special master for assignment to a special master under section 300aa–12(d)(1) of this title.

(2)(A) No person may bring a civil action for damages in an amount greater than $1,000 or in an unspecified amount against a vaccine administrator or manufacturer in a State or Federal court for damages arising from a vaccine-related injury or death associated with the administration of a vaccine after October 1, 1988, and no such court may award damages in an amount greater than $1,000 in a civil action for damages for such a vaccine-related injury or death, unless a petition has been filed, in accordance with section 300aa–16 of this title, for compensation under the Program for such injury or death and—

(i)(I) the United States Court of Federal Claims has issued a judgment under section 300aa–12 of this title on such petition, and

(II) such person elects under section 300aa–21(a) of this title to file such an action, or

(ii) such person elects to withdraw such petition under section 300aa–21(b) of this title or such petition is considered withdrawn under such section.

(B) If a civil action which is barred under subparagraph (A) is filed in a State or Federal court, the court shall dismiss the action. If a petition is filed under this section with respect to the injury or death for which such civil action was brought, the date such dismissed action was filed shall, for purposes of the limitations of actions prescribed by section 300aa–16 of this title, be considered the date the petition was filed if the petition was filed within one year of the date of the dismissal of the civil action.

(3) No vaccine administrator or manufacturer may be made a party to a civil action (other than a civil action which may be brought under paragraph (2)) for damages for a vaccine-related injury or death associated with the administration of a vaccine after October 1, 1988.

[The law then follows with a number of other restrictions against the filing of tort suits because of injuries from vaccinations.] . . .

(b) Petitioners

(1)(A) Except as provided in subparagraph (B), any person who has sustained a vaccine-related injury, the legal representative of such person if such person is a minor or is disabled, or the legal representative of any person who died as the result of the administration of a vaccine set forth in the Vaccine Injury Table may, if the person meets the requirements of subsection (c)(1) of this section, file a petition for compensation under the Program.

[The Vaccine Injury Table mentioned here lists a number of vaccines commonly in use, illnesses and injuries that may be associated with their use, and time periods associated with appearance of symptoms. The original Vaccine Injury Table has been revised and modified; the current form can be found online at http://www. hrsa.gov/vaccinecompensation/vaccineinjurytable.pdf.]

(B) No person may file a petition for a vaccine-related injury or death associated with a vaccine administered before October 1, 1988, if compensation has been paid under this part for 3500 petitions for such injuries or deaths.

(2) Only one petition may be filed with respect to each administration of a vaccine.

(c) Petition content

[This section contains detailed information about the material that must be included in a vaccine-injury petition.] . . .

§300aa–12. Court jurisdiction
(a) General rule

The United States Court of Federal Claims and the United States Court of Federal Claims special masters shall, in accordance with this section, have jurisdiction over proceedings to determine if a petitioner under section 300aa–11 of this title is entitled to compensation under the Program and the amount of such compensation. The United States Court of Federal Claims may issue and enforce such orders as the court deems necessary to assure the prompt payment of any compensation awarded.

(b) Parties

(1) In all proceedings brought by the filing of a petition under section 300aa–11(b) of this title, the Secretary shall be named as the respondent, shall participate, and shall be represented in accordance with section 518(a) of title 28.

(2) Within 30 days after the Secretary receives service of any petition filed under section 300aa–11 of this title the Secretary shall publish notice of such petition in the Federal Register. The special master designated with respect to such petition under subsection (c) of this section shall afford all interested persons an opportunity to submit relevant, written information—

(A) relating to the existence of the evidence described in section 300aa–13(a)(1)(B) of this title, or

(B) relating to any allegation in a petition with respect to the matters described in section 300aa–11(c)(1)(C)(ii) of this title.

(c) United States Court of Federal Claims special masters

(1) There is established within the United States Court of Federal Claims an office of special masters which shall consist of not more than 8 special masters. The judges of the United States Court of Federal Claims shall appoint the special

masters, 1 of whom, by designation of the judges of the United States Court of Federal Claims, shall serve as chief special master. The appointment and reappointment of the special masters shall be by the concurrence of a majority of the judges of the court.

(2) The chief special master and other special masters shall be subject to removal by the judges of the United States Court of Federal Claims for incompetency, misconduct, or neglect of duty or for physical or mental disability or for other good cause shown.

(3) A special master's office shall be terminated if the judges of the United States Court of Federal Claims determine, upon advice of the chief special master, that the services performed by that office are no longer needed. .

[Remaining portions of this section deal with the operation of the special masters program.]
[Remaining sections of the act discuss:
Determination of eligibility and compensation (§30011–13);
The Vaccine Injury Table (§30011–14);
Compensation (§30011–15);
Limitations of Actions (§30011–16);
Subrogation (§30011–17);
Repealed laws (§30011–18);
Creation of an Advisory Commission on Childhood Vaccines (§30011–19); and
Additional remedies (subpart b).

Source: "National Vaccine Injury Compensation Program." http://www.hrsa.gov/vaccinecompensation/authorizingleg-islation.pdf.

Measles Eradication Program (1996)

The first measles vaccine was licensed for use in the United States in 1963. Almost immediately, public health experts began imagining a world free of the disease. The U.S. Centers for Disease Control and Prevention has announced programs for eradicating measles in the United States in 1966, 1978, and 1996. The last of these eradication programs was developed in conjunction with the World Health Organization and the Pan American Health Organization. The target date for the elimination of measles worldwide was 2005–2010. Among the conclusions (C) and recommendations (R) made at the 1996 meeting were the following (deleted text is indicated by ellipses):

[C]: Based on the success of efforts to control measles in the Western Hemisphere and the United Kingdom, global measles eradication is technically feasible with available vaccines.

[R]: A goal of global measles eradication should be established, with a target date during 2005–2010. . . .

[C]: Existing vaccines are sufficient to eradicate measles, but eradication requires more than a routine one-dose vaccination strategy. However, no single two-dose approach is optimal for all countries.

[R]: Countries that adopt a strategy of measles elimination should implement some form of "catch-up" vaccination rather than simply adding a second dose to the routine vaccination schedule. All children must receive measles vaccine, and the "second dose" should also reach those who missed the first dose. . . .

[C]: Measles case surveillance is a critical component of any strategy to control measles, including strategies to eliminate or eradicate measles. The most important functions of surveillance are to assess the effectiveness of the strategy and to detect circulation of measles virus in a population. . . .

[R]: Surveillance for individual measles cases should be implemented at an early stage of the elimination program. . . .

[C]: Preventing measles outbreaks is more effective than trying to contain them. Mass vaccination campaigns undertaken in response to outbreaks are of limited usefulness in most countries because such efforts are costly, disruptive, and often ineffective by the time they are instituted.

[R]: Measles outbreaks should be treated as opportunities to reinforce surveillance, assess the health burden of continuing measles transmission, and identify appropriate measures to prevent future outbreaks. . . .

[C]: The major obstacles to measles eradication are perceptual, political, and financial. The full health impact of measles is often underestimated. Measles is frequently perceived as a minor illness of little consequence, particularly in industrialized countries. This perception may make it difficult to develop the political support necessary to carry out a successful global eradication effort.

[R]: Parents, medical practitioners, and public health professionals—particularly those in industrialized countries—must be educated about the global disease burden imposed by measles. . . .

Source: Centers for Disease Control and Prevention. "Measles Eradication: Recommendations from a Meeting Cosponsored by the World Health Organization, the Pan American Health Organization, and CDC." *MMWR* 46, RR-11 (1997): 15–18.

Project Bioshield Act, P.l. 108–276 (2004)

The U.S. Congress passed and President George W. Bush signed the Project Bioshield Act in 2004 as a means for increasing the nation's defensive capacity against possible terrorist attacks. The act authorized the Secretary of Health and Human Services to take a number of extraordinary steps to protect citizens against a variety of possible bioterrorist acts. Some major elements of the act are listed on the next page (deletions are indicated with ellipses). The selection that follows illustrates some problems involved in converting strategic planning for bioterrorism prevention into real-life programs.

An Act

To amend the Public Health Service Act to provide protections and countermeasures against chemical, radiological, or nuclear agents that may be used in a terrorist attack against the United States by giving the National Institutes of Health contracting flexibility, infrastructure improvements, and expediting the scientific peer review process, and streamlining the Food and Drug Administration approval process of countermeasures. . . .

"(c) AUTHORITY TO EXPEDITE PEER REVIEW.—

"(1) IN GENERAL.—The Secretary may, as the Secretary determines necessary to respond to pressing qualified countermeasure research and development needs under this section, employ such expedited peer review procedures (including consultation with appropriate scientific experts) as the Secretary, in consultation with the Director of NIH, deems appropriate to obtain assessment of scientific and technical merit and likely contribution to the field of qualified countermeasure research, in place of the peer review and advisory council review procedures that would be required under sections 301(a)(3), 405(b)(1)(B), 405(b)(2), 406(a)(3)(A), 492, and 494, as applicable to a grant, contract, or cooperative agreement—

[This provision allows the Secretary to bypass the normal peer-review process used by the Food and Drug Administration to approve the use of various drugs, vaccines, and other materials.] . . .

"(4) AVAILABILITY OF FACILITIES TO THE SECRETARY.— In any grant, contract, or cooperative agreement entered into under the authority provided in this section with respect to a biocontainment laboratory or other related or ancillary specialized research facility that the Secretary determines necessary for the purpose of performing, administering, or supporting qualified countermeasure research and development, the Secretary may provide that the facility that is the object of such grant, contract, or cooperative agreement shall be available as needed to the Secretary to respond to public health emergencies affecting national security.

[This section allows the Secretary to provide such funds as may be necessary to expand, remodel, renovate, or otherwise modify a research facility to conduct research on bioterrorism materials as he/she may deem necessary.] . . .

"(e) STREAMLINED PERSONNEL AUTHORITY.—

"(1) IN GENERAL.—In addition to any other personnel authorities, the Secretary may, as the Secretary determines necessary to respond to pressing qualified countermeasure research and development needs under this section, without regard to those provisions of title 5, United States Code, governing appointments in the competitive service, and without regard to the provisions of chapter 51 and subchapter III of chapter 53 of such title relating to classification and General Schedule pay rates, appoint professional and technical employees, not to exceed 30 such employees at any time, to positions in the National Institutes of Health to perform, administer, or support qualified countermeasure research and development activities in carrying out this section. .

[This section allows the Secretary to hire up to 30 additional employees to carry out the requirements of this act without following normal federal hiring procedures.]

Source: Public Law 108–276—July 21, 2004, 118 Stat. 835.   http://www.gpo.gov/fdsys/pkg/PLAW-108publ276/pdf/PLAW-108publ276.pdf.

Project Bioshield Assessment (2007)

In 2004, the U.S. Congress passed the Project Bioshield Act, allocating $5 billion for the development and purchases of vaccines that could be used in case of a bioterrorist attack on the United States. The Office of the Assistant Secretary for Preparedness and Response (ASPR) of the Department of Health and Human

Services awarded a contract to a small biomedical firm, VaxGen, to produce 25 million doses of a recombinant protective antigen (rPA) anthrax vaccine over the next two years. The company was unable to complete the terms of the contract, which was then cancelled in 2006. Congressional observers asked the U.S. General Accountability Office (GAO) to conduct a study to determine why this project failed. The GAO report highlights some of the political, social, economic, and other issues involved in the development of a vaccine for meeting an important national priority so clearly outlined in the Project Bioshield Act. The general conclusions reached by the GAO were as follows (citations and references are omitted):

Results in Brief

Three major factors contributed to the failure of the first Project BioShield procurement effort. First, ASPR awarded the first BioShield procurement contract to VaxGen when its product was at a very early stage of development and many critical manufacturing issues (such as stability and scale-up production) had not been addressed. ASPR officials told us that they felt a sense of urgency to demonstrate to the public that a new, improved vaccine was coming; they also stated that at the time of the award, they were 80 percent to 90 percent confident about VaxGen's chances of success. These officials based this confidence level on a subjective assessment and not on objective tools to determine a product's level of maturity. This award—several years before planned completion of earlier and uncompleted NIAID development contracts with VaxGen—preempted critical development work. Similarly, the requirement to deliver 75 million doses of rPA anthrax vaccine was not based on objective data. This requirement, according to the industry experts, would have been unrealistic for even a large pharmaceutical firm, given that the product was at an early stage of development.

Second, VaxGen took unrealistic risks in accepting the contract terms. According to VaxGen officials, they understood that their chances of success were limited. Nonetheless, they accepted the contract terms in spite of (1) the aggressive delivery time line, (2) their lack of in-house technical expertise in stability and vaccine formulation—a condition exacerbated by the attrition of key staff from the company as the contract progressed—and (3) their limited options for securing additional funding should the need arise for additional testing required to meet regulatory requirements.

Third, important FDA requirements regarding the type of data and testing required for the rPA anthrax vaccine to be eligible for use in an emergency were not known—to FDA [Food and Drug Administration], NIAID [National Institute of Allergy and Infectious Diseases], ASPR, and VaxGen—at the outset of the procurement contract. They were defined later when FDA introduced new guidance on emergency use authorization (EUA). In addition, ASPR's anticipated use of the rPA anthrax vaccine was not articulated to all parties clearly enough and evolved over time. Finally, according to VaxGen, the purchase of BioThrax for the stockpile as a stopgap measure raised the requirement for using the VaxGen rPA vaccine. All of these factors created confusion over the acceptance criteria for VaxGen's product and significantly diminished VaxGen's ability to meet contract time lines.

> **Source:** "PROJECT BIOSHIELD: Actions Needed to Avoid Repeating Past Problems with Procuring New Anthrax Vaccine and Managing the Stockpile of Licensed Vaccine." Washington, DC: General Accountability Office, October 2007. Project GAO-08–88. http://www.gao.gov/new.items/d0888.pdf.

———

Executive Order RP65 (State of Texas) (2007)

In 2007, the state of Texas became the first state in the United States to require vaccination against the human papillomavirus, an action taken by executive order of Governor Rick Perry. That order is reprinted on the following page. The order never took effect since the state legislature adopted a bill, H.B. 1098 (text follows), negating the executive order, an act that Perry chose not to veto.

BY THE
GOVERNOR OF THE STATE OF TEXAS
Executive Department
Austin, Texas

February 2, 2007

WHEREAS, immunization from vaccine-preventable diseases such as Human Papillomavirus (HPV) protects individuals who receive the vaccine; and

WHEREAS, HPV is the most common sexually transmitted infection-causing cancer in females in the United States; and

WHEREAS, the United States Food and Drug Administration estimates there are 9,710 new cases of cervical cancer, many of which are caused by HPV, and 3,700 deaths from cervical cancer each year in the United States; and

WHEREAS, the Texas Cancer Registry estimates there were 1,169 new cases and 391 deaths from cervical cancer in Texas in 2006; and

WHEREAS, research has shown that the HPV vaccine is highly effective in preventing the infections that are the cause of many of the cervical cancers; and

WHEREAS, HPV vaccine is only effective if administered before infection occurs; and

WHEREAS, the newly approved HPV vaccine is a great advance in the protection of women's health; and

WHEREAS, the Advisory Committee on Immunization Practices and Centers for Disease Control and Prevention recommend the HPV vaccine for females who are nine years through 26 years of age;

NOW THEREFORE, I, RICK PERRY, Governor of Texas, by virtue of the power and authority vested in me by the Constitution and laws of the State of Texas as the Chief Executive Officer, do hereby order the following:

Vaccine. The Department of State Health Services shall make the HPV vaccine available through the Texas Vaccines for Children program for eligible young females up to age 18, and the Health and Human Services Commission shall make the vaccine available to Medicaid-eligible young females from age 19 to 21.

Rules. The Health and Human Services Executive Commissioner shall adopt rules that mandate the age appropriate vaccination of all female children for HPV prior to admission to the sixth grade.

Availability. The Department of State Health Services and the Health and Human Services Commission will move expeditiously to make the vaccine available as soon as possible.

Public Information. The Department of State Health Services will implement a public awareness campaign to educate the public of the importance of vaccination, the availability of the vaccine, and the subsequent requirements under the rules that will be adopted.

Parents' Rights. The Department of State Health Services will, in order to protect the right of parents to be the final authority on their children's health care, modify the current process in order to allow parents to submit a request for a conscientious objection affidavit form via the Internet while maintaining privacy safeguards under current law.

This executive order supersedes all previous orders on this matter that are in conflict or inconsistent with its terms and this order shall remain in effect and in full force until modified, amended, rescinded, or superseded by me or by a succeeding governor.

Given under my hand this the 2nd day of February, 2007.

RICK PERRY (Signature)
Governor

Source: "RP65—Relating to the Immunization of Young Women from the Cancer-Causing Human Papillomavirus." Office of the Governor Rick Perry. http://governor.state. tx.us/news/executive-order/3455/.

Texas House Bill 1098 (2007)

The bill adopted by the Texas legislature overturning Governor Perry's executive order (above) was as follows (sections in brackets were deleted before final passage):

An Act

relating to immunization against human papillomavirus.

BE IT ENACTED BY THE LEGISLATURE OF THE STATE OF TEXAS:

SECTION 1. Section 38.001, Education Code, is amended by amending Subsection (b) and adding Subsection (b-1) to read as follows:

(b) Subject to Subsections (b-1) and [Subsection] (c), the executive commissioner of the Health and Human Services Commission [Texas Board of Health] may modify or delete any of the immunizations in Subsection (a) or may require immunizations against additional diseases as a requirement for admission to any elementary or secondary school.

(b-1) Immunization against human papillomavirus is not required for a person's admission to any elementary or secondary school; however, by using existing resources, the Health and Human Services Commission shall provide educational material about the human papillomavirus vaccine that is unbiased, medically and scientifically accurate, and peer reviewed, available to parents or legal guardians at the appropriate time in the immunization schedule by the appropriate school. This subsection preempts any contrary executive order issued by the governor. This subsection expires January 11, 2011.

SECTION 2. This Act takes effect immediately if it receives a vote of two-thirds of all the members elected to each house, as provided by Section 39, Article III, Texas Constitution. If this Act does not receive the vote necessary for immediate effect, this Act takes effect September 1, 2007.

Source: H.B. No. 1098. http://www.legis.state.tx.us/ tlodocs/80R/billtext/pdf/HB01098F.pdf#navpanes=0.

Cedillo and Cedillo vs. Secretary of Health and Human Services (2010)

As of 2009, approximately 5,000 cases had been filed in the Court of Federal Claims (the so-called Vaccine Court) claiming that children had developed autism and/or other medical conditions as a consequence of having received vaccinations. In attempting to deal with all these claims, the Special Masters of the Court of Federal Claims created the Omnibus Autism Proceeding (OAP), to determine the relationship, if any, between vaccines and autism and/or other medical conditions. The first test case under the OAP was a complaint brought by Theresa and Michael Cedillo under the National Childhood Vaccine Injury Act of 1986. The case was heard by Special Master George Hastings, Jr., who issued his decision on February 12, 2009, denying the Cedillo's claim for compensation. Special Master Hastings explained his decision in the following terms:

The petitioners in this case have advanced a causation theory that has several parts, including contentions (1) that thimerosal-containing vaccines can cause immune dysfunction, (2) that the MMR vaccine can cause autism, and (3) that the MMR vaccine can cause chronic gastrointestinal dysfunction. However, as to each of those issues, I concluded that the evidence was overwhelmingly contrary to the petitioners' contentions. The expert witnesses presented by the respondent were far better qualified, far more experienced, and far more persuasive than the petitioners' experts, concerning most of the key points. The numerous medical studies concerning these issues, performed by medical scientists worldwide, have come down strongly against the petitioners' contentions. Considering all of the evidence, I found that the petitioners have failed to demonstrate that thimerosal-containing vaccines can contribute to causing immune dysfunction, or that the MMR vaccine can contribute to causing either autism or gastrointestinal dysfunction. I further conclude that while Michelle Cedillo has tragically suffered from autism and other severe conditions, the petitioners have also failed to demonstrate that her vaccinations played any role at all in causing those problems. .

Source: Theresa Cedillo and Michael Cedillo, as parents and natural guardians of Michelle Cedillo, Petitioners v. Secretary of Health and Human Services. No. 98–916V. http://www.uscfc.uscourts.gov/sites/default/files/vaccine_files/Hastings-Cedillo.pdf.

Frequently Asked Questions about Thimerosal (Ethylmercury) (2011)

Since the late 1990s, a number of individuals have argued that the widespread use of vaccination may be associated with a rise in cases of autism spectrum disorder (ASD) among children. Most scientific studies have since demonstrated rather convincingly that no such correlation exists. The "culprit" in vaccines usually thought to be responsible for ASD symptoms is thimerosal, a mercury compound used as a preservative in some vaccines. The U.S. Centers for Disease Control and Prevention (CDC) has produced a fact sheet containing information about this compound that is reproduced here. References included in the original fact sheet are omitted here.

There are two, very different, types of mercury which people should know about: methylmercury and ethylmercury.

Mercury is a naturally occurring element found in the earth's crust, air, soil, and water. Since the earth's formation, volcanic eruptions, weathering of rocks and burning coal have caused mercury to be released into the environment. Once released, certain types of bacteria in the environment can change mercury into methylmercury. Methylmercury makes its way through the food chain in fish, animals, and humans. At high levels, it can be toxic to people. For more information about methylmercury: please read "What You Need to Know about Mercury in Fish and Shellfish" from the Environmental Protection Agency (EPA).

Thimerosal contains a different form of mercury called ethylmercury. Studies comparing ethylmercury and methylmercury suggest that they are processed differently in the human body. Ethylmercury is broken down and excreted much more rapidly than methylmercury. Therefore, ethylmercury (the type of mercury found in the influenza vaccine) is much less likely than methylmercury (the type of mercury in the environment) to accumulate in the body and cause harm.

What is thimerosal?

Thimerosal is a mercury-based preservative that has been used for decades in the United States in multi-dose vials (vials containing more than one dose) of medicines and vaccines.

Why is thimerosal used as a preservative in vaccines?

Thimerosal is added to vials of vaccine that contain more than one dose to prevent the growth of bacteria and fungi in the event that they get into the vaccine. This may occur when a syringe needle enters a vial as a vaccine is being prepared for administration. Contamination by germs in a vaccine could cause severe local reactions, serious illness or death. In some vaccines, preservatives are added during the manufacturing process to prevent microbial growth.

How does thimerosal work in the body?

Thimerosal does not stay in the body a long time so it does not build up and reach harmful levels. When thimerosal enters the body, it breaks down, to ethylmercury and thiosalicylate, which are easily eliminated.

Is thimerosal safe?

Thimerosal has a proven track record of being very safe. Data from many studies show no convincing evidence of harm caused by the low doses of thimerosal in vaccines.

What are the possible side-effects of thimerosal?

The most common side-effects are minor reactions like redness and swelling at the injection site. Although rare, some people may be allergic to thimerosal. Research shows that most people who are allergic to thimerosal will not have a reaction when thimerosal is injected under the skin.

Does thimerosal cause autism?

Research does not show any link between thimerosal in vaccines and autism, a neurodevelopmental disorder. Although thimerosal was taken out of childhood vaccines in 2001, autism rates have gone up, which is the opposite of what would be expected if thimerosal caused autism.

Do MMR vaccines contain thimerosal?

No, measles, mumps, and rubella (MMR) vaccines do not and never did contain thimerosal. Varicella (chickenpox), inactivated polio (IPV), and pneumococcal conjugate vaccines have also never contained thimerosal.

Do all flu vaccines contain thimerosal?

No. Influenza (flu) vaccines are currently available in both thimerosal-containing and thimerosal-free versions. The total amount of flu vaccine without thimerosal as a preservative at times has been limited, but availability will increase as vaccine manufacturing capabilities are expanded. In the meantime, it is important to keep in mind that the benefits of influenza vaccination outweigh the theoretical risk, if any, of exposure to thimerosal.

How can I find out if thimerosal is in a vaccine?

For a complete list of vaccines and their thimerosal content level, you may visit the U.S. Food and Drug Administration. Additionally, you may ask your health care provider or pharmacist for a copy of the vaccine package insert. It lists ingredients in the vaccine and discusses any known adverse reactions.

Source: "Frequently Asked Questions About Thimerosal (Ethylmercury)." http://www.cdc.gov/vaccinesafety/Concerns/thimerosal/thimerosal_faqs.html.

Exemption from Vaccination

Some of the earliest laws requiring that individuals be immunized included a section, often called a "conscience clause," permitting individuals to decline vaccination if the practice violated their religious or other philosophical beliefs. In the United States, all but two states (Mississippi and West Virginia) grant exemptions from vaccination laws if individuals attest that the practice offends their religious beliefs, and 20 allow exemptions for philosophical (that are not necessarily religious) beliefs. An example of such clauses is the one found in the laws of the state of California:

120365. Immunization of a person shall not be required for admission to a school or other institution listed in Section 120335 if the parent or guardian or adult who has assumed responsibility for his or her care and custody in the case of a minor, or the person seeking admission if an emancipated minor, files with the governing authority a letter or affidavit stating that the immunization is contrary to his or her beliefs. However, whenever there is good cause to believe that the person has been exposed to one of the communicable diseases listed in subdivision (a) of Section 120325, that person may be temporarily excluded from the school or institution until the local health officer is satisfied that the person is no longer at risk of developing the disease.

States may also designate the specific form that parents are required to execute in order to obtain a vaccination exemption. An example is the form used by the state of Delaware:

AFFIDAVIT OF RELIGIOUS BELIEF
STATE OF DELAWARE
_____COUNTY

1. (I) (We) (am) (are) the (parent(s)) (legal guardian(s)) of

_____

_____

Name of Child

2. (I) (We) hereby (swear) (affirm) that (I) (we) subscribe to a belief in a relation to a Supreme Being involving duties superior to those arising from any human relation.

3. (I) (We) further (swear) (affirm) that our belief is sincere and meaningful and occupies a place in (my) (our) life parallel to that filled by the orthodox belief in God.

4. This belief is not a political, sociological or philosophical view of a merely personal moral code.

5. This belief causes (me) (us) to request an exemption from the mandatory school vaccination program for.

_____

Name of Child

_____

Signature of Parent(s) or Legal Guardian(s)

SWORN TO AND SUBSCRIBED before me, a registered Notary Public, this_____day of._____

_____Seal)

Notary Public

My commission expires:

_____

In Mississippi and West Virginia, the sole reason for granting exemption from vaccinations for school entry are certain medical reasons that would put a child at risk. For example, the West Virginia law says that:

All children entering school for the first time in this state shall have been immunized against diphtheria, polio, rubeola, rubella, tetanus and whooping cough. Any person who cannot give satisfactory proof of having been immunized previously or a certificate from a reputable physician showing that an immunization for any or all diphtheria, polio, rubeola, rubella, tetanus and whooping cough is impossible or improper or sufficient reason why any or all immunizations should not be done, shall be immunized for diphtheria, polio, rubeola, rubella, tetanus and whooping cough prior to being admitted in any of the schools in the state. . . .

Any parent or guardian who refuses to permit his or her child to be immunized against diphtheria, polio, rubeola, rubella, tetanus and whooping cough, who cannot give satisfactory proof that the child or person has been immunized against diphtheria, polio, rubeola, rubella, tetanus and whooping cough previously, or a certificate from a reputable physician showing that immunization for any or all is impossible or improper, or sufficient reason why any or all immunizations should not be done, shall be guilty of a misdemeanor, and except as herein otherwise provided, shall, upon conviction, be punished by a fine of not less than ten nor more than fifty dollars for each offense.

Sources: [California] Health and Safety Code Section 120325–120380.http://www.leginfo.ca.gov/cgi-bin/displaycode?section=hsc&group=120001–121000&file=120325–120380; [Delaware] Title 14, Chapter 1, Sections 121–134. http://delcode.delaware.gov/title14/c001/sc02/index.shtml#P227_51758;

West Virginia Code. Chapter 16. Public Health. http://www.legis.state.wv.us/wvcode/ChapterEntire.cfm?chap=16&art=3.

If You Choose Not to Vaccinate Your Child,
Understand the Risks and Responsibilities.

Last updated October 2009

If you choose to delay some vaccines or reject some vaccines entirely, there can be risks. Please follow these steps to protect your child, your family, and others.

With the decision to delay or reject vaccines comes an important responsibility that could save your child's life, or the life of someone else.

Any time that your child is ill and you:

- call 911;
- ride in an ambulance;
- visit a hospital emergency room; or
- visit your child's doctor or any clinic

you must tell the medical staff that your child has not received all the vaccines recommended for his or her age.

Keep a vaccination record easily accessible so that you can report exactly which vaccines your child has received, even when you are under stress.

Telling healthcare professionals your child's vaccination status is essential for two reasons:

- When your child is being evaluated, the doctor will need to consider the possibility that your child has a vaccine-preventable disease. Many of these diseases are now uncommon, but they still occur, and the doctor will need to consider that your child may have a vaccine-preventable disease.

- The people who help your child can take precautions, such as isolating your child, so that the disease does not spread to others. One group at high risk for contracting disease is infants who are too young to be fully vaccinated. For example, the measles vaccine is not usually recommended for babies younger than 12 months. Very young babies who get measles are likely to be seriously ill, often requiring hospitalization. Other people at high risk for contracting disease are those with weaker immune systems, such as some people with cancer and transplant recipients.

Before an outbreak of a vaccine-preventable disease occurs in your community:

- Talk to your child's doctor or nurse to be sure your child's medical record is up to date regarding vaccination status. Ask for a copy of the updated record.

- Inform your child's school, childcare facility, and other caregivers about your child's vaccination status.

- Be aware that your child can catch diseases from people who don't have any symptoms. For example, Hib meningitis can be spread from people who have the bacteria in their body but are not ill. You can't tell who is contagious.

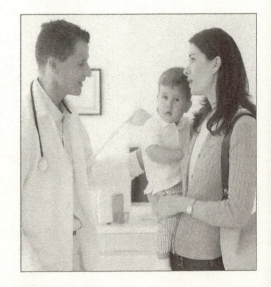

  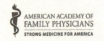 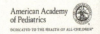

Immunization is the subject of a very large collection of books and print and electronic scientific and general articles. Space does not permit a complete or exhaustive listing of those resources. The items presented here do provide a general overview of the types of materials available on the subject. The resources are listed in four general categories: books, periodicals, reports, and Internet resources. Because some items are available in more than one format, they may be listed here in differing, but comparable, categories.

Books

Anderson, H. B. *The Facts Against Compulsory Vaccination.* New York: Citizens Medical Reference Bureau, 1929. Also available in full online at http://www.vaccinationawareness.com.au/Images/facts1.pdf.

> This book provides an example of the kind of anti-vaccination sentiment that has been popular in the United States and other countries in history.

Angelo, Lauren B. *APhA's Immunization Handbook.* Washington, DC: American Pharmacists Association, 2012.

> This publication contains all the technical details practicing pharmacists needed about vaccines and vaccinations,

First page of a CDC flyer advising parents on vaccination. (Centers for Disease Control and Prevention) including ordering, storage and handling, record keeping, travel requirements, and special needs.

Artenstein, Andrew W., ed. *Vaccines: A Biography.* New York; London: Springer, 2010.

This book provides an excellent introduction to the subject of infectious disease and immunization, with 20 of its 22 chapters dealing with one of the major infectious diseases, such as smallpox, hepatitis A, hepatitis B, and rotavirus.

Barrett, A. D. T., and Lawrence R. Stanberry, eds. *Vaccines for Biodefense and Emerging and Neglected Diseases.* Amsterdam; Boston: Academic Press, 2009.

The essays in this book focus on a group of diseases included under the rubrics of "emerging diseases," "neglected diseases," or potential bioterrorist weapons. They provide readers with a review of current information on these diseases and on current efforts to develop defensive vaccines for each such disease.

Bartolotti, Charles R. *The H1N1 Influenza Pandemic of 2009.* New York: Nova Science Publishers, 2010.

This book provides a comprehensive review of the 2009 H1N1 epidemic, the major events that occurred during that epidemic, and the steps that were taken by international, national, state, and other organization to deal with the consequences of the epidemic.

Bazin, Hervé. *Vaccination: A History from Lady Montagu to Genetic Engineering.* Montrouge, France: J. Libbey Eurotext, 2011.

This English translation of a 2008 French text actually expands the discussion of the history of vaccination, including a new chapter on yellow fever.

Belhorn, Thomas K. *100 Questions & Answers about Childhood Immunizations.* Sudbury, MA: Jones and Bartlett, 2009.

This book provides answers to 100 generally simple and direct questions about the nature of vaccines and vaccinations and issues associated with their use and practice.

Bona, Constantin A., and Adrian I. Bot. *Genetic Immunization.* New York: Kluwer Academic/Plenum Publishers, 2000.

This highly technical book proposes a new approach to immunization in which vaccines are developed with specific involvement of the genetic bases for various infectious diseases. One interesting chapter explores the use of this technology with neonates, whose immune system is so poorly developed that traditional vaccines are of little value.

Cave, Stephanie, and Deborah R. Mitchell. *What Your Doctor May Not Tell You about Children's Vaccinations*, rev. ed. New York: Wellness Central, 2010.

The authors suggest that we may be "overvaccinating" our children today, exposing them in the process to possible deleterious side effects, such as autism, asthma, learning disabilities, and diabetes.

Cochi, Stephen L., and Walter R. Dowdle, eds. *Disease Eradication in the 21st Century Implications for Global Health.* Cambridge, MA: MIT Press, 2011.

The chapters in this book discuss the hopes for eradicating a number of infectious diseases during the 21st century, including measles, rubella, and malaria, along with a discussion of the scientific, technical, social, and economic issues involved in campaigns designed to achieve this result.

Committee on the Review of Priorities in the National Vaccine Plan; Institute of Medicine. *Priorities for the National Vaccine Plan.* Washington, DC: National Academies Press, 2010.

The goal of the National Vaccine Plan is to provide a vision for the U.S. vaccine and immunization enterprise for the next decade. This book provides an introduction to the general subject of vaccines and vaccination, a summary of the problems faced by the United States in achieving adequate levels of vaccination for its populace, and an outline of the steps that can be taken to achieve that objective.

Committee on Special Immunizations Program for Laboratory Personnel Engaged in Research on Countermeasures for Select Agents; National Research Council. *Protecting the Frontline in Biodefense Research: The Special Immunizations Program.* Washington, DC: National Academies Press, 2011.

This report discusses the Special Immunizations Program (SIP) of the U.S. Army Medical Research Institute of Infectious Diseases at Fort Detrick, Maryland. SIP provides special immunization opportunities to individuals who are likely to be exposed to hazardous biomaterials, using vaccines that both have and have not been approved by the U.S. Food and Drug Administration.

Compans, Richard W., and Walter A. Orenstein. *Vaccines for Pandemic Influenza.* Dordrecht; New York: Springer, 2009.

The sections of this book are devoted to an overview of pandemic influenza, current approaches to the development of human and animal vaccines against influenza, novel vaccine approaches, and novel approaches for vaccine delivery.

Cournoyer, Cynthia. *What about Immunizations? Exposing the Vaccine Philosophy.* Avon, CT: Better Books, 2010.

The author argues that the "vaccine philosophy" that is pervasive in modern society drives many people to have their children vaccinated when it is not always clear that the benefits of vaccination outweigh the risks associated with the procedure.

Davies, Gwyn, ed. *Vaccine Adjuvants: Methods and Protocols.* New York: Humana Press, 2010.

The essays in this book review the development of vaccine adjuvants and discuss the practical issues involved in the development and use of adjuvants for new vaccines.

Dehner, George. *Influenza: A Century of Science and Public Health Response.* Pittsburgh: University of Pittsburgh Press, 2012.

> The author provides a comprehensive review of the nature of influenza and the way that societies have responded to the outbreak of pandemics, dating from the Russian flu of 1889 to the swine flu outbreak of 2009.

Dormitzer, Philip R., Christian W. Mandl, and Rino Rappuoli, eds. *Replicating Vaccines: A New Generation.* Basel: Springer, 2011.

> Live vaccines have always played a very important role in immunology. Modern technology has made possible a number of important adaptations and developments in the development and use of such vaccines. This book reviews some of the most important of those developments.

Eisenstein, Mayer, and Neil Z. Miller. *Making an Informed Vaccine Decision for the Health of Your Child: A Parent's Guide to Childhood Shots.* Santa Fe, NM: New Atlantean Press, 2010.

> The first 18 chapters in this book are all devoted to specific diseases for which vaccines are available. The final four chapters deal with related topics, such as multiple vaccines, aluminum, and other ingredients in vaccines.

Flower, Darren, R. *Bioinformatics for Vaccinology.* Hoboken, NJ: Wiley-Blackwell, 2008.

> This book provides a superb general introduction to the study of vaccinology, with an especially interesting and useful opening section on the history of the field.

Foege, William H. *House on Fire: The Fight to Eradicate Smallpox.* Berkeley: University of California Press, 2011.

> The author, who was involved in the fight to eradicate smallpox, provides a review of that interesting battle.

Griffin, Diane E., and Michael B. A. Oldstone. *Measles: Pathogenesis and Control.* Berlin: Springer, 2009.

The authors review worldwide efforts—now largely successful—to bring under control and eventually eradicate the disease of measles.

Habakus, Louise Kuo, and Mary Holland, eds. *Vaccine Epidemic: How Corporate Greed, Biased Science, and Coercive Government Threaten Our Human Rights, Our Health, and Our Children.* New York: Skyhorse Publishing, 2011.

Twenty-three contributors write about a variety of health, social, economic, and personal liberty issues that have arisen as a result of compulsory vaccination. Authors ascribe a host of health problems, including autism, Gulf War syndrome, and muscle deterioration, to forced vaccination programs in the United States and elsewhere.

Henderson, Donald A. *Smallpox: The Death of a Disease: The Inside Story of Eradicating a Worldwide Killer.* Amherst, NY: Prometheus Books, 2009.

The author tells the story of efforts by the World Health Organization to eradicate smallpox worldwide and the ultimate consequences of that effort.

Herlihy, Stacy Mintzer, and E. Allison Hagood. *Your Baby's Best Shot: Why Vaccines Are Safe and Save Lives.* Lanham, MD: Rowman & Littlefield, 2012.

The authors base this book on the assumption that parents of young children are faced with competing messages about the need for safety and efficacy of vaccinations. They review the evidence that confirms that shots for babies are both "safe" and that they "save lives."

Hoyt, Kendall. *Long Shot: Vaccines for National Defense.* Cambridge, MA: Harvard University Press, 2011.

The author reviews the history of vaccine development and focuses on the special problems created by the increasing concerns over possible bioterrorism attacks since the terrorist attacks of September 11, 2001. He outlines the new challenges to developing vaccines against such attacks and suggests ways in which those challenges can be met.

Joellenbeck, Lois M., Lee L. Zwanziger, Jane S. Durch, and Brian L. Strom, eds. *The Anthrax Vaccine: Is It Safe? Does It Work?* Washington, DC: National Academies Press, 2002.

This book is the result of a study conducted by a committee especially appointed for the purpose, the Committee to Assess the Safety and Efficacy of the Anthrax Vaccine of the Institute of Medicine. The committee concluded that the vaccine is both effective and "reasonably safe."

Kitta, Andrea. *Vaccinations and Public Concern in History: Legend, Rumor, and Risk Perception.* New York: Routledge, 2011.

For as long as vaccines have been available for the prevention of infectious diseases, there have been public concerns about possible serious side effects as a result of one's being vaccinated. This book reviews the long history of the objections that have been raised to vaccination up to the present day.

Link, Kurt. *The Vaccine Controversy: The History, Use, and Safety of Vaccinations.* Westport, CT: Praeger Publishers, 2005.

This book consists of a number of short essays on vaccines that are currently available or under development, with a discussion of the disease for which each vaccine is designed, its safety, and its potential side effects.

Mak, Tak W., Maya Chadda, and Mary E. Saunders. *Primer to the Immune Response.* Amsterdam; Boston: Elsevier, 2011.

This textbook provides a general introduction to the immune system and the theoretical and clinical principles underlying immunology.

Merino, Noël, ed. *Should Vaccinations Be Mandatory?* Detroit: Greenhaven Press, 2010.

> This book, written for young adults, provides a broad, general introduction to the subject of vaccinations and then offers both (all) sides of arguments for and against requiring vaccinations of all individuals.

Miller, Neil Z. *Vaccine Safety Manual for Concerned Families and Health Practitioners*, 2nd ed. Santa Fe, NM: New Atlantean Press, 2012.

> This book is divided into chapters devoted to a large number of infectious diseases, containing a description of each disease and vaccines available for prevention and treatment of the disease.

Mnookin, Seth. *The Panic Virus: A True Story of Medicine, Science, and Fear.* New York: Simon & Schuster, 2011.

> Mnookin provides a fascinating review of the recent controversy about the connection between autism and vaccination, only the most recent example of objections raised by some individuals and organizations against the widespread use of immunization for children.

Monsonégo, Joseph. *The End of a Cancer?: The Hopes Vested in Vaccination Against Papillomavirus.* Paris: ESKA Publishing, 2010.

> The author, a researcher who has worked on problems of HPV and cervical cancer, reviews the development and promise of the HPV vaccine and points out its potential value in eradicating cervical cancer in regions where it is widely employed.

Morrow, John H., et al., eds. *Vaccinology: Principles and Practice.* New York: Wiley-Blackwell, 2012.

> This book covers all aspects of vaccine development, production, and use, from theoretical design to implementation.

Offit, Paul A. *Deadly Choices: How the Anti-Vaccine Movement Threatens Us All.* New York: Basic Books, 2011.

> The author reviews the history of the anti-vaccine movement in the United States and elsewhere, the role played by its leaders, and some of the impacts the movement has had on the lives of everyday individuals.

Offit, Paul A., and Charlotte A. Moser. *Vaccines and Your Child: Separating Fact from Fiction.* New York: Columbia University Press, 2011.

> The short chapters in this book are arranged around specific questions that a parent might ask about the process of vaccination, such as "How do vaccines work?" "Should vaccines be mandated?" "Are vaccines safe?" "Do vaccines cause diabetes?" and "Who shouldn't get vaccines?"

O'Shea, Tim. *The Sanctity of Human Blood: Vaccination Is Not Immunization*, 14th ed. San Jose, CA: Two Trees, 2010.

> Now in its 14th edition, this book attempts to demonstrate that vaccination is neither safe nor effective and that, therefore, it should not be required of all children, let alone offered to the general public as a safe and effective medical option.

Petersen, Christine. *Frequently Asked Questions about Vaccines and Vaccinations.* New York: Rosen Classroom, 2011.

> This book is intended for young adult readers. It provides a general introduction to the subject of immunization, with a review of some of the issues that surround the use of the procedure.

Plotkin, Stanley A. *History of Vaccine Development*, 2nd ed. New York; London: Springer, 2010.

> The 30 essays in this book cover most of the major developments in the history of immunization, including the use of variolation and vaccination in early Chinese history; Edward Jenner's contributions to the development

of immunization; a history of toxoids; the invention of vaccines for a variety of specific diseases, including typhoid fever, pertussis, yellow fever, influenza, rubella, hepatitis, HPV, and rotavirus; and the development and deployment of veterinary vaccines.

Plotkin, Stanley A., Walter Orenstein, and Paul A. Offit. *Vaccines: Expert Consult*, 6th ed. Philadelphia: Saunders, 2012.

This highly regarded publication deals with virtually every imaginable issue relating to the design, production, and use of vaccines worldwide.

Scherr, George H. *Why Millions Died: Before the War on Infectious Diseases*. Lanham, MD: University Press of America, 2012.

The author reviews the history of the slow and somewhat idiosyncratic development of vaccines for a variety of infectious diseases.

Sears, Robert. *The Vaccine Book: Making the Right Decision for Your Child*. New York: Little, Brown, 2011.

This book provides fundamental information about the nature of infectious diseases and the vaccines available for use against them.

Selgelid, Michael J., et al., eds. *Infectious Disease Ethics: Limiting Liberty in Contexts of Contagion*. Dordrecht; New York: Springer, 2011.

The papers published in this book come from a conference held on the topic that included top researchers and theoreticians in the fields of law, philosophy, medicine, and bioethics. Their primary theme is the conflict that often arises in modern society between the rights of individuals (such as the right to decline vaccination) versus social goods and needs (such as the need to prevent pandemics and epidemics).

Singh, Manmohan, and Indresh K. Srivasta, eds. *Development of Vaccines: From Discovery to Clinical Testing.* Hoboken, NJ: John Wiley & Sons, 2011.

> The chapters in this book deal with every aspect of vaccine development, from theoretical analysis, through testing, to final industrial development stages.

Smith, Michael Joseph, and Laurie Bouck. *The Complete Idiot's Guide to Vaccinations.* New York: Alpha Books, 2009.

> As with other books in the Complete Idiot's series, this book provides a comprehensive and straightforward approach to its subject, providing a concise and adequate review of the history of vaccines, an explanation as to how they work, a description of vaccines currently available for major infectious diseases, and special issues relating to the use of vaccines.

State of the World's Vaccines and Immunization, 3rd ed. Geneva: World Health Organization, 2010.

> This publication consists of three major parts, the first of which provides a broad general overview of the status of immunization programs in all parts of the world. Part two is devoted to a review of vaccines currently available and the diseases for which they can be used. The final section deals with financial issues associated with the broader use of vaccines around the world.

Steen, David G., and Howard L. Dyson, eds. *Vaccinations: Types, Potential Complications, and Health Effects.* Hauppauge, NY: Nova Science Publishers, 2009.

> This book is especially valuable because, in addition to the general introduction to immunization that it provides, it also discusses in some detail current research on the development of new vaccines for diseases such as cancer, bacterial meningitis, multiple sclerosis, hepatitis B, and tuberculosis.

Studer, Hans-Peter and Geoffrey Douch. *Vaccination: A Guide for Making Personal Choices*, 2nd ed. Edinburgh: Floris, 2010.

The authors point out that many parents prefer not to follow recommendations or requirements established by governmental authorities for vaccination of their children. They offer a review of the vaccines currently available, along with risks they believe may be associated with the use of those vaccines.

Thiel, Andreas, ed. *Immunosenescence*. Basel: Springer, 2012.

Immunosenescence is the process by which a person's immune system becomes less effective as she or he ages. This effect poses problems for individuals who are concerned about maintaining a person's ability to fight off infectious diseases and to develop vaccines that are more effective as individuals age. This collection of essays deals with a number of topics related to that problem.

Teunissen, Marcel B. M., ed. *Intradermal Immunization*. Heidelberg: Springer, 2012.

This book offers a collection of technical papers on a method of immunization that is currently not in wide use, but that has the potential for increasing the efficiency and efficacy of vaccination for many diseases.

Valenta, Rudolf, and Robert L. Coffman, eds. *Vaccines against Allergies*. Heidelberg: Springer, 2011.

The 10 contributed papers that make up this book provide technical discussions of a variety of topics related to the use of immunization for the prevention and treatment of so-called IgE-mediated allergies, which may affect as many as a quarter of all Americans.

Vashishtha, Vipin M., Kalra Ajay, and Thacker Naveen. *FAQs on Vaccines and Immunization Practices*. New Delhi: Jaypee Brothers Medical Publishers, 2011.

This book contains chapters on basics of vaccine immunology, elementary epidemiology, vaccination schedules, vaccination in special situations, adverse events associated with vaccination, vaccine storage, and adolescent immunization.

Wailoo, Keith, et al. eds. *Three Shots at Prevention: the HPV Vaccine and the Politics of Medicine's Simple Solutions.* Baltimore: Johns Hopkins University Press, 2010.

This book provides a comprehensive introduction to the availability of HPV vaccination and the medical, social, economic, ethical, and other issues associated with the practice. The 15 essays that make up the book deal with topics such as The Great Undiscussable: Anal Cancer, HPV, and Gay Men's Health; Producing and Protecting Risky Girlhoods; Decision Psychology and HPV Vaccine; and Vaccination as Governance: HPV Skepticism in the United States and Africa, and the North-South Divide.

Wertheim, Heiman F. L., Peter Horby, and John P. Woodall, eds. *Atlas of Human Infectious Diseases.* Hoboken, NJ: John Wiley & Sons, 2012.

Arguably the most comprehensive and detailed reference book on the nature, causes, and treatment of infectious diseases in humans.

Williams, Tony. *The Pox and the Covenant: Mather, Franklin, and the Epidemic That Changed America's Destiny.* Naperville, IL: Sourcebooks, 2010.

The author tells the story of how the smallpox virus arrived by ships from England in the early 17th century; swept through Boston, the Massachusetts Bay Colony, and other regions; and was eventually brought under control by the use of vaccination.

Willrich, Michael. *Pox: An American History.* New York: Penguin Press, 2011.

Willrich explains how the effort to eradicate smallpox in the United States collided with a growing antigovernment movement that objected to the imposition of vaccination on Americans, whether they wanted it or agreed with it or not.

Periodicals

Achong, M. Natalie. "What Women Need to Know about HPV and Cervical Cancer: The HPV Vaccination Is a New Weapon in the Fight." *Ebony* 62, no. 9 (2007): 146.

> The author, a practicing gynecologist, discusses the problems of HPV and cervical cancer and provides basic information about the role that the HPV vaccine can play in reducing the risk of that disease.

Amorij, Jean-Pierre, et al. "Needle-free Influenza Vaccination." *The Lancet Infectious Diseases* 10, no. 10 (2010): 699–711.

> The authors point out that, although immunization by needle is by far the most common procedure, vaccination can also be given without the use of a needle. Some advantages are that needle-free vaccination is less painful, easier to administer in a wide range of circumstances, and generally less costly than vaccination by needle.

Campbell, James B., Jason W. Busse, and H. Stephen Injeyan. "Chiropractors and Vaccination: A Historical Perspective." *Pediatrics* 105, no. 4 (April 1, 2000): e43. Available online at http://www.pediatricsdigest.mobi/content/105/4/e43.full.

> The authors provide an excellent review of the positions taken by chiropractors over the past century or more about the safety and efficacy of vaccinations, and the alternatives they propose to the conventional vaccination schedule.

Castillo-Solórzano, Carlos, et al. "Elimination of Rubella and Congenital Rubella Syndrome in the Americas." *Journal of Infectious Diseases* 204, suppl. 2 (2011): S571–S578.

> The authors describe the process by which rubella and congenital rubella syndrome were eradicated from the

Western Hemisphere during the first decade of the 21st century.

"Catch-Up Immunization Schedule for Persons Aged 4 Months Through 18 Years Who Start Late or Who Are More than 1 Month Behind." *AAP News* 31, no. 1 (2010): 19.

> The chart provided here helps practitioners and parents to catch up on vaccinations for children whose immunization schedule has otherwise been disrupted for some reason.

Centers for Disease Control and Prevention. "Measles Eradication: Recommendations from a Meeting Cosponsored by the World Health Organization, the Pan American Health Organization, and CDC." *MMWR* 46, no. RR-11 (2007): i–vi; 1–22.

> This article summarizes the conclusions and recommendations agreed upon at a meeting of the World Health Organization, Pan American Health Organization, and Centers for Disease Control and Prevention on the feasibility of eradicating measles worldwide.

Connolly, Terry, and Jochen Reb. "Toward Interactive, Internet-Based Decision Aid for Vaccination Decisions: Better Information Alone Is Not Enough." *Vaccine,* 2012. Epub ahead of publication. http://www.ncbi.nlm.nih.gov/pubmed/22234264?dopt=Abstract.

Crosbie, E. J. "Global Human Papillomavirus Vaccination: Can It Be Cost-effective?" *BJOG* 119, no. 2 (2012): 125–128.

> The author points out that widespread vaccination for the human papillomavirus (HPV) could save up to five million lives annually worldwide. He then explores the mitigating factors that might or might not make a concerted effort to promote HPV vaccinations worthwhile.

De Gregorio, Ennio, and Rino Rappuoli. "Vaccines for the Future: Learning from Human Immunology." *Microbial Biotechnology* 5, no. 2 (2012): 149–155.

The authors discuss the success of vaccines in eradicating and reducing the effects of infectious diseases and then point out that a number of diseases are resistant to the use of traditional vaccines. They point out new technologies that may make these diseases susceptible to treatment by immunization also.

Derhovanessian, Evelyna, and Graham Pawelec. "Vaccination in the Elderly." *Microbial Biotechnology* 5, no. 2 (2012): 226–232.

The authors review evidence that immunization in the elderly tends to be less effective than it is in younger individuals. They suggest some changes in immunization practices that might improve the effectiveness of vaccinations among the elderly.

Geier, David, and Mark Geier. "The True Story of Pertussis Vaccination: A Sordid Legacy?" *Journal of the History of Medicine* 57, no. 3 (2002): 249–284.

The authors provide a detailed review of the history of the development of the pertussis vaccine, along with some unfortunate consequences of the research and testing involved.

Gladstone, R. A., et al. "Continued Control of Pneumococcal Disease in the UK—The Impact of Vaccination." *Journal of Medical Microbiology* 60, part 1 (2011): 1–8.

The authors explore the challenges of devising a vaccine against the many forms of pneumococcal diseases, the vaccines that have thus far been developed, and their successes and limitations.

Glass, Roger I. "Unexpected Benefits of Rotavirus Vaccination in the United States." *Journal of Infectious Diseases* 204, no. 7 (2011): 975–977.

The author comments on recent research findings that the immunization of young children against rotaviruses appears to have decreased the incidence of rotavirus-related disease among older children and adults in the United States. For details of this research, see the following article: Lopman, Ben A., et al.. "Infant Rotavirus Vaccination May Provide Indirect Protection to Older Children and Adults in the United States." *Journal of Infectious Diseases* 204, no. 7 (2011): 980–986.

Gnann, John N. "Varicella-zoster Virus: Prevention through Vaccination." *Clinical Obstetrics and Gynecology.* 55, no. 2 (2012): 560–570.

The author discusses the success of the varicella-zoster vaccine in reducing the incidence of chickenpox, but points out that many adult women are still susceptible to the disease. He recommends an aggressive program of vaccinating these women to reduce the risk of complications from the disease during pregnancy.

Hansen, Steffi, and Claus-Michael Lehr. "Nanoparticles for Transcutaneous Vaccination." *Microbial Biotechnology* 5, no. 2 (2012): 156–167.

The authors discuss progress in research on the use of nanoparticles for the production of vaccines that can be applied directly on the skin, thus avoiding the use of injection by needle.

Hennock, E. P. "Vaccination Policy Against Smallpox, 1835–1914: A Comparison of England with Prussia and Imperial Germany." *Social History of Medicine* 11, no. 1 (1998): 49–71.

Governmental policies with regard to smallpox vaccination, actual practice, and the results of such policies all differed substantially in Great Britain, Prussia, and Germany during the last half of the 19th and early 20th centuries. This excellent article reviews and analyzes those differences.

Hoyt, Kendall L. "Vaccine Innovation: Lessons from World War II." *Journal of Public Health Policy* 27, no. 1 (2006): 38–57.

> The author points out that the 1940s were an unusually rich period for the development of vaccines, largely in response to the increased risk posed by diseases that became more common during the war. He reviews the history of that period and the implications for further research on new vaccines.

"Immunization of Health-Care Personnel: Recommendations of the Advisory Committee on Immunization Practices (ACIP)." *MMWR* 60, no. 7 (2011): whole.

> This issue of *MMWR* discusses in detail issues involved with providing healthcare workers with all necessary immunizations. It also includes a bibliography of more than 300 references and a chart summarizing its recommendations.

Jones, Dan. "Reverse Vaccinology on the Cusp." *Nature Reviews: Drug Discovery* 11, no. 3 (2012): 175–176.

> The author reviews an exciting new technology for the development of vaccines, called reverse vaccinology, a process in which proteomics is used to design protein sequences that have the potential for producing immune responses to antigens. He discusses the first vaccine produced by this method, Bexsero, designed for use against the pathogen meningococcus B.

Katz, Jenna A., Talia Capua, and Joseph A. Bocchini, Jr. "Update on Child and Adolescent Immunizations: Selected Review of Us Recommendations and Literature." *Current Opinion in Pediatrics* 24, no. 3 (2012): 407–421.

> The authors provide an up-to-date and comprehensive review of research on childhood and adolescent vaccinations and the effect they have had on infectious diseases around the world. They also review the most recent recommendations about vaccinations from the American

Academy of Pediatrics and the Advisory Committee on Immunization Practices.

Kilgore, Christine. "How to Meet the Challenges of HPV Vaccination." *Obstetrics and Gynecology News* 62, no. 1 (2011): 18+.

> The author reviews the potential benefits of using HPV vaccination to reduce the risk of cervical cancer, some of the objections that have been raised to using the procedure, and some ways of dealing with those objections.

Kumar, Sameer. "Planning for Avian Flu Disruptions on Global Operations: a Dmaic Case Study." *International Journal of Health Care Quality Assurance* 25, no. 3 (2012): 197–215.

> The author uses computer models to explore the potential effects of a worldwide avian flu epidemic, using Wal-Mart and Dell Computers as two representative businesses that might be seriously affected by such an event.

Kutscher, Sarah, et al. Design of Therapeutic Vaccines: Hepatitis B as an Example. *Microbial Biotechnology* 5, no. 2 (2012): 270–282.

> Therapeutic vaccines are vaccines designed to reduce the severity of symptoms of a disease that has already developed. This paper reviews the underlying concepts involved in the development and use of such vaccines, with special emphasis on the hepatitis B vaccine.

Lee, Bruce Y., et al. "The Potential Economic Value of a 'Universal' (Multi-year) Influenza Vaccine." *Influenza and Other Respiratory Viruses* 6, no. 3 (2012): 167–175.

> The authors report on an analysis of the relative economic benefits of developing an influenza vaccine that could be used year after year compared to the current practice of developing a new vaccine against the disease each year.

Li, Ni, et al. "Transcutaneous Vaccines: Novel Advances in Technology and Delivery for Overcoming the Barriers." *Vaccine* 29, no. 37 (2011): 6179–6190.

> This article discusses the process of transcutaneous vaccination, in which a vaccine administered to the skin enters the body transdermally, thus avoiding the pain and inconvenience of needle injections as a means of administration.

Malone, Kevin M., and Alan R. Hinman. "Vaccination Mandates: The Public Health Imperative and Individual Rights." In Hoffman, Richard E., et al., eds. *Law in Public Health Practice.* New York: Oxford University Press, 2003, Chapter 13.

> This essay analyzes the competition between individual rights and the need to ensure adequate public health practices in the practice of vaccination, with an excellent review of current state laws on the topic.

Marette, Stéphan, Brian E. Roe, and Mario Teisl. "The Welfare Impact of Food Pathogen Vaccines." *Food Policy* 37, no. 1 (2012): 86–93.

> The authors explore possible economic effects of dealing with food-borne illnesses by one of two methods: developing vaccines against such illnesses and tightening regulatory provisions to reduce the risk of such pathogens in the nation's food supply. They discuss the effects of using one approach, the other approach, or both approaches on consumer food choices and the economics of the food industry.

Nakaya, H. I., and B. Pulendran. "Systems Vaccinology: Its Promise and Challenge for HIV Vaccine Development." *Current Opinion in HIV and AIDS* 7, no. 1 (2012): 24–31.

> The authors explain that vaccine development has traditionally been an empirical effort that involved finding elements of an antigen that could be used to evoke an immune response. They point out that systems biology

permits a new and more rational approach to vaccine development that takes into consideration all elements of the immune system in designing vaccines that will stimulate the system's response.

Napoli, Denise. "Widespread HPV Vaccination May Require School Mandate." *Obstetrics and Gynecology News* 44, no. 9 (2009): 32–33.

The author points out that the availability of a vaccine against the HPV virus raised hopes of drastically reducing the rate of cervical cancer, but the reluctance of parents to have their children vaccinated means that mandatory programs may be necessary to achieve this end.

Neutra, Marian R., and Pamela A. Kozlowski. "Mucosal Vaccines: The Promise and the Challenge." *Nature Reviews Immunology* 6, no. 2 (2007): 148–158.

Most infectious agents enter the body through body openings, such as the mouth or nose, by way of mucosal surfaces. Yet, almost every vaccine currently available is administered by injection or orally. The authors explore the possibilities of developing vaccines that can be applied directly to mucosal surfaces, and the problems associated with this approach.

Omer, Saad B., et al. "Vaccine Refusal, Mandatory Immunization, and the Risks of Vaccine-Preventable Diseases." *New England Journal of Medicine* 360, no. 19 (2009): 1981–1988.

The authors point out that the rate of "vaccination-refusal" in the United States is increasing, a trend that appears to be reflected in outbreaks of preventable infectious diseases in certain parts of the country. They discuss the problems facing pediatricians who have to deal with children who have not been vaccinated and suggest an approach that might be helpful in encouraging a greater rate of vaccination.

Orenstein, Walter, A., Alan R. Hinman, and Peter M. Strebel. "Eradicating Measles: A Feasible Goal?" *Pediatric Health* 1, no. 2 (2007): 183–190.

> The authors review earlier efforts to eradicate measles from various parts of the world and review the elements needed in order to achieve worldwide eradication of the disease.

Perry, Robert T., et al. "Progress in Global Measles Control, 2000–2010." *MMWR* 61, no. 4 (2012): 73–78.

> This report reviews global efforts to eradicate measles in the first decade of the 21st century, with death rates from the disease dropping from about 2.6 million worldwide in 1980 to about 164,000 in 2008.

Plotkin, Stanley A., and Susan L. Plotkin. "The Development of Vaccines: How the Past Led to the Future." *Nature Reviews. Microbiology* 9, no. 12 (2011): 889–893.

> The authors provide a brief review of the development of vaccines in the past, some theoretical concepts upon which that development was based, and the implications for past vaccine safety for future development of new vaccines.

Plotkin, Stanley A. "Six Revolutions in Vaccinology." *The Pediatric Infectious Disease Journal* 24, no. 1 (2005): 1–9.

> The author divides the history of vaccinology into five periods, characterized by the development of technologies in attenuation, inactivation, cell culture of viruses, genetic engineering, and methods to induce cellular immune responses. He then predicts a six revolution that will arise from technologies in combination vaccines, new adjuvants, proteomics, reverse vaccinology, and vaccines for noninfectious diseases.

Porter, Dorothy, and Roy Porter. "The Politics of Prevention: Anti-vaccinationism and Public Health in Nineteenth-century England." *Medical History* 32, no. 3 (1988): 231–252.

The authors provide a concise and incisive review of the social and political factors involved in the development of the anti-vaccination movement in the last half of the 19th century in Great Britain.

Raupach, Tobias, et al. "Nicotine Vaccines to Assist with Smoking Cessation: Current Status of Research." *Drugs* 72, no. 4 (2012): e1–e16.

The authors review the social and health problems associated with smoking and methods available for withdrawing from the habit. They point out that some researchers have suggested the development of a vaccine against tobacco components as a way of reducing the desire to smoke. Although recent such efforts have been relatively unsuccessful, the authors still see some potential for anti-tobacco vaccines in the future.

Roukens, A. H., L. B. Gelinck, and L. G. Visser. "Intradermal Vaccination to Protect Against Yellow Fever and Influenza." *Current Topics in Microbiology and Immunology* 351 (2012): 159–179.

The authors review the histories of both yellow fever and influenza vaccines and discuss current research on the development of intradermal vaccines for both diseases.

Tucker, Mirian E. "ACIP Recommends HPV Vaccine for Older Boys." *Family Practice News* 41, no. 18 (2011): 8–9.

The author reports on the decision of the Advisory Committee on Immunization Practices (ACIP) to recommend HPV vaccination for males as well as for females.

"Vaccines." *Nature* 473, no. 7348 (2011): whole. Also available online at http://www.nature.com/news/specials/vaccines/index.html.

This special issue of the journal *Nature* includes articles on a wide variety of vaccine-related topics, such as Modern Heroes, Polio Clings on in Pakistan, The Case of Measles,

The Real Issues in Vaccine Safety, Target the Fence-Sitters, and Persistence Pays Off (the AIDS vaccine).

Reports

Harris, Katherine M., et al. *A Blueprint for Improving the Promotion and Delivery of Adult Vaccination in the United States.* Santa Monica, CA: Rand Corporation, 2012.

The authors of this report conducted a comprehensive review of the published literature on adult immunization, held a workshop for individuals with an interest in the topic, and carried out follow-up interviews with meeting participants and additional experts to determine the current status of adult immunization in the United States and to develop recommendations for possible changes that would result in expanding the availability of vaccinations for adults.

Smith, Philip J., and James A. Singleton. "County-Level Trends in Vaccination Coverage among Children Aged 19–35 Months—United States, 1995–2008." *MMWR* 60, no. 4 (2011): whole.

This report is the first of its kind, providing very detailed statistics on the rate of vaccination in counties throughout the United States, with correlations with other relevant variables, such as access to health care, economic conditions, and demographic characteristics.

Internet Resources

"Anthrax." National Network for Immunization Information. http://www.immunizationinfo.org/vaccines/anthrax. Accessed on April 2, 2012.

This comprehensive and detailed website provides extensive information on the disease, the history of the vaccine's development, recommendations as to who should and should not have the vaccine, proper dosage, effectiveness of the vaccine, known side effects, and related issues.

"Anthrax: Vaccination." Centers for Disease Control and Prevention. http://www.bt.cdc.gov/agent/anthrax/vaccination/. Accessed on April 2, 2012.

This CDC fact sheet provides a broad range of articles dealing with many aspects of the disease and the vaccine currently available to protect against it.

"Anthrax Vaccine Immunization Program." http://www.anthrax.osd.mil/. Accessed on April 2, 2012.

This website provides details on the Anthrax Vaccine Immunization Program, a long and somewhat troubled effort by the U.S. Department of Defense to supply anthrax vaccines to all members of the U.S. military.

"Anthrax Vaccine: What You Need to Know." http://www.cdc.gov/vaccines/pubs/vis/downloads/vis-anthrax.pdf. Accessed on April 2, 2012.

This brief publication provides basic information on the anthrax vaccine that is currently available in the United States, including the purposes for which it is intended, potential side effects, and compensation in case of unexpected adverse effects.

Atwood, Kimball C., IV, and Stephen Barrett. "Naturopathic Opposition to Immunization." http://www.quackwatch.com/01QuackeryRelatedTopics/Naturopathy/immu.html. Accessed on April 1, 2012.

The authors discuss naturopathic arguments against immunization and point out some flaws in this argument.

"Autism Decisions and Background Information." U.S. Court of Federal Claims. http://www.uscfc.uscourts.gov/node/5026. Accessed on April 7, 2012.

This web page provides links to a number of cases dealing with the relationship between autism and vaccines heard by Special Masters of the court. The page also provides a number of useful links to related topics.

Barrett, Stephen. "Chiropractors and Immunization." Chirobase. http://www.chirobase.org/06DD/chiroimmu.html. Accessed on April 1, 2012.

Chirobase is a division of Quackwatch, an organization whose goal it is to correct misinformation on a number of topics, immunization being one. The author presents the argument against immunization offered by some chiropractors and explains the errors in that argument.

Bill and Melinda Gates Foundation. "Vaccines." http://www.gatesfoundation.org/vaccines/pages/default.aspx. Accessed on May 12, 2012.

One of the strongest supporters of vaccination programs worldwide, the Gates Foundation supports this website, which provides extensive basic information on vaccines and vaccinations, along with resources on a host of related topics.

Boylston, A. W. "The Origins of Inoculation." 2012. http://www.jameslindlibrary.org/illustrating/articles/the-origins-of-inoculation. Accessed on March 11, 2012.

This website provides a very interesting introduction to the history of inoculation, as practiced in the Middle and Far East prior to and during the 18th century.

Brunk, Doug. "Making the Case for Universal HPV Vaccination." http://www.obgynnews.com/news/gynecology/single-article/making-the-case-for-universal-hpv-vaccination/63abcef13c637e66b49d2e0ea6905291.html. Accessed on May 11, 2012.

This article presents the views of Dr. Eduardo L. Franco about mandatory vaccinations with the HPV vaccine to reduce the risk of cancer among both males and females.

"Cancer Vaccines." National Cancer Institute. http://www.cancer.gov/cancertopics/factsheet/Therapy/cancer-vaccines. Accessed on March 31, 2012.

This website provides information on vaccines that have been developed or are under development that will aid the human immune system in protecting against the development of cancerous growths. Reports on clinical trials now under way for a variety of potential cancer vaccines are also available on the site.

"Diphtheria, Tetanus, Pertussis (DtaP)." National Network for Immunization Information. http://www.immunizationinfo. org/vaccines/diphtheria. Accessed on March 25, 2012.

This article provides a complete and lucid explanation of the combination vaccine, the forms in which it is available, side effects, and other relevant information about the vaccine.

"The History of Vaccines." The College of Physicians of Philadelphia. http://www.historyofvaccines.org/. Accessed on March 11, 2012.

This website offers a very attractive and informative interactive introduction to the history of vaccines, providing detailed information on both the vaccines themselves as well as the diseases for which they were developed.

"H1N1 and Pandemic Influenza." MERLIN (Military Education Research Library Network). http://merln.ndu.edu/index. cfm?type=section&secid=266&pageid=35#congress. Accessed on March 28, 2012.

This website provides one of the most (if not *the* most) complete sources of information on the H1N1 pandemic that struck the United States and other parts of the world in 2009.

Harris, Gardiner. "Panel Endorses HPV Vaccine for Boys of 11." *New York Times.* http://www.nytimes.com/2011/10/26/ health/policy/26vaccine.html. Accessed on April 2, 2012.

Gardiner reports on a decision by the Advisory Committee on Immunization Practices of the Centers for Disease Control and Prevention to recommend vaccination of male children at age 11 to protect against certain throat and anal cancers.

"Historic Dates and Events Related to Vaccines and Immunization." Immunization Action Coalition. http://www.immunize.org/timeline/. Accessed on March 25, 2012.

This website provides one of the most detailed histories of the development and use of vaccines currently available on the Internet.

"History of Epidemics and Plagues." http://uhavax.hartford.edu/bugl/histepi.htm. Accessed on April 9, 2012.

This superb website provides extensive detail on major epidemics and pandemics that have afflicted human civilization, along with a detailed description of the diseases involved.

"History of Vaccine Safety." Centers for Disease Control and Prevention. http://www.cdc.gov/vaccinesafety/Vaccine_Monitoring/history.html. Accessed on March 25, 2012.

This website focuses on vaccine safety issues and history dating to the 1970s.

"HPV Vaccine." National Conference of State Legislatures. http://www.ncsl.org/issues-research/health/hpv-vaccine-state-legislation-and-statutes.aspx. Accessed on April 2, 2012.

This web page provides detailed information on policies on HPV vaccination in all 50 states as of mid-2012.

"HPV Vaccines." WebMD. http://www.webmd.com/sexual-conditions/hpv-genital-warts/hpv-vaccines-human-papillomavirus. Accessed on April 2, 2012.

This website provides basic information on the human papillomavirus, genital warts, cervical cancer, and topics related to the HPV virus. It also discusses vaccines available for prevention of the disease.

"HPV Vaccine Information for Young Women—Fact Sheet." Centers for Disease Control and Prevention. http://www.cdc.

gov/std/hpv/stdfact-hpv-vaccine-young-women.htm. Accessed on April 2, 2012.

This fact sheet provides basic information about the human papillomavirus, the diseases for which it is responsible, and the vaccine that is available for its prevention. It discusses the individuals for whom HPV vaccination is appropriate and the safety and efficacy of the vaccine.

"Human Papillomavirus (HPV) Vaccines." National Cancer Institute. http://www.cancer.gov/cancertopics/factsheet/prevention/HPV-vaccine. Accessed on April 2, 2012.

In addition to providing basic information about the human papillomavirus and the diseases it causes, this web page also describes in some detail the two vaccines available for the virus, Gardasil and Cervarix.

"Human Vaccines and Immunotherapeutics." http://www.landesbioscience.com/journals/vaccines/. Accessed on May 12, 2012.

This website provides access to the online version of this important research journal. Most of the articles are of a technical nature and available only by subscription, but a number of general interest articles are also available, many by free use.

Huth, E. J. "Quantitative Evidence for Judgments on the Efficacy of Inoculation for the Prevention of Smallpox: England and New England in the 1700s." 2005. http://www.jameslindlibrary.org/illustrating/articles/quantitative-evidence-for-judgments-on-the-efficacy-of-inoculati. Accessed on March 12, 2012.

This fascinating commentary describes in detail the efforts made by researchers in the 18th century to determine how effective immunization was in the prevention of smallpox.

"Immunization." Medline Plus. http://www.nlm.nih.gov/medlineplus/immunization.html. Accessed on April 1, 2012.

Medline Plus is one of the most dependable sources of medical information on the Internet. This site provides detailed information on the basics of immunization, ongoing research in the field, law and policy, statistics, references, latest news, and individualized information on the topic.

"Immunization." UNICEF. http://www.unicef.org/immuniza tion/index_2819.html. Accessed on April 1, 2012.

This website provides comprehensive information on many aspects of immunization, with subsections on the eradication of polio, worldwide statistics on immunization, resources on the topic, and news on current developments in the field.

"Immunization." World Health Organization. http://www. who.int/topics/immunization/en/. Accessed on April 1, 2012.

This comprehensive and detailed site covers a variety of immunization-related topics, including frequently asked questions about the procedure, current news on immunization, vaccine quality, WHO programs and activities, statistics, and publications.

"Immunizations." Missouri Department of Health & Senior Services. http://health.mo.gov/living/wellness/immunizations/. Accessed on April 1, 2012.

All state departments of health (or comparable topics) offer web pages with detailed information about vaccinations and vaccines in general, along with specific requirements for that state. This website is an example of the type of offering provided by all states.

International Vaccine Access Center. Johns Hopkins University, Bloomberg School of Public Health. http://www.jhsph. edu/ivac. Accessed on May 12, 2012.

The purpose of this program is to promote the use of vaccination to reduce the rate of infectious diseases among children worldwide. It bases its work on the simple equation:

Evidence→Policy→Access.

Kidd, Devy. "Mandatory Vaccinations? Tell Feds and States to 'Stick It'." http://www.newswithviews.com/Devvy/kidd463.htm. Accessed on April 7, 2012.

> The author describes her own experience in being diagnosed with "Peking flu," how she dealt with that diagnosis, and what the medical mindset that led to that diagnosis means for Americans' choice in having or not having vaccinations.

Kirby, David. "Government Concedes Vaccine-Autism Case in Federal Court—Now What?" http://www.huffingtonpost.com/david-kirby/government-concedes-vacci_b_88323.html. Accessed on April 7, 2012.

> Kirby reports on a case in which the federal government concedes a connection between vaccine use and autism and, as the title suggests, asks what the significance of this decision will be for the future of the vaccine-autism dispute.

Knox, Richard. "HPV Vaccine: The Science Behind the Controversy." http://www.npr.org/2011/09/19/140543977/hpv-vaccine-the-science-behind-the-controversy. Accessed on April 2, 2012.

> This transcript of an NPR radio broadcast reviews the debate as to whether girls (and, perhaps, boys) at the age of 11 should be vaccinated against the HPV virus.

Koleva, Gergana. "Revised Recommendations for Vaccines Are Being Phased In, CDC Report Says." http://www.forbes.com/sites/gerganakoleva/2012/05/11/revised-recommendations-for-vaccines-are-being-phased-in-cdc-report-says/. Accessed on May 12, 2012.

> The U.S. Centers for Disease Control and Prevention have come to the conclusion that vaccination schedule

recommendations need to be developed with more subtlety, acknowledging differences in scientific evidence about vaccines and individual differences among potential recipients of a vaccine.

Koleva, Gergana. "Vaccine Debate Acknowledged, Explained at Global Conference." Forbes. http://www.forbes.com/sites/gerganakoleva/2012/03/14/vaccine-debate-acknowledged-explained-at-global-conference/. Accessed on May 12, 2012.

> Journalist Seth Mnookin addresses the International Conference on Emerging Infectious Diseases about the ongoing debate about the relationship (or lack of it) between vaccines and autism and provides a fascinating description of the way in which social, political, psychological, and other types of issues trump scientific evidence on the topic.

Lendman, Stephen. "Readying Americans for Dangerous, Mandatory Vaccinations." http://www.globalresearch.ca/index.php?context=va&aid=13925. Accessed on April 7, 2012.

> The author warns that legislation recently passed by the U.S. Congress will make it possible for the Food and Drug Administration and the Secretaries of Health and Human Services and Defense to order mandatory immunization against diseases that they believe to be threats to the safety of American citizens.

Marks, H. M. "The Kendrick-Eldering-(Frost) Pertussis Vaccine Field Trial." 2006. http://www.jameslindlibrary.org/illustrating/articles/the-kendrick-eldering-frost-pertussis-vaccine-field-trial. Accessed on March 25, 2012.

> This article reviews the complex and fascinating history of the development and testing of vaccines against pertussis.

Martini, Betty. "Anthrax Vaccine Is Dangerous." http://www.naturodoc.com/library/public_health/anthrax_vaccine.htm. Accessed on April 2, 2012.

> The author argues that the anthrax vaccine is neither efficacious nor safe.

"Medications and Drugs." emedicinehealth. http://www.emedi
cinehealth.com/drug-anthrax_vaccine/article_em.htm. Accessed
on April 2, 2012.

This website provides a long and very detailed article
about Biothrax, an anthrax vaccine developed by Emer-
gent BioSolutions for use with the U.S. military.

"Michigan Opposing Mandatory Vaccines." http://www.mom
vaccines.org/. Accessed on April 7, 2012.

Michigan Opposing Mandatory Vaccines is a nonprofit
organization founded in 1993 to provide information
about vaccinations and to promote the rights of individuals to choose whether or not to be vaccinated and, if so,
against which diseases.

"Misconceptions about Immunization." Quackwatch. http://
www.quackwatch.com/03HealthPromotion/immu/immu00.
html. Accessed on April 1, 2012.

The goal of Quackwatch is to provide accurate information on a wide variety of topics about which intentional
or unintentional information has been provided. Immunization is one such topic, and the website counters 12
such misconceptions, including the belief that vaccines
cause autism, thimerosal causes autism, and children get
too many immunizations.

National Vaccine Injury Compensation Program. U.S. Depart-
ment of Health and Human Resources. Health Resources and
Services. http://www.hrsa.gov/vaccinecompensation/index.html.
Accessed on May 12, 2012.

This web page provides a complete description of the National Vaccine Injury Compensation Program established
by an act of the U.S. Congress in 1988. The page provides
instructions as to how one files a claim for injury under
the provisions of this act.

Nelson, Kenrad E., and Carolyn F. Williams. "Early History of Infectious Disease." http://www.jblearning.com/samples/

0763728799/28799_CH01_001_022.pdf. Accessed on April 7, 2012.

> This document is Chapter One of Nelson and Williams' book *Infectious Disease Epidemiology: Theory and Practice.* It provides an excellent introduction to the status of infectious diseases from the earliest history of human society to (despite the title) the present day, with projections for the future of vaccinology.

"New Decade of Vaccines." *The Lancet.* http://www.thelancet.com/series/new-decade-of-vaccines. Accessed on May 12, 2012.

> This special issue of the medical journal, *The Lancet,* discusses a number of features of the future of vaccine design, production, and use, including articles on "Will the Decade of Vaccines Mean Business as Usual?" "Is Immunisation Child Protection?" "Public-Private Collaboration in Vaccine Research," and "Addressing the Vaccine Confidence Gap."

Perrone, Matthew. "Truvada for HIV Prevention: FDA Review Is Favorable." http://healthland.time.com/2012/05/09/truvada-for-hiv-prevention-fda-review-favors-approval/. Accessed on May 12, 2012.

> The U.S. Food and Drug Administration (FDA) announces that a drug long used for the treatment of HIV/AIDS is also safe and effective as a preventative for the disease, suggesting that it may soon be licensed for use for that purpose.

Post, Keith. "Alternatives to Vaccines." http://newconnexion.net/articles/index.cfm/2004/11/vaccinations.html. Accessed on May 10, 2012.

> The author focuses on the use of homeopathic vaccinations as an alternative to the conventional vaccine schedule used in the United States and other parts of the world.

Prescott, Bonnie. "Researchers Develop Novel Antibodies to Diagnose and Treat Alzheimer's Disease at Early Stages." Beth Israel Deaconess Medical Center. http://www.bidmc.org/News/InResearch/2012/March/Lu_Alzheimers.aspx. Accessed on March 31, 2012.

> The author reports on a breakthrough in the design of a vaccine that might be useful in treating the early stages of Alzheimer's disease.

Rempfer, Thomas L. "Anthrax Vaccine as a Component of the Strategic National Stockpile: A Dilemma for Homeland Security." http://www.dtic.mil/dtic/tr/fulltext/u2/a514307.pdf. Accessed on April 3, 2012.

> This doctoral thesis was written at the Naval Postgraduate School at Monterey, California. It explores the history of the U.S. government's development and use of the anthrax vaccine, especially following the 2001 terrorist attacks in the United States. The author suggests a policy for use of the vaccine against possible future bioterrorist attacks.

"Shingles Vaccine." WebMD. http://www.webmd.com/skin-problems-and-treatments/shingles/shingles-vaccine. Accessed on April 2, 2012.

> This website reminds readers that anyone over the age of 50 should consider being immunized against shingles, a painful disease that is a special problem for the elderly.

"Smallpox: A Great and Terrible Scourge." U.S. National Library of Medicine. http://www.nlm.nih.gov/exhibition/smallpox/sp_threat.html. Accessed on March 12, 2012.

> This website provides a well-illustrated and very informative history of smallpox, including a review of methods for inoculating against the disease (variolation and vaccination), as well as the story of its ultimate eradication.

Smith, Rebecca. "Vaccine to Stop Heart Attacks Could Be Developed." *The Telegraph.* http://www.telegraph.co.uk/health/healthnews/9173043/Vaccine-to-stop-heart-attacks-could-be-developed.html. Accessed on March 31, 2012.

> The author reports on an announcement at the Frontiers in CardioVascular Biology meeting in London about work on vaccines designed to prevent the buildup of plaque on arteries, thus reducing the risk of heart attacks.

Spuls, Phyllis I., Jan D. Box, and Donald Rudikoff. "Smallpox: What the Dermatologist Should Know." http://www.medscape.com/viewarticle/483590. Accessed on March 14, 2012.

> This article provides a very readable and complete description of all aspects of smallpox, including a brief history of the disease, symptoms, and available treatments.

Steckelberg, James M. "Shingles." Mayo Clinic. http://www.mayoclinic.com/health/shingles-vaccine/AN01738. Accessed on April 2, 2012.

> The author provides an excellent overview of the shingles disease and provides information to help readers decide whether or not they should be vaccinated against the disease.

Trim, Kristina, et al. "Parental Knowledge, Attitudes, and Behaviours towards Human Papillomavirus Vaccination for Their Children: A Systematic Review from 2001 to 2011." *Obstetrics and Gynecology International.* http://www.hindawi.com/journals/ogi/2012/921236/. Accessed on March 27, 2012.

> The authors report on an exhaustive review of studies dealing with parental attitudes toward HPV vaccination of their children.

"Vaccination: A Crime against Humanity." http://www.ajwrb.org/science/vaccinat.html. Accessed on May 10, 2012.

> This website discussed in some detail the long campaign against conventional vaccination carried out in the pages

of the *Watchtower* magazine, a publication of the Jehovah's Witnesses religious denomination.

"Vaccination and Vaccine Safety." FLU.gov. http://www.flu.gov/prevention-vaccination/vaccination/index.html. Accessed on March 30, 2012.

> This U.S. government website provides extensive basic information about vaccines and vaccination for influenza, including symptoms, prevention, populations at risk, planning and preparedness, and planning for pandemics.

"Vaccination Liberation—Home." http://www.vaclib.org/. Accessed on March 30, 2012.

> This website provides information on the anti-vaccination movements, whose position is expressed in the website masthead: Mandatory vaccination programs are "A violation of the Nuremburg Code."

"Vaccination News." http://www.vaccinationnews.com/homepage. Accessed on March 30, 2012.

> Vaccination News claims that it presents all sides of the dispute over mandatory vaccination of children. Its stated position is that it is "not against an informed parent choosing to vaccinate his or her child. Vaccination News is against bad science being used to justify forcing parents to vaccinate. It is against bad science being used to convince a parent to vaccinate." The site contains a number of useful sections, including pages on daily vaccine news, adverse reactions, relevant books, medical journal articles, political action, and state laws on vaccination.

"Vaccination News, Articles, and Information." Natural News.com. http://www.naturalnews.com/vaccination.html. Accessed on March 30, 2012.

> This page is a section of the Natural News.com website, which claims to be a "non-profit collection of public education websites covering topics that empower individuals

to make positive changes in their health, environmental sensitivity, consumer choices and informed skepticism." Recent articles include reports on hepatitis B immunizations as "crimes against newborns," newly raised doubts about scientific theories of immunity, proposed changes in Vermont's laws on required immunizations, and use by the Australian government of "dangerous flu vaccine."

"Vaccinations for Adults." Immunization Action Coalition. http://www.immunize.org/catg.d/p4030.pdf. Accessed on April 2, 2012.

This short publication argues that "You're never too old to get immunized." It consists of an easy-to-read chart listing the immunizations that individuals should get between the ages of 19 and 49, 50 and 64, and 65 years and older.

Vaccine. http://www.sciencedirect.com/science/journal/02644 10X. Accessed on May 12, 2012.

This website provides online access to the journal *Vaccine,* which contains very technical articles on the design, production, and use of vaccines, as well as topics of more general interest to the public about vaccinations. Subscription is required for access to articles.

"Vaccine Adverse Reporting Center." http://vaers.hhs.gov/ index. Accessed on March 31, 2012.

The Vaccine Adverse Reporting Center is a service of the U.S. government designed to record and evaluate reports of adverse results of vaccination. This web page provides the form necessary for individuals to report on such events as well as access to the service's database on adverse events associated with vaccinations.

"Vaccine Education Center." Children's Hospital of Philadelphia. http://www.chop.edu/service/vaccine-education-center/ home.html. Accessed on March 31, 2012.

The Children's Hospital of Philadelphia provides a complete list of topics designed for the average reader on the most important topics relevant to vaccination.

"The Vaccine Page." http://www.vaccines.org/. Accessed on March 31, 2012.

This page attempts to provide a broad range of useful information on all aspects of vaccines, including vaccine pages by country, lists of vaccine and vaccination organizations, vaccination information for travel, general and professional information on various topics related to vaccines, and lists of vaccine-related journals.

"Vaccine Safety Website." http://www.vaccines.net/newpage 114.htm. Accessed on May 12, 2012.

This website is based on the assumption that vaccines are, in general, not nearly as safe as they are claimed to be. The site has sections on safety testing, risks associated with vaccination, cancer, immune mechanisms, autoimmunity, Gulf War Syndrome, diabetes, and useful references.

"Vaccines." GlaxoSmithKline. http://www.gsk.com/products/ vaccines/index.htm. Accessed on May 12, 2012.

GlaxoSmithKline Pharmaceuticals markets about 30 different vaccines. This website provides detailed information on all of those vaccines—an interesting page for those who want to know a lot of technical detail about specific vaccine products.

"Vaccines." *Los Angeles Times.* http://www.latimes.com/topic/ health/vaccines-HEDAR00000154.topic. Accessed on May 12, 2012.

This website contains a large number (nearly 3,000, as of mid-2012) of news articles dealing with current developments in the field of vaccine design and use, and vaccination and controversies surrounding the practice.

"Vaccines." Vaccines.gov. http://www.vaccines.gov/. Accessed on March 31, 2012.

> This web page is maintained by the U.S. Department of Health and Human Services. It contains sections on most important topics related to vaccination, including a review of infectious diseases, the basics of immunization, who should get vaccinated and at what stage of their lives, and special concerns related to travel.

"Vaccines." World Health Organization. http://www.who.int/topics/vaccines/en/. Accessed on March 31, 2012.

> This website is especially valuable because it provides links to a number of other important related topics and organizations, such as infection safety, immunization financing, vaccine research and development, new vaccines, and the HIV Vaccine Initiative.

"Vaccines and Immunizations." Centers for Disease Control and Prevention. http://www.cdc.gov/vaccines/. Accessed on March 27, 2012.

> This website contains information on virtually every aspect of immunization that one might imagine, including sections on immunization schedules, recommendations, vaccines available in the United States, preventable diseases, and side effects.

"Vaccines, Bloods, & Biologics." U.S. Food and Drug Administration. http://www.fda.gov/biologicsbloodvaccines/vaccines/default.htm. Accessed on March 31, 2012.

> This web page provides extensive information on all aspects of vaccines and related biologics, including vaccine safety and availability, counterterrorism information, pandemics, and seasonal information on the current status of infectious diseases.

"What Are Vaccines?" News Medical. http://www.news-medical.net/health/What-are-Vaccines.aspx. Accessed on March 31, 2012.

This web page provides an extensive review of many aspects of the subject of vaccination.

Yeung, Miriam, and Amanda Allen. "Eliminating HPV Vaccine Mandate for Immigrant Women: A Victory on the Road to Reproductive Justice." RH Reality Check. http://www.rhrealitycheck.org/blog/2009/12/13/eliminating-hpv-vaccine-mandate-for-immigrant-women-one-victory-on-road-toward-reproductive-justice. Accessed on April 6, 2012.

In July 2008, the U.S. Citizenship and Immigration Services announced that it would require all immigrant women and girls to be vaccinated against HPV. In December 2009, the service reversed that decision. This article discusses the issue of requiring females' immigrants to have immunizations that citizens of the United States are not required to have.

"Your Child's Immunizations." Kids Health. http://kidshealth.org/parent/infections/immunizations/vaccine.html. Accessed on April 1, 2012.

This website provides an extensive review and discussion of all immunizations recommended for children and adolescents. It also includes information on related topics, such as immunization schedules, immunizations for travel, and helping children deal with fears about immunization.

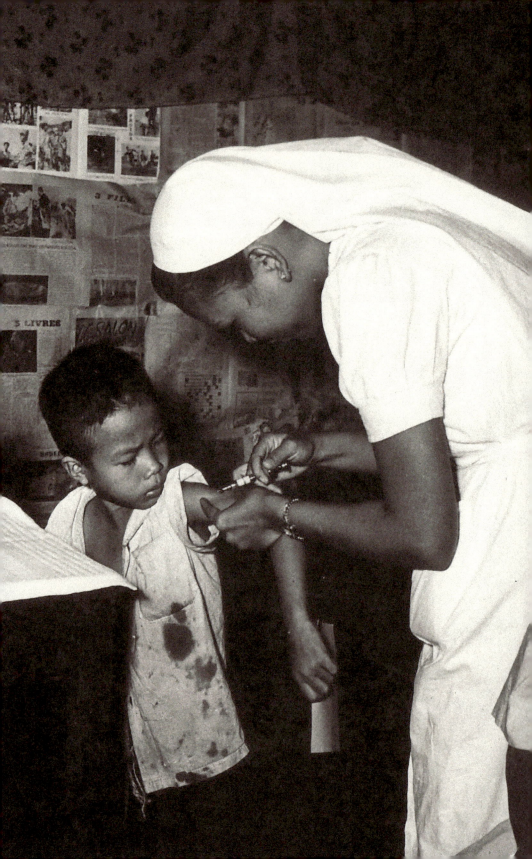

The history of immunization dates back more than two millennia. This chapter lists some of the most important events that have occurred in the discovery, development, and application of immunological knowledge over that period.

ca. 3000–2400 BCE   Analysis of the spines of Egyptian mummies dating to this period suggests that death was caused by complications of tuberculosis, the earliest evidence of the existence of infectious disease in humans.

ca. 1500 BCE   Some scholars trace the beginning of immunological techniques to the early Vedic physician Dhanvantari, who lived during this period in India. He is reputed to have described the symptoms of smallpox and methods for protecting against the disease by using variolation.

1157 BCE   Modern research suggests that Egyptian pharaoh Ramses V died of smallpox, the first documented death resulting from that disease.

ca. 500–300 BCE   Sanskrit medical records describe a disease by which individuals die through "draining of water," a disease that was almost certainly cholera.

A nurse working for UNICEF vaccinates a young boy against tuberculosis in Vietnam. The organization launched its International Tuberculosis Campaign in 1948. (World Health Organization/UNICEF)

429 BCE Greek historian Thucydides describes a horrible plague (smallpox) that swept through Athens and noted that survivors of the plague appeared to have developed a resistance to the disease.

ca. 8th century CE Mention of smallpox and the method of variolation occur in a long medical treatise, Nidāna, by the Indian physician Madhava-Kara. Uncertainty exists, however, as to the authenticity of this oft-quoted work, with some scholars believing that it was actually written more than a thousand years later.

910 In his book, al-Judari wa al-Hasbah (On Smallpox and Measles), Persian physician Muhammad ibn Zakariya Razi (Rhazes) first describes the difference between smallpox and measles.

ca. 1000 Variolation appears to have been used among upper class and noble families in India, Tibet, and China. The method involves collecting scabs from a smallpox infection, grinding them into a powder, and then introducing them into a person's nose to provide immunity against the disease.

ca. 1500 Increasing availability of means of transportation leads to the spread of smallpox across large regions of India and China. Spread of the disease apparently leads to greater use of variolation to immunize people against smallpox.

ca. 1500 Spanish conquistadores bring smallpox to the Western Hemisphere for the first time. Death rates are very high, with half the population of Hispaniola, for example, dying from the disease.

1563 Portuguese physician Garcia de Orta provides the first modern scientific description of cholera as a result of his visit to the Portuguese colony, Goa, in India.

1584 Italian physicist Girolamo Fracastoro provides the first accurate scientific description of rabies and gave the disease its name which, in Latin, means "to rage."

ca. 1610 European explorers introduce a number of nonnative diseases to North America, including smallpox, measles, and influenza. The diseases kill up to 90 percent of the Native American Indian population in some areas even before the first permanent European settlements are established.

1661 The Chinese emperor K'ang ascends to the throne after his father, Fu-lin, dies of smallpox. K'ang understands the importance of immunization against the disease and orders that all members of his family also be inoculated against smallpox.

1675 Danish physician Thomas Bartholin provides the first detailed description of variolation in Western Europe, although his work draws relatively little interest for nearly half a century.

1676 English physician Thomas Sydenham provides the first medical description of measles that clearly distinguishes the disease from smallpox.

1699 The first confirmed episodes of yellow fever are reported in the colonies, with the greatest number of deaths reported in Philadelphia and Charleston.

1706 Boston cleric Cotton Mather receives the gift of a slave named Onesimus, originally from Libya, who had been immunized for smallpox with variolation. The slave's story prompts Mather to research both the disease and the method of immunization, prompting him to promote use of the technique in the Massachusetts Bay Colony.

1715 Lady Mary Montagu, wife of the British ambassador to the Ottoman Empire, is disfigured by a case of smallpox. She learns of the use of variolation by local residents to prevent the disease and has her own son variolated against the disease. Her letters to friends in Great Britain increases knowledge of and interest in variolation as a preventative treatment for smallpox.

1721 Six convicts sentenced to death by hanging are promised a reprieve if they will take part in a "Royal Experiment" that involves their being inoculated against smallpox by variolation. They agree to participate, are treated, survive, and are freed, as promised.

1721   Variolation is introduced to the United States during a smallpox epidemic that eventually killed 844 residents of Boston. Largely at the impetus of Reverend Cotton Mather, many people are variolated against the disease, reducing their risk of death by a factor of about 5.

1731   The first well-documented scientific description of smallpox and its treatment by variolation appears in a letter written by an English physician serving in the Bengal, India, Robert Coult, to a colleague in Great Britain.

1738   A smallpox epidemic strikes Charleston, South Carolina, killing more than 440 residents. Eighteen percent of those who were not variolated died, compared to four percent who were treated.

1740   German physician Friedrich Hoffman provides the first scientific description of the disease now known as German measles, or rubella.

1759   At the behest of Benjamin Franklin, English physician William Heberden writes a pamphlet entitled "Some account of the success of the inoculation for the smallpox in England and America, together with plain instructions by which any person may be enabled to perform the operation and conduct the patient through the distemper," describing the use of variolation for inoculation against smallpox by a procedure that can be used by anyone. Franklin distributed the pamphlet at no cost throughout the colonies.

1765   English physician John Fewster reads a paper before the London Medical Society entitled "Cowpox and Its Ability to Prevent Smallpox," describing a fact apparently well known among rural folks that individuals who had been exposed to cowpox were far less likely to develop the more serious disease of smallpox.

1774   English farmer Benjamin Jesty inoculates his wife and two oldest sons with cowpox to protect them against smallpox. He had earlier inoculated himself and two servants. Jesty is generally considered to be the first person to intentionally infect someone with cowpox to provide resistance to smallpox.

1768   English physicians Patrick and Alexander Russell publish a paper in the Philosophical Transactions of the Royal Society providing detailed information and a history of the use of variolation to immunize against smallpox among Bedouin tribespeople living in the area of modern-day Aleppo, Syria. Russell's paper suggests that the practice has been in use among Arabs for many centuries and was probably brought to the region by tradesmen traveling from India and China.

1796   English physician Edward Jenner inoculates eight-year-old James Phipps with pus taken from the cowpox sore of milkmaid Sarah Nelmes. He then exposes the boy to variolous material that normally causes smallpox, but that produces no effect on the boy. Jenner's experiments are responsible for his being known today as the father of immunization.

1800   American physician and Harvard professor Benjamin Waterhouse becomes the first American to test smallpox immunization in the United States, using his own family as subjects. Waterhouse later attempts to maintain a monopoly over the procedure, but eventually fails and decides to freely distribute vaccine and the procedures for immunization among his colleagues.

1803   English physician Richard Dunning suggests the term vaccination for immunization with cowpox materials, the name deriving from the Latin word vacca for "cow."

1803   King Charles V of Spain decides to introduce smallpox inoculation into his American colonies. He sends a ship carrying five orphans from Madrid who are serially vaccinated en route to the New World, providing fresh vaccine for natives upon the ship's arrival.

1805   The Italian physician Michele Troja institutes the practice of retrovaccination, in which viral material taken from a patient with smallpox is injected into a cow. After the cow develops an immunity to the disease, fluid is removed from its lymph glands for use as a vaccine with other humans.

1805   The practice of variolation is banned in Russia.

1813   The U.S. Congress creates the National Vaccine Agency, designed to encourage and facilitate vaccination.

1817   The first of seven cholera pandemics breaks out in the Bengal region of India.

1819   French epidemiologist Pierre Bretonneau distinguishes between typhus and typhoid fever, two diseases that had previously been confused.

1822   The U.S. Congress repeals the act creating the National Vaccine Agency when the director, Dr. James Smith, accidentally sends smallpox material rather than cowpox material, resulting in the death of at least ten individuals.

1826   Pierre Bretonneau provides the first scientific description of diphtheria and gives the disease its name, which means "leathery" (which describes its appearance in the throat).

1835   Variolation is banned in Prussia.

1840   Variolation is banned in Great Britain.

1853   The British Parliament passes a law requiring all infants born in England and Wales to be vaccinated against smallpox, with the exception of those who were "unfit" to be vaccinated.

1854   Italian anatomist Filippo Pacini identifies the causative agent of cholera, a microbe named 82 years later in his honor, *Vibrio cholerae Pacini 1854*.

1855   The Massachusetts state legislature passes the first law in the United States mandating that all children must be vaccinated before attending school.

1870–1871   The effectiveness of vaccination is illustrated in the Franco-Prussian War when 500 soldiers from Prussia (where vaccination is required) die of smallpox, while 23,000 soldiers from France (where vaccination is not required) die of the disease.

1879   French chemist and microbiologist Louis Pasteur develops the first vaccine produced in a laboratory, an attenuated bacterium for use against chicken cholera.

1879   Inspired by a visit from British anti-vaccinationist William Tebb, opponents of vaccination in the United States form the Anti-Vaccination Society of America. Shortly thereafter the New England Anti-Compulsory Vaccination League (1882) and the Anti-Vaccination League of New York City (1885) also come into existence.

1882   German physician Robert Koch discovers the bacterium, *Bacillus anthracis*, that causes tuberculosis. A year later he discovers the causative agent for cholera, *Vibrio cholerae*.

1883   Swiss-German pathologist Edwin Klebs identifies the bacterium that causes diphtheria, now called *Corynebacterium diphtheriae*.

1884   Louis Pasteur produces the first attenuated vaccine for use against rabies.

1885   Pasteur successfully vaccinates nine-year-old Joseph Meister against rabies after the boy has been bitten by a rabid dog.

1894   The first major polio epidemic in the United States occurs in Rutland County, Vermont, with a total of 18 deaths and more than 130 cases of permanent paralysis being reported.

1898   The British Vaccination Act of 1898 includes for the first time a "conscience clause" that allows individuals opposed to vaccination to be excused from provisions of the law. Within the first year, more than 200,000 requests for exemption had been approved.

1898   Arm-to-arm vaccination is banned in Great Britain.

1900   A medical commission led by Major Walter Reed studying yellow fever in the Canal Zone of Panama discovers the method by which the disease is spread by means of mosquitoes.

1902 In response to the death of two children from contaminated vaccines, the U.S. Congress passes the Biologics Control Act, intended to guarantee the purity of a variety of medical products.

1905 A total of 452 individuals die in New Orleans in the last yellow fever epidemic to strike the United States.

1905 Swedish physician Ivar Wickman discovers that polio is a contagious disease.

1905 The United State Supreme Court finds that states may require residents to be vaccinated against infectious diseases.

1908 Austrian physicians Karl Landsteiner and Erwin Popper discover that polio is caused by a virus, later called the poliovirus.

1913 Hungarian-American pediatrician Béla Schick develops a test for determining whether or not a person has been exposed to diphtheria, thereby determining whether or not one needed to be vaccinated against the disease.

1923 French veterinarian Gaston Ramon develops a diphtheria toxoid by treating the diphtheria toxin with heat and formaldehyde, providing a safe and effective vaccine against the disease.

1931 The U.S. Food and Drug Administration licenses the first smallpox vaccine, called Dryvax®.

1936 South African-American virologist Max Theiler develops a live, attenuated vaccine for use against yellow fever.

1939 American bacteriologists Pearl Kendrick and Grace Elderling report the results of a long and comprehensive study on the effectiveness of a vaccine against pertussis.

1948 The Executive Board of the United Nations International Children's Emergency Fund (UNICEF) creates the International Tuberculosis Campaign, designed to test and immunize children around the world against the disease.

Eventually, a total of 37,694,983 persons were given tuberculin tests and 16,650,624 individuals were vaccinated against the disease.

1948   The first combined diphtheria-pertussis-tetanus (DPT) vaccine becomes available for use in the United States.

1949   The last smallpox case in the United States is reported in the town of Elsa, Texas.

1953   American physician Thomas C. Peebles isolates the measles virus.

1955   The U.S. Food and Drug Administration (FDA) licenses the first polio vaccine, an inactivated form of the polio virus. Use of the vaccine is temporarily suspended later in the year when two batches of the vaccine are found to have been contaminated.

1955   The U.S. Congress passes the Polio Vaccination Assistance Act, designed to provide financial support to help states and communities acquire and distribute the polio vaccine.

1957–1958   A pandemic caused by the H2N2 influenza virus kills more than two million people worldwide and about 70,000 individuals in the United States.

1962   The FDA licenses an oral polio vaccine developed by American physician Albert Sabin.

1963   The FDA licenses the first measles vaccine for use in the United States.

1963   American microbiologist Maurice Hilleman isolates the mumps virus.

1964   The U.S. Surgeon General establishes the Immunization Practices Advisory Committee to provide advice and recommendations on the control of infectious diseases.

1966   The Centers for Disease Control and Prevention announce a program for eradicating measles from the United States. The program is not entirely successful, although the incidence of the disease drops by more than 90 percent in following years. (Also see 1978 and 1996.)

1967   The FDA licenses the first mumps vaccine, MumpsVax (produced by Merck), developed by Maurice Hilleman.

1967   The World Health Organization (WHO) initiates a worldwide program, Smallpox Eradication Programme (SEP), designed to eliminate the disease from the planet.

1971   The FDA licenses a combined measles-mumps-rubella (MMR) vaccine, produced by Merck.

1977   The last smallpox case in the world is reported in Somalia.

1977   The FDA licenses the first vaccine against pneumonia, effective against 14 of the 83 serotypes then known, responsible for about 80 percent of reported cases of bacterial pneumonia.

1978   The Centers for Disease Control and Prevention announce a second program for the eradication of measles in the United States. (Also see 1966 and 1996.)

1979   The last cases of wild type polio in the United States were reported among unvaccinated Amish individuals who had refused vaccination. The cases were later found to have been transmitted from unvaccinated visitors from the Netherlands.

1980   The World Health Assembly officially announces that smallpox has been eradicated worldwide.

1981   The FDA licenses the first hepatitis B vaccine.

1985   The FDA licenses the first Hib (Haemophilus influenzae type b) vaccine.

1988   The World Health Assembly passes a resolution calling for the eradication of polio by the year 2000.

1991   The last case of poliomyelitis is recorded in the Western Hemisphere.

1994   The Pan American Health Organization and the World Health Organization certify that polio has been eradicated from the Western Hemisphere.

1995   The Advisory Committee on Immunization Practices, American Academy of Pediatrics, and American Association of

Family Physicians issue a joint statement on a recommended schedule for immunization of infants and children from birth to age 16.

1995 The FDA licenses a vaccine for hepatitis A.

1996 The International AIDS Vaccine Initiative (IAVI) is founded to promote the development of a vaccine to prevent HIV/AIDS disease.

1996 The World Health Organization, Centers for Disease Control, and Pan American Health Organization announce a joint effort to eradicate measles worldwide.

2000 Endemic measles in the United States is declared to have been eliminated.

2000 The Regional Commission for the Certification of Poliomyelitis Eradication certifies that the Western Pacific Region of the World Health Organization is free of indigenous wild poliovirus transmission.

2002 President George W. Bush announces a program to vaccinate nearly half a million public health and healthcare workers against a terrorist attack using smallpox virus. The program is cancelled when less than 10 percent of those workers are actually vaccinated.

2002 The European Regional Commission for the Certification of Poliomyelitis Eradication announces that Europe is free of indigenous wild poliovirus transmission.

2004 The U.S. Congress passes the Project BioShield Act, designed to expedite research on vaccines and other products to protect U.S. citizens against possible bioterrorist attacks on the country.

2004 A committee convened by the CDC concludes that rubella is no longer endemic in the United States.

2005 The FDA approves the first meningococcal vaccine, designed for use with adolescents aged 11–12 years and for individuals at special risk for meningococcal infections.

2006   The Advisory Committee on Immunization Practices (ACIP) recommends hepatitis A vaccination for all children older than the age one. In the same year, the ACIP recommends immunization of infants with the new rotavirus vaccine.

2006   The FDA approves a vaccine against shingles, of special value to the elderly.

2007   The FDA approves the first vaccine against avian influenza virus H5N1.

2009   The Office of Special Masters of the U.S. Court of Federal Claims (the so-called Vaccine Court) rules that the MMR vaccine does not cause autism, invalidating more than 5,000 claims based on that claim.

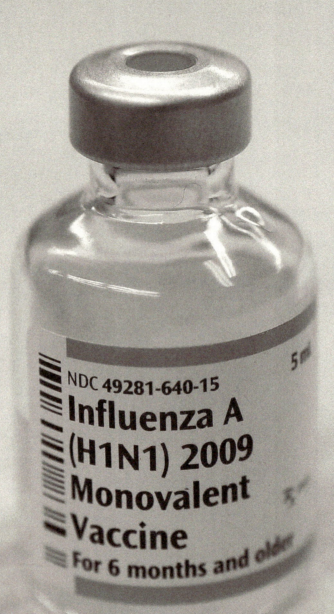

NDC 49281-640-15

Influenza A (H1N1) 2009 Monovalent Vaccine

For 6 months and older

5 mL

Discussions of immunization involve the use of many terms that are somewhat familiar to the average reader, but many of which are relatively technical. The purpose of this chapter is to review some of the most common of those terms, with their most commonly accepted meanings.

abortive infection   An infection in which a virus is present, but not effective in producing an actual infection. Also known as **nonproductive infection.**

active immunity   The production of antibodies against a specific disease by the immune system, either by having contracted the disease or by having been immunized against the disease with a vaccine. *See also* **passive immunity.**

adjuvant   A substance added to a vaccine to increase the body's immune response to the vaccine.

adverse event   An undesirable experience produced as the result of exposure to a vaccine.

anatoxin   *See* **toxoid.**

antigen   Any substance that produces an immune response in an organism.

A vial of H1N1 vaccine, an example of a monovalent vaccine, or one used to protect an individual against a single pathogen. (AP Photo/Paul Sancya)

antitoxin   A substance that responds to and neutralizes the effect of a specific toxin.

arm-to-arm vaccination   A process by which one person is inoculated with a vaccine, after which material taken from the pustule thus formed is transferred to a second person, and so on through many repetitions of the practice. The process is no longer used.

attenuated   Weakened; an attenuated vaccine is one that consists of an infectious agent that is less virulent that normal.

B-cell   A type of white blood cell produced in the bone marrow involved in the immune process. B-cells eventually develop into plasma cells, which produce antibodies. Also known as **B-lymphocytes.**

B-lymphocyte   *See* **B-cell.**

booster shot   Supplementary immunizations given at some time after an initial vaccination or series of vaccinations in order to maintain an appropriate level of defense by the immune system.

breakthrough infection   An infectious disease that develops in spite of a person's having been vaccinated against that disease.

community immunity   Immunity to an infectious disease that is sufficiently widespread in a population of individuals that the chance of transmission of the disease between individuals is very low. Also known as **herd immunity.**

conjugate vaccine   A vaccine consisting of two components, often a protein and a polysaccharide, whose efficacy is greater than that of a simple vaccine.

contagious   Transmissible by either direct or indirect means between two organisms.

endemic   A disease that occurs commonly and predictably in a particular region without input from some external source, such as another region.

epidemic Outbreak of a disease that spreads through a large part of a population.

gamma globulin *See* **immune globin.**

herd immunity *See* **community immunity.**

immune globin A protein in blood that fights infection. Also known as **gamma globulin.**

inactivated vaccine A vaccine made from bacteria or viruses that have been killed and that are, therefore, incapable of producing a disease.

incidence The number of new disease cases reported in a population over a certain period of time.

infectious Capable of being transmitted from one organism to another organism.

innate immunity An immune response that occurs naturally in the body and that does not develop as the result of the response to an antigen.

memory cell A cellular component of the immune system with the ability to "remember" antigens to which it has previously been exposed, thus making it possible for the cell to respond when exposed to the antigens upon later exposure.

monovalent vaccine A vaccine designed to immunize a person against a single pathogen. Also called **univalent vaccine.**

multivalent vaccine A vaccine designed to immunize a person against two or more pathogens. Also called **polyvalent vaccine.**

nonproductive infection *See* **abortive infection.**

pandemic Outbreak of a disease that is prevalent throughout the world.

passive immunity Protection gained against a disease by means of antibodies obtained from another human being or from an animal. *See also* **active immunity.**

pathogen A bacterium, virus, or other organism capable of producing a disease.

placebo   A substance or treatment that has no biological, psychological, or other effect on an organism to which it has been given.

potency   A measure of the strength of a substance or treatment.

prevalence   The number of disease cases (both new and existing) present in a population over a given period of time.

prodromal   An early symptom indicating the onset of an attack or a disease.

prophylactic vaccination   Vaccination undertaken for the purpose of preventing the development of an infectious disease. *Also see* **therapeutic vaccination.**

quarantine   The isolation of a person or animal who has, or is suspected of having, a disease, carried out for the purpose of preventing further spread of the disease.

rotavirus   Any one of a group of viruses that cause diarrhea in children.

seroconversion   Appearance of antibodies in the body of an animal that previously did not have those antibodies.

serotypes   Various forms of bacterium, virus, or other organism that can be identified in the blood.

strain   A taxonomic subtype of organisms within a species that are distinguishable from each other, but not to the extent to constitute distinct species.

therapeutic vaccination   Vaccination undertaken for the purpose of reducing the severity of symptoms associated with a disease that has already developed. *Also see* **prophylactic vaccination.**

toxin   Any poisonous substance produced by a plant, animal, or other organism.

toxoid   A substance that has been treated to destroy its toxic properties, but retains the ability to stimulate production of antitoxins. Originally (and still sometimes) called an **anatoxin** or **anti-toxin.**

vaccine   A biological material that provides an organism with immunity to some specific infectious disease, such as smallpox or measles.

vaccinology   The science that deals with the design and development of vaccines.

variolation   A form of immunization in which scabs taken from a smallpox infection are dried and ground to a powder, which is then introduced into the nose of the person to be immunized or spread into an open wound on the person's skin created for that purpose.

variolous   Having to do with smallpox.

virulence   The degree to which a pathogen is capable of producing a disease.

active immunity, 339
active immunization, 32
active infection, 339
adjuvant, 37–38, 105–110, 339
adverse event, 339
alternatives to vaccination, 100–102
aluminum compounds (as adjuvants), 106–108
American Medical Liberty League, 70
An Act to Secure General Vaccination (1855), 253–255
Anti-Compulsory Vaccination League (Great Britain), 63, 147
Anti-Vaccination League (Great Britain), 62, 147
Anti-Vaccination League (United States), 67
Anti-Vaccination League of America, 69–70

Anti-Vaccination League of New York City, 66, 331
Anti-Vaccination Society of America, 66, 331
anti-vaccinationism, modern, 85–101
Anti-Vaccinator (journal), 64
antibodies, 27
antigen, 339
antigen presentation, 30
antitoxin, 340
Antonine Plague, 8
arm-to-arm vaccination, 340
Association of Parents of Vaccine Damaged Children, 82
Atharva Veda (manuscript), 6
attenuated vaccine, 33, 340
attenuation, 33
autism, connection to vaccination, 90–93
autistic enterocolitis (hypothesized disease), 90

B-cell, 29–31, 340
B-lymphocytes. *See* B-cell
Balmis Expedition, 44
Barr, Richard, 91
Bartholin, Thomas, 327
Biologics Act (United States), 80
Biologics Control Act of 1902, 332
Blaylock, Russell, 94
Blumberg, Baruch S., 167–170
booster shot, 340
Bordet, Jules, 188
Boylston, Zabdiel, 57, 251–253
breakthrough infection, 340
Bretonneau, Pierre, 330
British Medical Research Council, 92
bubonic plague, 9, 12
Bumpers, Betty, 170, 172
Burnett, James Compton, 72
Bush, George W., 155, 335

Callahan, Joan R., 158–164
Carlson, Bruce, 99
Carrey, Jim, 103
Carter, Rosalyn, 172
Cedillo and Cedillo vs. Secretary of Health and Human Services (2010), 275–276
Cervaris®, 177
Charles IV (Spain), 44

Charles V (Spain), 329
chiropractic, views toward vaccination, 71
cholera, 45–46
Citizens Medical Reference Bureau, 70
combination vaccine. *See* multivalent vaccine
community immunity, 340
conjugate vaccine, 35, 340
Constitutional Liberty League of America, 70
contagious, 340
Coult, Robert, 40
cowpox, 42–43

Dale and Betty Bumpers Vaccine Research Center, 170–172
de Orta, Garcia, 326
Deer, Brian, 92, 230–232
dengue fever, 23–24
Dhanvantari, 40, 325
Dryvax, 45, 332
Dunning, Richard, 329

Ebers Papyrus, 6
eldering, 187–190, 332
endemic disease, 9, 340
epidemic, 7–14, 341
Epidemic of Galen. *See* Antonine Plague
Every Child By Two (organization), 172–175

Executive Order RP65 (State of Texas) (2007), 271–274

Exemption from Vaccination (document), 279–281

"The Fallacy of Vaccination" (pamphlet), 67

Feinstone, Stephen, 186

Fewster, John, 328

Fisher, Barbara Loe, 199–200

Fracastoro, Girolamo, 326

Franklin, Benjamin, 328

Frazer, Ian, 175–177

Frequently Asked Questions about Thimerosal (Ethylmercury) (2011) (factsheet), 276–279

gamma globulin. *See immune globin*

Gardasil®, 112, 133–141, 177, 193

Gengou, Octave, 188

GenVac (company), 36

the great pox. *See* smallpox

Gulf War Syndrome, 93–95

Habakus, Louise Kuo, 148–154

Haemophilus influenzae type B (Hib) vaccine, 35

Haffkine, Waldemar Mordecai Wolff, 46

Harper, Diane M., 137–141

Haycock, Dean A., 141–144

Healey, Bernadine, 148–149

Heberden, William, 328

hepatitis A, 25

hepatitis B, 25

hepatitis C, 25–26

herd immunity, 102, 340

Higgins, Charles M., 67

Hilleman, 177–180, 333, 334

Hippocrates, 6–7, 25

HIV/AIDS, 12–14

Hoffman, Friedrich, 328

homeopathy, views toward vaccination, 72

homeoprophylaxis, 101

Hopkins, Donald R., 4

human papillomavirus (HPV), 111–114

human papillomavirus (HPV) vaccine, 76

Hume-Rothery, Mrs., 98

immune globin, 341

immune system (human), 26–31

immunization: definition, 32

Immunization Action Coalition, 180–182

Immunization Practices Advisory Committee, 333

Immunization schedule, recommended (United States), 237, 241

use (worldwide), 242, 244–249

inactivated vaccine, 341
Incao, Philip, 97
incidence, 341
infection disease, major
    diseases, 16–26
  nature of, 14–16
infectious, 341
innate immune response,
    28
innate immunity, 341
inoculation, 32
insufflation, 39
International AIDS Vaccine
    Initiative, 335
International Anti-Vaccination
    League, 60
International Tuberculosis
    Campaign, 332

Jacobson v. Massachusetts
    (court case), 68–69,
    255–258
Jacobson, Henning, 67–68
Jenner, Edward, 32, 43–44,
    182–185, 329
Jensen, Mr., 43
Jesty, Benjamin, 43, 329

Kapikian, Albert Z., 185–187
Kendrick, Pearl, 187–190,
    332
killed vaccine, 34
Kitasato, Shibasaburo,
    190–192
Klebs, Edwin, 331
Koch, Robert, 190–191, 331

Kyoto vaccine epidemic
    (1948), 81

Landsteiner, Karl, 22, 332
Law of Mandatory Vaccine
    (Brazil), 73
Ledingham, J.C.G., 20
Leicester Anti-Vaccination
    League, 62
Lendman, Stephen, 154–158
live vaccines, 33
Lowy, Douglas R., 192–194
Lust, Benedict, 72

macrophage, 28
Madhava-Kara, 326
Mather, Cotton, 42, 65, 327,
    328
Matusmoto, Gary, 94–95,
    108–109
Measles Eradication Program
    (1996), 265–267
Meister, Joseph, 206, 331
memory cell, 31, 341
Miller, Jacques, 195–197
mixed vaccine. *See* multiva-
    lent vaccine
MMR vaccine, 35, 90–93,
    334
Model State Emergency
    Health Powers Act of
    2009, 156
monovalent vaccine, 35, 341
Muhammad Ali, 58
Muhammad ibn Zakariya
    Razi. *See* Rhazes

multiple sclerosis (association with vaccination), 158–164
multivalent vaccine, 35, 341
mumps Vax, 334
Myers, Martin, 114

Nabel, Gary J., 172
National Anti-Compulsory Vaccination Reporter (journal), 64
National Childhood Vaccine Injury Act of 1986, 198, 261–265
National League for Medical Freedom, 70
National Vaccine Agency, 330
National Vaccine Information Center, 197–200
naturopathy, views toward vaccination, 72
Nelmes, Sarah, 43, 329
New England Anti-Compulsory Vaccination League, 66, 331
Novella, Steven, 145
Nussenzweig, Ruth S., 200–202

Obomsawin, Raymond, 95–97
Office of Special Masters of the U.S. Court of Federal Claims, 92, 336

Offit, Paul, 149–150, 202–204
O'Leary, John, 91
On Airs, Water, and Places (book), 6
Onesimus, 42, 327

Pacini, Filippo, 330
Palmer, Batlett Joshua, 71
Palmer, David D., 71
Pandemic, 7, 341
Pandemic and All-Hazards Preparedness Act of 2006, 154
Paschen, Enrique, 20
passive immunity, 341
Pasteur, Louis. 45, 205–208, 331
pathogen, 341
Patient Protection and Affordable Care Act of 2010, 70
Peebles, Thomas C., 333
Perry, Rick, 113
phagocytosis, 28
Phipps, James, 43, 183, 239
Pitcairn, John, 66–67
placebo, 342
Plague of Athens, 8
Plett, Peter, 43
Plotkin, Stanley A., 208–210
Polio Global Eradication Initiative, 23
Polio Vaccination Assistance Act, 333

polio vaccine epidemic
(1955), 82–83
poliomyelitis, 21–23
Poliomyelitis Vaccination
Assistance Act (1955),
258–259
polyvalent vaccine. *See* multivalent vaccine
Poor Law Commission, 61
Popper, Erwin, 22, 332
potency, 342
poxvirus, 4
prevalence, 342
primary immune response,
27–30
prodromal, 342
Project Bio Shield Act of
2004, 154, 267–269, 335
Project Bioshield Assessment
(2007), 269–271
prophylactic vaccination, 342
Public Readiness and Emergency Preparedness
(PREP) Act, 154
Purcell, Robert, 186

quarantine, 342
Queen Caroline, 41–42

Radford, Benjamin, 144–148
Ramon, Gaston, 210–231,
332
Ramses V, xv, 4, 325
Reed, Walter, 331–332
religious objections to vaccination, 110–111

Rendall, Mrs., 43
reverse vaccinology, 36
Revolta da Vacina, 73
Rhazes, 326
Roehr, Bob, 133–137
RotaShield (vaccine), 83–84
rotavirus vaccine epidemic
(1999), 83–84, 342
Rubin, Benjamin A.,
213–215
Russell, Alexander, 329
Russell, Patrick, 329

Sabin, Albert, 22, 215–218,
333
Salk, Jonas, 22, 218–220
Scheibner, Viera, 221–223
Schick, Béla, 332
Schiller, John T., 192–194
Scott, Sir Walter, 21
Sears, Robert W., 104
secondary immune response,
30–31
seroconversion, 342
serotypes, 342
Sevel, Mrs., 43
smallpox, 18–20, 42–45,
328
Smallpox Eradication Pro-
gramme, 334
Smith, James, 330
squalene (as an adjuvant),
108–109
strain, 342
sub-unit vaccine, 34
Syndenham, Thomas, 327

T-cells, 29–31
Tebb, William, 66, 331
Texas House Bill 1098
    (2007), 274–275
Theiler, Max, 332
therapeutic vaccination, 342
thimerosal, 105–108
Thucydides, 326
Timmoni, Emmanuel, 42
toxin, 342
toxoid, 34, 342
Troja, Michele, 330

vaccination, alternatives to,
    100–103
  data, 237, 238–240
  definition, 31, 32, 329
  epidemics, 73–77
  history, 38–47
  laws (Great Britain), 61–65
  laws (United States), 73–77
  laws (worldwide), 77–78
  legal status, history, 84–85
  named, 44
  opposition to, 58–73
  schedules, 103
Vaccination Act of 1853
    (Great Britain), 62, 330
Vaccination Act of 1898
    (Great Britain), 45, 331
Vaccination Assistance Act of
    1962, 259–261
Vaccination Inquirer (journal),
    64
Vaccination Risk Awareness
    Network, Inc., 225–227

vaccine(s), 32, 343
  approved for use (United
    States), 242
  attenuated vaccine, 33
  conjugate vaccine, 35
  killed vaccine, 34
  monovalent vaccine, 35
  multivalent vaccine, 35
  name, 44
  shortages, 141–144
  sub-unit vaccine, 34
*Vaccine A: The Covert Govern-
    ment Experiment That's
    Killing Our Soldiers and
    Why GI's Are Only the
    First Victims* (book),
    94–95
Vaccine Act of 1813 (United
    States), 80
vaccine court. *See* Office of
    Special Masters of the U.S.
    Court of Federal Claims
Vaccine Education Center,
    223–225
Vaccine Injury Compensa-
    tion Program, 151
vaccine-derived polio, 33
vaccinology, 32–38, 343
vaccinosis, 72–73
*Vaccinosis and Its Cure by
    Thuja* (book), 72–73
van Mansvelt, C. G., 190
variola. *See* smallpox
variola major, 19
variola minor, 19
variola vera. See smallpox

variolation, 19, 250–251,
    326, 328, 330, 343
  history, 38–42
variolous, 343
virulence, 343
von Behring, Emil, 191,
    227–229

Wakefield, Andrew, 90–93,
    147, 229–232
Waterhouse, Benjamin, 74,
    79
Wharton, Melinda, 113

whooping cough, 144–148
Wickman, Ivar, 332
Wortley Montagu, Lady
    Mary, 41–42, 232–235,
    250–251, 327

Xiao-Yi Sun, 176–177

Yersin, Alexandre, 192
Yu Mao Kun, 39

Zucht v. King (court case),
    69

About the Author

David E. Newton holds an associate degree in science from Grand Rapids (Michigan) Junior College, a BA in chemistry (with high distinction) and an MA in education from the University of Michigan, and an EdD in science education from Harvard University. He is the author of more than 400 textbooks, encyclopedias, resource books, research manuals, laboratory manuals, trade books, and other educational materials. He taught mathematics, chemistry, and physical science in Grand Rapids, Michigan, for 13 years; was professor of chemistry and physics at Salem State College in Massachusetts for 15 years; and was adjunct professor in the College of Professional Studies at the University of San Francisco for 10 years. Previous books for ABC-CLIO include *Global Warming* (1993), *Gay and Lesbian Rights–A Resource Handbook* (1994, 2009), *The Ozone Dilemma* (1995), *Violence and the Mass Media* (1996), *Environmental Justice* (1996, 2009), *Encyclopedia of Cryptology* (1997), *Social Issues in Science and Technology: An Encyclopedia* (1999), *DNA Technology* (2009), and *Sexual Health* (2010). Other recent books include *Physics: Oryx Frontiers of Science Series* (2000), *Sick!* (4 volumes; 2000), *Science, Technology, and Society: The Impact of Science in the 19th Century* (2 volumes; 2001), *Encyclopedia of Fire* (2002), *Molecular Nanotechnology: Oryx Frontiers of Science Series* (2002), *Encyclopedia of Water* (2003), *Encyclopedia of Air* (2004), *The New Chemistry* (6 volumes; 2007), *Nuclear Power* (2005), *Stem Cell Research* (2006), *Latinos in the Sciences, Math, and Professions*

(2007), and *DNA Evidence and Forensic Science* (2008). He has also been an updating and consulting editor on a number of books and reference works, including *Chemical Compounds* (2005), *Chemical Elements* (2006), *Encyclopedia of Endangered Species* (2006), *World of Mathematics* (2006), *World of Chemistry* (2006), *World of Health* (2006), *UXL Encyclopedia of Science* (2007), *Alternative Medicine* (2008), *Grzimek's Animal Life Encyclopedia* (2009), *Community Health* (2009), and *Genetic Medicine* (2009).